Improve Gut Health

And Mental Health Too

Daniel Dennis

ISBN: 978-1-77961-989-1
Imprint: Telephasic Workshop
Copyright © 2024 Daniel Dennis.
All Rights Reserved.

Contents

Historical Context of Mental Health 13
The Social Determinants of Mental Health 37
The Impact of Technology on Mental Health 52
Historical Perspectives on Mental Health Care 66

Chapter 2: Understanding Psychological Challenges **81**
Chapter 2: Understanding Psychological Challenges 81
Common Mental Health Disorders 84
Trauma and Post-Traumatic Stress Disorder (PTSD) 106
Addiction and Mental Health 119
Neurodevelopmental Disorders 132
Personality Disorders 145
Eating Disorders 161
Psychosomatic Disorders 172
Sleep Disorders 186
Other Psychological Challenges 199
Historical Perspectives on Mental Illness 217

Chapter 3: Promoting Holistic Health **231**
Chapter 3: Promoting Holistic Health 231
Holistic Approaches to Mental Health 234
Nutrition and Mental Health 247
Exercise and Mental Health 258
Mind-Body Practices for Mental Wellbeing 272
Art and Music Therapy 282
Animal-Assisted Therapy 295
Spirituality and Mental Health 309
Social Support and Mental Health 319
Workplace Mental Health 333

Promoting Holistic Mental Health Policy 348

Chapter 4: Building Resilience for Overall Sustainability 363
Chapter 4: Building Resilience for Overall Sustainability 363
The Concept of Resilience 366
Personal Strengths and Resources 374
Chapter 4: Building Resilience for Overall Sustainability 380
Social Support Networks 385
Access to Mental Health Care 397
Positive Coping Strategies 410
Chapter 4: Building Resilience for Overall Sustainability 410
Promoting Resilience in Children and Adolescents 420
Resilience in Adulthood 433
Resilience and Aging 445
Chapter 4: Building Resilience for Overall Sustainability 448
Intersectionality and Resilience 455
Resilient Communities and Societies 464

Chapter 5: Conclusion: Towards a Sustainable Mental Health Future 477
Chapter 5:
Conclusion: Towards a Sustainable Mental Health Future 477
The Evolution of Mental Health Care 478
Advancing Mental Health Research and Training 485
5.3.2 The Importance of Interdisciplinary Collaboration 489
Strengthening Mental Health Policies and Systems 498
Promoting Mental Health Advocacy and Awareness 513
A Call to Action: Building a Sustainable Mental Health Future 526
Reflecting on our Journey: Mental Health and Wellbeing in Contemporary History 539

Index 551

Definition and Scope of Mental Health

Definition and Scope of Mental Health

Mental health refers to a person's emotional, psychological, and social well-being. It affects how individuals think, feel, and act, and it also determines how they handle stress, relate to others, and make choices. Mental health is essential at every stage of life, from childhood and adolescence through adulthood. While mental health is often discussed in the context of mental illness, it is important to understand that mental health is more than just the absence of mental disorders.

The scope of mental health encompasses a wide range of factors that contribute to an individual's well-being. It includes emotional well-being, which involves understanding and managing one's feelings and emotions in a healthy way. It also includes psychological well-being, which involves having a positive outlook on life, feeling a sense of purpose, and being able to manage stress effectively.

Furthermore, mental health encompasses social well-being, which involves having positive relationships and a strong support network. It also involves being able to contribute to society and engage in meaningful activities. Lastly, mental health includes cognitive well-being, which involves having a sharp mind, good memory, and the ability to think critically and problem-solve.

The definition and scope of mental health have evolved over time as our understanding of human behavior and the factors that influence mental well-being has deepened. Initially, mental health was primarily viewed in a negative light, focusing on the absence of mental illness. However, the concept has now shifted towards a more positive perspective, emphasizing the importance of promoting and maintaining mental well-being.

Contemporary understandings of mental health emphasize the holistic nature of well-being, recognizing that mental health is influenced by various biological, psychological, social, and environmental factors. It acknowledges that mental health exists on a continuum, with individuals experiencing different levels of well-being and resilience.

Culture plays a significant role in shaping mental health definitions and practices. People from different cultural backgrounds may have distinct beliefs, values, and norms regarding mental health. These cultural factors influence how mental health is perceived, diagnosed, and treated. It is crucial to consider cultural context when addressing mental health issues to ensure that interventions and support are culturally sensitive and relevant.

Stigma is another critical aspect of mental health. Stigma refers to the negative attitudes, beliefs, and stereotypes associated with mental illness. It often leads to discrimination and social exclusion, contributing to the perpetuation of mental health disparities. Addressing stigma is crucial for promoting mental health and ensuring that individuals feel comfortable seeking help and support when needed.

Mental health is a global issue that affects people of all backgrounds, ages, and socio-economic statuses. It is not limited to specific regions or populations, and its impact extends beyond individual well-being to include families, communities, and societies as a whole. Global efforts are necessary to address mental health challenges and ensure that everyone has access to quality mental health care and support.

Research plays a vital role in advancing our understanding of mental health and developing effective interventions. By conducting rigorous studies, researchers can identify risk factors, protective factors, and evidence-based treatments for mental health disorders. Research also helps to shape mental health policies and programs, ensuring that resources are directed towards evidence-based practices.

In summary, the definition and scope of mental health encompass various aspects of a person's well-being, including emotional, psychological, social, and cognitive factors. It takes a holistic approach, recognizing the influence of culture, stigma, and social determinants on mental health. Mental health is a global issue that requires interdisciplinary research, effective policies, and community support to promote and maintain overall well-being.

Contemporary Understanding of Mental Health

In recent years, our understanding of mental health has evolved significantly, moving away from a purely pathological view towards a more holistic and person-centered approach. This contemporary understanding acknowledges the complex interplay of biological, psychological, social, and environmental factors in influencing mental well-being. By recognizing the multidimensionality of mental health, we are better equipped to promote and support individuals in their journey towards overall well-being.

Bio-Psycho-Social Model of Mental Health

At the core of the contemporary understanding of mental health is the bio-psycho-social model. This model recognizes that mental health is not solely determined by biological factors (e.g., genetics, brain chemistry) but is also influenced by psychological (e.g., thoughts, emotions, behaviors) and social factors (e.g., relationships, socio-cultural context).

According to the bio-psycho-social model, mental health disorders are not simply a result of biological abnormalities but arise from a complex interaction of biological, psychological, and social factors. For example, while someone may have a genetic predisposition to depression, the manifestation of the disorder may be influenced by psychological factors such as stress and social factors such as lack of social support.

This model emphasizes the need for a comprehensive understanding of an individual's circumstances and experiences in order to provide effective mental health care. It highlights the importance of addressing not only the symptoms of mental disorders but also the underlying causes and contextual factors that contribute to an individual's mental health.

Person-Centered Approach

Another key aspect of the contemporary understanding of mental health is the shift towards a person-centered approach. This approach recognizes that each individual's experience of mental health is unique and should be respected and valued. It emphasizes the importance of empowering individuals to actively participate in decisions regarding their mental health care.

In a person-centered approach, mental health professionals collaborate with individuals, taking into account their preferences, values, and goals. This approach challenges the traditional therapeutic model that focuses solely on symptom reduction and places more emphasis on the individual's overall well-being and quality of life.

A person-centered approach also acknowledges the importance of cultural, social, and contextual factors in shaping an individual's understanding of mental health. It recognizes the need for culturally sensitive care that respects and embraces diversity, ensuring that mental health services are accessible and inclusive for all.

Holistic Well-being

Contemporary understanding of mental health goes beyond the absence of mental illness and emphasizes the importance of holistic well-being. It recognizes that mental health is not just about the absence of symptoms but encompasses a state of complete physical, mental, and social well-being.

Promoting holistic well-being involves addressing all dimensions of a person's life, including physical health, emotional well-being, social connectedness, and spiritual fulfillment. This approach recognizes the interconnectedness of these dimensions and the impact they have on an individual's overall mental health.

For example, physical exercise has been shown to have a positive impact on mental health by reducing symptoms of depression and anxiety, improving sleep quality, and boosting overall well-being. Similarly, nurturing social connections and maintaining a sense of belonging and support can enhance mental resilience and well-being.

In summary, the contemporary understanding of mental health emphasizes the bio-psycho-social model, the person-centered approach, and holistic well-being. By recognizing the complexity of mental health and embracing individual uniqueness, we can provide more effective and inclusive mental health care that promotes overall sustainability and well-being.

The Impact of Culture on Mental Health Definitions

Culture plays a significant role in shaping our understanding and definitions of mental health. It influences how mental health is perceived, diagnosed, treated, and experienced within a given society. Cultural beliefs, values, norms, and practices shape the way individuals, families, communities, and larger societies conceptualize and respond to mental health issues.

Cultural Relativism and Mental Health

One key concept in understanding the impact of culture on mental health definitions is cultural relativism. Cultural relativism recognizes that different cultures have distinct ways of conceptualizing and addressing mental health. It emphasizes the importance of understanding mental health within its cultural context, rather than imposing a universal definition or perspective.

Cultural relativism challenges the idea that mental health disorders and symptoms are universally understood and experienced. Instead, it suggests that mental health should be understood through the lens of cultural norms and values. For example, in some cultures, experiences such as hearing voices or having visions may be considered normal or even spiritual, while in other cultures, they may be seen as symptoms of mental illness.

Cultural Factors Influencing Mental Health Definitions

Various cultural factors can influence mental health definitions, including:

1. **Language and Communication:** Language shapes our understanding and expression of mental health. Different cultures may have unique words, concepts,

and metaphors to describe mental health states and psychological distress. For example, in some cultures, depression may be described as "heartache" or "soul sadness," emphasizing the emotional aspect of the condition.

2. **Cultural Beliefs and Values:** Cultural beliefs and values shape how mental health disorders are perceived and understood. In some cultures, mental illness may not be recognized as a medical condition but rather attributed to supernatural or spiritual causes. Stigma may also be associated with mental health issues, preventing individuals from seeking help.

3. **Social Support Systems:** Cultural norms regarding social support and interpersonal relationships influence how individuals with mental health issues are perceived and supported. In collectivist cultures, community support and family cohesion may play a crucial role in recovery, while individualistic cultures may emphasize self-reliance and personal responsibility.

4. **Help-Seeking Behavior:** Cultural factors also influence help-seeking behaviors for mental health issues. Stigma, availability of mental health services, and cultural beliefs about the effectiveness of different treatments may influence whether individuals seek professional help or rely on informal support networks.

Cultural Competence in Mental Health Care

Recognizing and addressing the impact of culture on mental health is essential for providing culturally competent care. Cultural competence refers to the ability of mental health professionals to understand and respond to the unique needs of individuals from diverse cultural backgrounds. It involves:

1. **Cultural Awareness:** Mental health professionals must develop an understanding of their own cultural values, biases, and assumptions. They need to be aware of how their own cultural background may influence their interactions with clients.

2. **Knowledge of Cultural Practices and Beliefs:** Mental health professionals should acquire knowledge about the cultural practices, beliefs, and values of the populations they serve. This knowledge enables them to provide appropriate and effective care that is respectful of cultural differences.

3. Adaptation of Treatment Approaches: Mental health professionals need to adapt their treatment approaches to align with the cultural beliefs, practices, and preferences of the individuals they serve. This may include incorporating traditional healing practices, involving family members in treatment, or using culturally relevant metaphors and language.

4. Collaborative Approach: Collaboration between mental health professionals and individuals from diverse cultural backgrounds is crucial for effective care. It involves valuing the expertise and perspectives of the individual and their community, and working together to develop mutually agreed-upon treatment plans.

Cultural competence also extends beyond individual interactions to inform mental health policies and systems. It helps promote equity, reduce disparities, and ensure that mental health services are accessible and appropriate for diverse populations.

Example: Cultural Factors and Mental Health in Indigenous Communities

An example of the impact of culture on mental health definitions can be seen in Indigenous communities. Indigenous peoples often have unique cultural beliefs, values, and experiences that shape their understanding and expression of mental health.

For instance, historical trauma, colonization, and ongoing experiences of racism and discrimination have profoundly affected the mental health of many Indigenous individuals and communities. The impact of these factors may not be adequately captured by traditional mental health definitions derived from Western perspectives.

Indigenous cultures often have holistic views of health that encompass physical, mental, emotional, and spiritual well-being. Mental health may be understood in relation to cultural identity, connection to land and community, and intergenerational trauma. Traditional healing practices, such as ceremony, storytelling, and connection with nature, play significant roles in promoting healing and resilience.

Addressing mental health disparities in Indigenous communities requires a comprehensive understanding of cultural values, practices, and experiences. Mental health interventions must be culturally sensitive, empowering, and grounded in collaboration with Indigenous communities.

Resources and Challenges

Culturally sensitive mental health research, training, and policies are essential for addressing the impact of culture on mental health definitions. Efforts should be made to include diverse cultural perspectives, narratives, and experiences in mental health literature and education. Resources such as cultural competency training programs, ethnographic studies, and community partnerships can enhance cultural understanding and inform mental health practices.

However, challenges exist in balancing cultural relativism with the need for evidence-based practices. Some cultural practices may conflict with ethical and legal standards or may not have sufficient empirical support. It is imperative to navigate these challenges carefully, ensuring cultural sensitivity while upholding ethical principles and providing effective care.

Conclusion

The impact of culture on mental health definitions is profound. Cultural beliefs, values, practices, and experiences influence how mental health is understood, diagnosed, and treated. Recognizing and addressing cultural factors in mental health care is critical for providing culturally competent and effective support to individuals from diverse backgrounds. Cultural sensitivity should be integrated into mental health policies, research, training, and service delivery to promote equitable and holistic mental health care for all.

The Role of Stigma in Mental Health

Stigma is a powerful force that can significantly impact individuals with mental health challenges. It refers to the negative attitudes, beliefs, and stereotypes that society holds towards those with mental illnesses. Stigma can manifest in various ways, including social exclusion, discrimination, and prejudice. In the context of mental health, stigma can be particularly detrimental, as it can create barriers to seeking help, accessing treatment, and integrating into society.

1. Understanding Stigma: Stigma towards mental health stems from misinformation, fear, and a lack of understanding. It often leads to the perception that individuals with mental illnesses are weak, dangerous, or morally flawed. This social stigma perpetuates negative stereotypes and prejudices, making it difficult for individuals to seek help and talk openly about their struggles.

2. Impact on Help-Seeking Behavior: The stigma surrounding mental health can be a significant deterrent for individuals to seek help and support. They may fear being judged, labeled, or ostracized by others. This fear can prevent individuals

from reaching out to healthcare professionals, disclosing their condition to family and friends, or seeking appropriate resources and treatment. As a result, individuals may suffer in silence and experience prolonged distress.

3. Barriers to Accessing Treatment: Stigma contributes to the existing barriers in accessing mental health services. Negative attitudes lead to underfunding of mental health resources, limited availability of mental health professionals, and a lack of insurance coverage for mental health conditions. This not only makes it difficult for individuals with mental illnesses to access care but also perpetuates the notion that mental health is less important than physical health.

4. Consequences of Stigma: The consequences of stigma can be pervasive, impacting various aspects of an individual's life. Social isolation, compromised relationships, limited employment opportunities, and reduced self-esteem are common experiences for individuals who face stigma related to their mental health. The cumulative effects of stigma can exacerbate mental health symptoms and hinder recovery.

5. Strategies to Address Stigma: Addressing stigma is crucial for promoting mental health and well-being. Education and awareness campaigns can challenge stereotypes and disseminate accurate information about mental illnesses. Encouraging open conversations and creating safe spaces for discussions can help combat the shame and silence associated with mental health. Media portrayals that humanize mental health struggles and highlight recovery stories can also play a key role in reducing stigma.

6. Advocacy and Support: Individuals, communities, and organizations must advocate for policy changes that protect the rights of individuals with mental illnesses and promote mental health equality. Laws that prohibit discrimination based on mental health status, promote equal access to healthcare, and ensure workplace accommodations are essential. Support systems, such as mental health support groups and peer-led initiatives, can provide a sense of belonging and empowerment for individuals affected by stigma.

In conclusion, stigma remains a significant barrier to mental health and well-being. It negatively affects individuals with mental illnesses, hindering their access to care, support, and social inclusion. Addressing stigma requires a collective effort from society, involving education, advocacy, and the creation of supportive environments. By challenging stereotypes, promoting understanding, and fostering acceptance, we can create a future where mental health is destigmatized, and individuals feel empowered to seek help without fear of judgment or discrimination.

Mental Health as a Global Issue

Mental health is not only an individual concern, but also a global issue that affects societies and communities on a large scale. The understanding and treatment of mental health disorders have evolved over time, and it is important to recognize the impact of these disorders on a global scale. In this section, we will explore the global perspective of mental health, including its prevalence, challenges, and the need for a comprehensive approach to address mental health issues worldwide.

Prevalence of Mental Health Disorders

Mental health disorders are a significant global health burden, affecting people of all ages and backgrounds. According to the World Health Organization (WHO), around 1 in 4 people worldwide will experience a mental health disorder at some point in their lives. This means that millions of individuals and their families are affected by mental health issues, leading to decreased quality of life, disability, and even premature death.

The prevalence of mental health disorders varies across different regions and countries, but it is important to note that no nation is immune to this issue. Low and middle-income countries often face greater challenges in accessing mental health services and have fewer resources allocated to mental health care. Additionally, population growth, urbanization, and socioeconomic disparities can further exacerbate mental health issues in these regions.

Challenges in Global Mental Health

Addressing mental health as a global issue comes with several challenges that need to be overcome. These challenges include:

1. Stigma and Discrimination: Stigma and discrimination surrounding mental health remain pervasive globally. Many cultures and societies still hold misconceptions and negative attitudes towards mental health disorders, leading to social exclusion, isolation, and limited access to proper care.

2. Lack of Resources: Many countries, especially low and middle-income countries, face a lack of resources and infrastructure to effectively address mental health. This includes a shortage of trained mental health professionals, limited access to medication and treatment options, and inadequate funding for mental health programs.

3. Inequitable Distribution of Mental Health Services: There is an inequitable distribution of mental health services within and between countries. Many rural and underserved areas have limited or no access to mental health care, resulting in a significant treatment gap.

4. Cultural and Contextual Factors: Mental health is heavily influenced by cultural, social, and contextual factors. Different cultural beliefs, attitudes, and practices can shape people's perceptions of mental health disorders, affecting help-seeking behaviors and treatment outcomes. It is crucial to approach mental health holistically, taking into account cultural diversity and individual experiences.

5. Conflict and Disasters: Conflict and disasters, both natural and man-made, have a profound impact on mental health. The displacement of communities, loss of livelihoods, and exposure to violence or trauma can lead to a higher prevalence of mental health disorders. In such situations, the provision of mental health services becomes even more challenging.

A Comprehensive Approach to Global Mental Health

Addressing mental health as a global issue requires a comprehensive and multi-faceted approach that takes into account the complexity and interconnectedness of various factors. This approach should focus on the following key areas:

1. Promotion and Prevention: Prevention plays a crucial role in reducing the burden of mental health disorders. Promoting mental well-being, raising awareness, and reducing stigma are essential components of preventive efforts. This can be achieved through educational campaigns, community-based initiatives, and early intervention programs.

2. Access to Treatment: Ensuring universal access to mental health care is a priority. This includes increasing the availability of mental health services, training more mental health professionals, and integrating mental health care into primary health care systems. Telemedicine and digital health platforms can also play a significant role in improving access to mental health services, especially in remote and underserved areas.

3. Integration with Primary Health Care: Integrating mental health care into primary health care systems is crucial for early detection and intervention. By providing mental health services at the community level, individuals can

receive timely and appropriate care, reducing the burden on specialized mental health services.

4. Collaboration and Partnerships: Addressing global mental health requires collaboration and partnerships between governments, non-governmental organizations, researchers, and communities. Sharing knowledge, expertise, and resources can strengthen mental health programs and policies, ultimately leading to better outcomes for individuals and communities.

5. Research and Innovation: Investing in mental health research is essential for advancing our understanding of mental health disorders and developing effective interventions. Research can help identify risk factors, inform evidence-based treatment approaches, and drive policy change. Innovations in technology, such as mobile mental health applications and artificial intelligence, also hold promise for improving mental health care delivery on a global scale.

Conclusion

Mental health is a global issue that requires collective efforts to address effectively. By recognizing the prevalence of mental health disorders, understanding the challenges they present, and promoting a comprehensive approach to mental health care, we can work towards creating a sustainable mental health future. By prioritizing mental health, allocating resources, and engaging in global collaborations, we can reduce the burden of mental health disorders, promote well-being, and ensure that individuals and communities around the world have access to the care they need.

The Importance of Research in Mental Health

In order to understand and address the complex nature of mental health, extensive research is essential. Research in mental health plays a crucial role in advancing our knowledge, improving diagnosis and treatment methods, promoting prevention strategies, and ultimately enhancing overall mental health outcomes.

1. Advancing Knowledge and Understanding: Research in mental health helps to expand our understanding of the complexities of the human mind and behavior. It provides insights into the underlying causes, risk factors, and mechanisms involved in mental health disorders. By investigating the biological, psychological, and social factors that contribute to mental health, researchers can uncover new information that can lead to breakthroughs in treatment and prevention.

For example, recent studies have identified specific genetic markers associated with certain mental disorders, providing a better understanding of the biological basis of these conditions. Likewise, research on the impact of adverse childhood experiences (ACEs) has highlighted the long-term effects of trauma on mental health, leading to the development of trauma-informed interventions.

2. Improving Diagnosis and Treatment: Accurate diagnosis is crucial for effective mental health care. Research helps to identify reliable and valid assessment tools, diagnostic criteria, and screening measures for various mental health conditions. This enables healthcare professionals to make more accurate diagnoses, leading to appropriate and timely treatment interventions.

Moreover, research plays a vital role in evaluating the effectiveness of different treatment approaches. Through rigorous scientific studies, researchers can determine which interventions are most successful in alleviating symptoms, improving functioning, and promoting recovery.

For instance, randomized controlled trials have demonstrated the efficacy of cognitive-behavioral therapy (CBT) in treating anxiety and depression. This research has led to the widespread adoption of CBT as a first-line treatment for these conditions.

3. Preventing Mental Illness: Research is crucial for developing effective prevention strategies to reduce the incidence and prevalence of mental health disorders. By identifying risk and protective factors, researchers can target specific populations or individuals at risk and implement preventive interventions.

For example, research on the impact of early childhood experiences on mental health outcomes has highlighted the importance of early intervention and support. This knowledge has informed the development of programs aimed at promoting positive parenting, enhancing resilience in children, and preventing the onset of mental health disorders later in life.

4. Informing Policy and Practice: Research serves as a foundation for evidence-based policy and practice in mental health. Policymakers rely on research findings to make informed decisions about resource allocation, service provision, and the implementation of mental health programs.

In addition, research contributes to the development of clinical practice guidelines and treatment protocols. These guidelines help to ensure that healthcare providers are using the most effective and up-to-date interventions for their patients.

5. Addressing Mental Health Disparities: Research has the power to shed light on mental health disparities and inequities in healthcare access and delivery. By investigating factors such as socioeconomic status, race, ethnicity, gender, and

geography, researchers can identify the barriers that prevent marginalized populations from accessing quality mental health care.

This knowledge can inform the development of targeted interventions and policies aimed at reducing disparities and promoting equitable access to mental health services.

In summary, research is essential in the field of mental health as it advances our knowledge, improves diagnosis and treatment, promotes prevention strategies, informs policy and practice, and addresses mental health disparities. By prioritizing and supporting research efforts, we can foster innovation, improve outcomes, and work toward a more sustainable mental health future.

Historical Context of Mental Health

Early Perspectives on Mental Health

In order to understand the historical context of mental health, it is crucial to explore the early perspectives and beliefs surrounding mental health. Throughout history, different cultures and civilizations have had varying interpretations and explanations for mental illness. These early perspectives provide valuable insights into the evolution of mental health care and highlight the progress that has been made in our understanding of mental health.

1. Ancient Egyptian Perspective: The ancient Egyptians believed that mental illnesses were caused by supernatural forces and spiritual disturbances. They attributed mental disorders to the actions of evil spirits or the displeasure of the gods. Treatment for mental illness often involved rituals, exorcisms, and amulets to ward off the evil spirits. This perspective demonstrates the significant impact of religious beliefs and cultural practices on early understandings of mental health.

2. Ancient Greek Perspective: Greek philosophers, such as Hippocrates, considered mental illness to be a result of imbalances in the body's humors (bodily fluids). According to the humoral theory, an excess or deficiency of blood, phlegm, yellow bile, or black bile led to various mental disorders. Treatment involved restoring the balance of humors through techniques such as bloodletting, purging, and dietary changes. This perspective laid the foundation for a more physiological understanding of mental health.

3. Traditional Chinese Medicine Perspective: In ancient China, mental health was understood within the framework of traditional Chinese medicine. Mental illnesses were believed to arise from imbalances or blockages in the flow of vital energy (Qi) and the harmony between Yin and Yang. Treatment involved practices

such as acupuncture, herbal medicine, and Qigong exercises to restore the balance of energy within the body. This perspective highlights the holistic approach of traditional Chinese medicine and the significance of energy flow in mental health.

4. Islamic Perspective: During the Islamic Golden Age, scholars like Ibn Sina (Avicenna) made significant contributions to the field of mental health. They believed that mental disorders were caused by physiological imbalances, as well as social and environmental factors. Treatment involved a combination of pharmacological interventions, psychotherapy, and spiritual practices. Islamic perspectives on mental health emphasized the importance of psychological well-being and the interconnectedness of mind, body, and soul.

5. Indigenous Perspectives: Indigenous cultures around the world have their own unique perspectives on mental health. They often view mental illness as a spiritual imbalance or disharmony with nature and the community. Healing practices may involve ceremonies, rituals, and connection with the natural world. These perspectives highlight the cultural diversity in understanding and addressing mental health issues.

It is important to acknowledge that these early perspectives on mental health were influenced by the limited scientific knowledge and cultural beliefs prevalent at the time. However, they laid the foundation for subsequent advancements in understanding and treating mental illness. Through the centuries, these perspectives have contributed to shaping the field of mental health and have paved the way for more evidence-based approaches to care.

As we delve further into the historical evolution of mental health, it becomes evident that early perspectives on mental health were shaped by a combination of cultural, religious, and philosophical beliefs. These perspectives provide a lens through which we can examine the roots of societal attitudes towards mental health and the significant progress that has been made in the field. By understanding the early perspectives, we can appreciate the importance of cultural competency and diverse approaches to mental health care in contemporary society.

In the next section, we will explore the ancient Greek and Roman views on mental health, shedding light on the influence of these civilizations on our current understanding of mental well-being.

Ancient Greek and Roman Views on Mental Health

In ancient times, the understanding and treatment of mental health issues were shaped by the beliefs and practices of the Greek and Roman civilizations. The Greeks and Romans had their distinct approaches to mental health, influenced by their cultural, philosophical, and medical frameworks. Exploring these ancient perspectives can provide valuable insights into the historical context of mental health and help us understand the foundations of contemporary practices.

Greek Views on Mental Health

In ancient Greece, mental health was closely associated with the concept of the soul or psyche. The Greeks believed that imbalances in the four bodily humors (blood, phlegm, yellow bile, and black bile) could affect mental well-being. Hippocrates, the renowned Greek physician often referred to as the "Father of Medicine," proposed the theory of humoral imbalance and categorized mental disorders accordingly.

Hippocrates believed that mental illnesses resulted from an excess or deficiency of certain humors. For example, an excess of black bile was thought to cause melancholia, a condition characterized by sadness and depression. Treatment involved restoring the balance of humors through dietary adjustments, exercise, and purging.

Greek philosophers such as Plato and Aristotle also contributed to the understanding of mental health. Plato emphasized the harmony of the soul, suggesting that mental disorders arose from a disruption in this harmony. He advocated for a balanced and virtuous life as a means of maintaining mental well-being.

Aristotle, on the other hand, focused on the connection between the mind and body. He believed that the mind could influence physical health and vice versa. Aristotle's holistic approach was an early precursor to the biopsychosocial model of mental health.

Roman Views on Mental Health

The Romans inherited much of their knowledge on mental health from the Greeks but developed their distinct approaches. They recognized the influence of external factors such as lifestyle, environment, and personal experiences on mental well-being. Roman physicians like Galen built upon the humoral theory, expanding it to include the impact of external factors.

Roman society placed great importance on the concept of virtue and mental stability. The Stoic philosophy, championed by prominent figures like Seneca and Marcus Aurelius, emphasized self-control, resilience, and rationality. Followers of Stoicism believed that individuals could cultivate mental strength and endure suffering through philosophical practices.

However, the Romans also attributed mental illnesses to supernatural causes. They believed in spiritual possession and the influence of evil spirits on mental health. Rituals like exorcism and offerings were performed to address these spiritual causes.

Roman physicians employed various therapeutic approaches, including medicinal treatments, bathing, massage, and physical exercises. They recognized the value of public baths and built expansive bathing complexes to promote mental and physical well-being.

Comparisons and Contrasts

While both the Greeks and Romans acknowledged the role of bodily humors in mental health, the Romans expanded the understanding to include external factors. The emphasis on holistic approaches, including lifestyle, environment, and philosophy, reflected a broader perspective on mental well-being.

In contrast, the Greeks had a more medicalized approach, focusing on humoral imbalances and bodily interventions. The philosophical perspectives of Plato and Aristotle introduced psychological and philosophical dimensions to the understanding of mental health.

Both civilizations recognized the societal impact of mental health and the importance of maintaining balance and virtue in individual and communal life. The teachings of Stoicism echo modern concepts of resilience and self-care.

Relevance to Contemporary Mental Health

The ancient Greek and Roman views on mental health laid the foundation for modern understandings and treatments. The holistic approaches and recognition of the mind-body connection align with contemporary biopsychosocial models of mental health. The emphasis on maintaining balance, practicing self-control, and promoting well-being align with current psychological and wellness practices.

Moreover, the historical context of mental health reminds us that cultural beliefs and societal factors significantly influence mental health perspectives and treatments. It underscores the importance of cultural competence and the need to consider diverse perspectives in contemporary mental health care.

While the ancient Greek and Roman views on mental health may differ from current scientific understandings, they provide valuable insights into the historical evolution of mental health practices. Exploring these ancient perspectives allows us to reflect on how far we have come and prompts us to continue advancing our understanding and treatment of mental health issues.

Key Takeaways

- Ancient Greek views on mental health centered around the theory of humoral imbalance, with Hippocrates proposing the concept and categorizing mental disorders based on an excess or deficiency of bodily humors.

- Greek philosophers such as Plato and Aristotle contributed to the understanding of mental health, emphasizing the harmony of the soul and the connection between the mind and body.

- Roman views on mental health built upon the Greek foundation and expanded to include external factors such as lifestyle and environment. Stoicism, a popular philosophy, emphasized self-control, resilience, and rationality for mental well-being.

- Comparisons and contrasts between Greek and Roman views highlight both medical and psychological dimensions in understanding mental health and the significance of societal and philosophical influences.

- The ancient perspectives on mental health remain relevant today, providing insights into the historical evolution of mental health practices and emphasizing the importance of cultural competence and holistic approaches.

Religious and Spiritual Beliefs in Mental Health

In the context of mental health, religious and spiritual beliefs can play a significant role in people's lives. Many individuals find solace, meaning, and purpose in their faith traditions, and these beliefs can provide a framework for understanding and coping with psychological challenges. This section explores the relationship between religious and spiritual beliefs and mental health, highlighting their potential benefits and challenges.

The Influence of Religion and Spirituality on Mental Health

Religious and spiritual beliefs can have a profound impact on mental health and wellbeing. For many individuals, their faith provides a sense of hope, comfort, and support during difficult times. Religious practices, such as prayer, meditation, and attending religious services, can offer a sense of connection, community, and a source of strength.

Research has shown that religious and spiritual beliefs are associated with a range of positive mental health outcomes. For example, studies have found that individuals who regularly engage in religious or spiritual practices tend to experience lower levels of depressive symptoms, anxiety, and stress. They also report higher levels of life satisfaction and overall wellbeing.

One explanation for these positive associations is that religious and spiritual beliefs and practices provide individuals with a sense of meaning and purpose in life. These beliefs often offer a framework for understanding suffering and provide guidance on how to cope with adversity. Additionally, religious communities can provide social support and a sense of belonging, which are protective factors for mental health.

Religion and the Treatment of Mental Illness

Religious and spiritual beliefs can also influence the perception and treatment of mental illness. In some cultures and faith traditions, mental health problems are viewed through a religious or spiritual lens. For example, in certain religious contexts, symptoms of mental illness may be interpreted as possession by evil spirits, moral shortcomings, or divine punishment.

The intersection of religion and mental health treatment can be complex and raise ethical considerations. While for some individuals, religious and spiritual practices may complement and enhance treatment outcomes, for others, these beliefs may interfere with seeking professional help or adhering to evidence-based treatments.

It is crucial for mental health professionals to approach religious and spiritual beliefs with cultural sensitivity and respect. Collaboration between mental health providers and religious leaders can be beneficial in ensuring holistic care that respects both the individual's faith and their mental health needs.

Challenges and Limitations

While religious and spiritual beliefs have the potential to promote mental health and wellbeing, they can also present challenges and limitations. In some cases, religious beliefs may contribute to stigma and discrimination towards individuals with mental illness. Misunderstandings or misinterpretations of religious teachings can lead to negative attitudes and beliefs, further isolating individuals who need support.

Moreover, religious and spiritual beliefs are not a panacea for mental health problems. While faith can provide comfort and support, it is essential to recognize that mental illnesses are complex conditions that may require professional help, including therapy and medication.

It is also crucial to respect individuals' autonomy and their right to choose their religious or spiritual beliefs. Mental health professionals should engage in open and non-judgmental discussions around religion and spirituality, ensuring that individuals feel heard and understood.

Integrating Religion and Spirituality in Mental Health Care

To promote holistic and culturally competent mental health care, it is essential for mental health professionals to be knowledgeable about various religious and spiritual beliefs and their potential impact on mental health. This knowledge can help professionals engage in respectful conversations, address spiritual and existential concerns, and identify potential sources of support within an individual's faith community.

Adopting a collaborative and integrated approach that acknowledges the role of religion and spirituality in mental health can lead to more comprehensive and effective care. Mental health providers can actively involve individuals' religious leaders or counselors in their treatment plans, when appropriate, to support their overall well-being.

Additionally, mental health professionals can draw upon the positive aspects of religion and spirituality by incorporating evidence-based strategies and interventions that align with an individual's beliefs. Mindfulness-based approaches, for example, have been adapted to include religious or spiritual elements and have shown promising results in promoting mental health.

Case Study: Faith-Based Outreach Program

To illustrate the potential benefits of integrating religious and spiritual beliefs in mental health care, let's consider the example of a faith-based outreach program aimed at addressing mental health issues in a diverse community.

The program brings together mental health professionals and religious leaders to provide education, support, and resources to community members. It offers workshops on mental health awareness, destigmatization, and coping strategies, drawing upon both psychological interventions and religious teachings.

The program promotes collaboration and dialogue between mental health providers and religious leaders, aiming to create a supportive and inclusive environment for individuals experiencing mental health challenges. It also emphasizes the importance of an interdisciplinary approach, recognizing that mental health care involves the integration of biological, psychological, social, and spiritual factors.

By combining evidence-based practices with religious and spiritual perspectives, this program creates a safe space for individuals to explore their mental health concerns within the context of their faith traditions. It empowers individuals to seek help, access appropriate resources, and promotes overall mental health and wellbeing within the community.

Conclusion

Religious and spiritual beliefs can significantly impact mental health and wellbeing. They offer solace, meaning, and support, while also presenting challenges and ethical considerations. Mental health professionals can enhance their practice by understanding and respecting the role religion and spirituality play in individuals' lives.

Through a collaborative and integrated approach, mental health care can address the unique needs of individuals while supporting their religious or spiritual beliefs. By promoting open dialogue, cultural competence, and collaboration between mental health providers and faith communities, holistic and sustainable mental health care can be achieved.

As we move forward, it is essential to continue exploring the intersection of religion, spirituality, and mental health, promoting research, education, and policies that foster inclusivity, respect, and wellbeing for all individuals, regardless of their religious or spiritual beliefs.

The Emergence of Psychiatry

Psychiatry is a branch of medicine that focuses on the diagnosis, treatment, and prevention of mental disorders. The field of psychiatry has evolved over centuries, influenced by various historical, cultural, and scientific factors. In this section, we will explore the emergence of psychiatry, tracing its roots from ancient times to the modern era.

Early Perspectives on Mental Health

The earliest known records of mental illness date back to ancient civilizations, such as those of Egypt, Mesopotamia, and Greece. In these societies, mental illnesses were often attributed to supernatural causes or seen as divine punishment. The treatment of mental disorders was largely based on religious rituals, incantations, and exorcisms.

Ancient Greek and Roman Views on Mental Health

In ancient Greece, mental health was associated with the balance of bodily fluids, known as humors. Greek physician Hippocrates believed that mental disorders were caused by imbalances in these humors and advocated for a more naturalistic approach to treatment. He emphasized the importance of environmental and social factors in mental well-being.

The Roman Empire built upon the Greek ideas and developed institutions known as asylums to house the mentally ill. However, these institutions were often overcrowded and lacked proper care for patients.

The Influence of Freudian Psychoanalysis

The late 19th and early 20th centuries witnessed significant advancements in the field of psychiatry, thanks to the pioneering work of Sigmund Freud. Freud's psychoanalytic theory revolutionized the understanding and treatment of mental disorders. He emphasized the role of the unconscious mind, childhood experiences, and repressed desires in shaping human behavior.

Freud's theories paved the way for the development of talk therapy, or psychotherapy, as a prominent treatment modality. The Freudian approach to psychiatry greatly impacted the field, leading to further exploration of unconscious processes and the development of different psychotherapeutic techniques.

The Medicalization of Mental Illness

The emergence of psychiatry as a medical specialty can be traced back to the 19th century. During this time, there was a shift toward medicalizing mental illness, which involved framing mental disorders as medical conditions requiring scientific diagnosis and treatment.

With advancements in neuroscience and the discovery of psychotropic medications, psychiatry began to adopt a more biological approach. The development of the first generation of antipsychotic and antidepressant medications in the mid-20th century revolutionized the treatment of mental disorders, providing relief for many individuals.

The Deinstitutionalization Movement

In the mid-20th century, there was a push to move away from the institutionalization of individuals with mental illness. The deinstitutionalization movement aimed to shift the focus from long-term hospitalization to community-based care. It was driven by the belief that people with mental disorders could lead fulfilling lives when provided with proper support and treatment outside of institutions.

The Impact of Deinstitutionalization on Mental Health Care

While deinstitutionalization led to the closure of many psychiatric hospitals and the integration of individuals with mental illness into the community, it also created challenges. The lack of adequate community-based resources and support services often left individuals without proper care, leading to homelessness, incarceration, and increased burden on families.

Challenges and Controversies in Deinstitutionalization

The deinstitutionalization movement faced numerous challenges and controversies. One of the main challenges was the lack of funding and resources for community-based mental health services. The closure of psychiatric hospitals sometimes resulted in a shortage of beds and specialized care, leading to a strain on the mental health system.

There were also concerns about the appropriate balance between individual rights and public safety. The fear of violence and harm associated with mental illness often led to debates surrounding involuntary commitment and the use of psychiatric medications without the individual's consent.

The Biopsychosocial Model of Mental Health

In recent years, psychiatry has embraced a more holistic approach to mental health care: the biopsychosocial model. This model recognizes that mental disorders are multifaceted and result from complex interactions between biological, psychological, and social factors.

The biopsychosocial model emphasizes the importance of a comprehensive assessment of individual needs, taking into account biological factors (such as genetics and brain chemistry), psychological factors (such as thoughts, emotions, and behavior), and social factors (such as family support, socioeconomic status, and cultural influences).

This model has influenced contemporary psychiatric practice, leading to personalized treatment plans that address the diverse needs of individuals with mental disorders.

Contemporary Approaches to Mental Health Care

In the present day, psychiatry continues to evolve and adapt to the changing landscape of mental health care. The field incorporates evidence-based practices and integrates various treatment modalities, including psychopharmacology, psychotherapy, and psychosocial interventions.

Collaborative models of care involving interdisciplinary teams are becoming more common, recognizing the value of a holistic approach to mental health. Mental health professionals, including psychiatrists, psychologists, social workers, and counselors, work together to provide comprehensive care and support for individuals with mental disorders.

Conclusion

The emergence of psychiatry as a medical specialty has been shaped by historical, cultural, and scientific influences. From ancient beliefs in supernatural causes to the medicalization of mental illness and the advent of psychoanalysis, psychiatry has undergone significant transformations.

The shift towards community-based care and the adoption of a biopsychosocial model have further expanded the understanding and treatment of mental disorders. Contemporary psychiatry emphasizes personalized care, evidence-based practices, and collaborative approaches.

As we move forward, it is crucial to recognize the challenges faced by individuals with mental disorders and work towards a sustainable mental health future. This involves advancing research, strengthening mental health policies, promoting awareness and advocacy, and fostering resilient communities that support the well-being of all.

The Influence of Freudian Psychoanalysis

Freudian psychoanalysis, developed by Sigmund Freud in the late 19th and early 20th centuries, has had a profound impact on the fields of psychology, psychiatry, and mental health. Freud's theories revolutionized our understanding of the human mind, paving the way for new perspectives on mental disorders and treatment approaches. In this section, we will explore the key concepts of Freudian psychoanalysis and its influence on the field of mental health.

The Unconscious Mind

One of Freud's central ideas is the concept of the unconscious mind. According to Freud, our behavior and experiences are influenced by unconscious thoughts, desires, and memories that are inaccessible to our conscious awareness. These unconscious processes shape our personality, motivations, and emotional experiences.

Freud proposed that the mind is divided into three parts: the conscious, preconscious, and unconscious. The conscious mind contains thoughts and feelings that we are currently aware of. The preconscious mind holds information that can be easily accessed with attention. The unconscious mind, on the other hand, contains repressed memories, traumatic experiences, and unacceptable desires that have been pushed out of conscious awareness.

Understanding the role of the unconscious mind is essential in psychoanalysis. Through techniques such as free association and dream analysis, Freud believed that individuals could gain insight into their unconscious conflicts and eventually resolve them.

Psychosexual Development

Another significant contribution of Freudian psychoanalysis is the theory of psychosexual development. According to Freud, individuals pass through distinct stages of psychosexual development, each characterized by a focus on different erogenous zones.

The stages of psychosexual development are the oral, anal, phallic, latency, and genital stages. In each stage, children face conflicts that shape their psychological development. For example, during the phallic stage, children experience the Oedipus complex (in boys) or the Electra complex (in girls), which involve unconscious sexual desires for the opposite-sex parent and rivalry with the same-sex parent.

Freud believed that unresolved conflicts during psychosexual development could lead to fixations at specific stages, resulting in psychological disturbances in adulthood. For example, an individual fixated at the oral stage may exhibit behaviors such as excessive dependency or aggression.

Defense Mechanisms

Freud proposed the concept of defense mechanisms as psychological strategies that individuals employ to cope with anxiety and protect their ego. These defense mechanisms operate unconsciously and act as a way to reduce emotional distress.

Some common defense mechanisms identified by Freud include repression, denial, projection, and displacement. Repression involves pushing unacceptable thoughts or memories into the unconscious. Denial is the refusal to accept painful realities. Projection involves attributing one's own unacceptable thoughts or feelings onto others. Displacement is redirecting emotions or impulses from their original source to a less threatening target.

Understanding defense mechanisms plays a crucial role in psychoanalysis. By uncovering and exploring these defense mechanisms, individuals can gain insight into their unconscious conflicts and develop healthier coping strategies.

Critiques and Contemporary Relevance

Freudian psychoanalysis has received both praise and criticism over the years. While Freud made significant contributions to the field of mental health, some of his ideas have been challenged by modern research and theoretical perspectives. For example, Freud's emphasis on early childhood experiences and sexual instincts has been seen as overly deterministic and limited in scope.

However, Freudian concepts continue to influence contemporary approaches to psychotherapy and our understanding of human behavior. Many therapeutic techniques, such as free association and dream analysis, trace their roots back to Freudian psychoanalysis. Additionally, the emphasis on the unconscious mind and the exploration of underlying conflicts are still relevant in contemporary psychodynamic therapies.

In conclusion, Freudian psychoanalysis has left an indelible mark on the field of mental health. By introducing groundbreaking concepts such as the unconscious mind, psychosexual development, and defense mechanisms, Freud paved the way for a deeper understanding of human psychology. While some of Freud's ideas have been refined or challenged, his contributions continue to shape our approach to mental health treatment and research.

The Medicalization of Mental Illness

In the field of mental health, the medicalization of mental illness refers to the process by which psychiatric disorders are understood and treated primarily from a biomedical perspective. This approach emphasizes the physiological and neurological aspects of mental health disorders and often relies on pharmacological interventions.

Historical Context

The medicalization of mental illness can be traced back to the late 18th and early 19th centuries when advancements in medical knowledge and understanding of the human body led to the emergence of psychiatry as a medical specialty. Prior to this, mental health conditions were often viewed through a moral or religious lens, with individuals being blamed for their own suffering.

The influence of Sigmund Freud and his psychoanalytic theory in the late 19th and early 20th centuries also played a significant role in shaping the medicalization of mental illness. Freud emphasized the importance of the unconscious mind and the role of early childhood experiences in the development of mental disorders. His theories introduced a new understanding of mental health rooted in psychological processes.

Biological Psychiatry

Biological psychiatry, also known as biopsychiatry or the medical model, became dominant in the mid-20th century. This approach considers mental health disorders as primarily caused by biological factors, such as genetics, neurochemical imbalances, or structural abnormalities in the brain.

The development of psychotropic medications, such as antidepressants and antipsychotics, further reinforced the medicalization of mental illness. These medications target specific neurotransmitters in the brain to alleviate symptoms and are often used as a first-line treatment for many mental health conditions.

Critiques of the Medicalization Approach

While the medicalization of mental illness has led to significant advancements in treatment and understanding, it has also faced criticism from various quarters.

One critique is that the medical model tends to oversimplify mental health conditions by reducing them to purely biological factors. This reductionism overlooks the complex interplay between biological, psychological, and social factors in the development and maintenance of mental disorders.

The medicalization approach also runs the risk of over-reliance on pharmacological treatments, potentially neglecting the effectiveness of other interventions, such as psychotherapy or lifestyle modifications. This narrow focus on medication as the primary treatment modality may limit the individual's autonomy and agency in managing their mental health.

Furthermore, the medicalization of mental illness raises ethical concerns surrounding the use of psychotropic medications. This includes issues related to informed consent, potential side effects, long-term effects, and the influence of pharmaceutical companies on psychiatric research and practice.

A Holistic Approach

In recent years, there has been a growing recognition of the importance of a holistic approach to mental health care. This approach acknowledges the multidimensional nature of mental health and emphasizes the integration of biological, psychological, and social factors in understanding and treating mental health disorders.

A holistic approach recognizes that mental health is not solely determined by biological factors but is also influenced by social determinants, such as socioeconomic status, culture, and environmental factors. It acknowledges the importance of psychosocial interventions, such as psychotherapy, counseling, and lifestyle modifications, in promoting mental wellbeing.

Integrative psychiatry is an emerging field that combines conventional psychiatric treatments with complementary and alternative therapies. These therapies may include mindfulness-based practices, yoga, acupuncture, and nutritional interventions. Integrative psychiatry seeks to address the limitations of the medical model by offering a more comprehensive and personalized approach to mental health care.

Case Study: Attention-Deficit/Hyperactivity Disorder (ADHD)

Attention-Deficit/Hyperactivity Disorder (ADHD) provides an example of how the medicalization of mental illness has evolved over time. Initially, ADHD was understood primarily as a behavioral issue and was not widely recognized as a medical condition. However, with advances in neuroscience and the development of stimulant medications, ADHD became increasingly medicalized.

Critics argue that the medicalization of ADHD has led to an overreliance on medication as the primary treatment and has neglected the importance of addressing environmental and psychosocial factors. Alternative approaches, such as behavioral interventions, psychoeducation, and lifestyle modifications, are increasingly being recognized as important components of a holistic treatment plan for individuals with ADHD.

Conclusion

The medicalization of mental illness has significantly shaped our understanding and treatment of psychiatric disorders. While it has led to important advancements in the field, the medical model is not without its limitations and critiques. A holistic approach that incorporates biological, psychological, and social factors is essential for comprehensive and individualized mental health care. By recognizing the complexities of mental health and the diverse needs of individuals, we can move towards a more sustainable and inclusive future for mental health.

The Deinstitutionalization Movement

The deinstitutionalization movement was a significant shift in mental health care during the late 20th century. It aimed to move individuals with mental illnesses out of large, centralized psychiatric institutions and towards community-based care. This section explores the historical context, goals, challenges, and impact of the deinstitutionalization movement.

Historical Context of Deinstitutionalization

To understand the deinstitutionalization movement, it is crucial to consider the historical context that led to the establishment of large psychiatric institutions in the first place. During the 18th and 19th centuries, the rise of the asylums marked the era of institutionalization. At that time, society's understanding of mental illness was limited, and individuals with mental health conditions were often considered dangerous or incurable. As a result, they were confined to asylums, which aimed to provide care but often became overcrowded and neglectful institutions.

Goals of Deinstitutionalization

The deinstitutionalization movement emerged as a response to the failings of the asylum system. Its primary goals were to:

- Provide more humane and individualized care for individuals with mental illnesses.

- Promote community integration and eliminate the isolation associated with institutionalization.

- Shift the focus from custodial care to recovery-oriented treatment approaches.

- Increase the availability of mental health services in community settings.

- Reduce the economic burden of large psychiatric institutions.

Challenges and Criticisms

The deinstitutionalization movement faced significant challenges and criticisms that affected its implementation and outcomes. Some of the key challenges include:

- Inadequate community-based mental health services: The closure of psychiatric institutions often occurred without proper planning and investment in community-based services. This led to a lack of adequate resources, including housing, outpatient clinics, and social support networks.

- Homelessness and incarceration: Many individuals who were discharged from psychiatric institutions ended up homeless or incarcerated due to the lack of community support. This highlighted the need for comprehensive support systems to ensure successful transitions.

- Stigma and discrimination: Despite the shift towards community-based care, mental health stigma persisted, making it difficult for individuals to access employment, housing, and other societal opportunities.

- Lack of coordination and collaboration: The fragmented nature of mental health services, with different agencies responsible for different aspects of care, hindered effective collaboration and coordination.

Impact of Deinstitutionalization

The impact of the deinstitutionalization movement has been mixed. On one hand, it has led to positive changes, including:

- Increased autonomy and freedom for individuals with mental illnesses.
- Greater focus on recovery and community integration.
- Encouragement of person-centered care and respect for individuals' rights.
- Improved treatment approaches, such as the development of psychosocial interventions and community support programs.

However, there have also been negative consequences, including:

- Increased burden on families and caregivers to provide support and care.
- Rise in homelessness and incarceration rates among individuals with mental illnesses.
- Overwhelmed community mental health services, leading to long waiting lists and limited access to care.
- Lack of coordination and continuity in care, resulting in individuals falling through the cracks of the system.

Lessons Learned and Future Directions

The deinstitutionalization movement has highlighted several important lessons and considerations for the future of mental health care. These include:

- The need for comprehensive and integrated community-based mental health services that offer a range of evidence-based treatments and supports.
- Collaborative approaches involving multiple stakeholders, including healthcare providers, community organizations, policymakers, and individuals with lived experience.
- Addressing social determinants of mental health, such as housing, employment, and education, to promote overall wellbeing and successful community integration.
- Implementing robust evaluation and monitoring systems to assess the effectiveness and outcomes of community-based mental health programs.
- Advocating for adequate funding and resources to support mental health initiatives and address disparities in access to care.

Overall, the deinstitutionalization movement represented a significant paradigm shift in mental health care. While it aimed to provide more humane and community-focused care, it also faced significant challenges. By learning from past experiences, addressing critical gaps, and promoting collaborative approaches, we can strive towards a more sustainable and inclusive mental health future.

The Impact of Deinstitutionalization on Mental Health Care

Deinstitutionalization refers to the process of transitioning individuals with mental illness from long-term psychiatric institutions to community-based settings. This movement gained momentum in the second half of the 20th century, driven by various factors such as advancements in psychiatric treatment, evolving societal attitudes towards mental health, and budgetary considerations.

1. Background on Deinstitutionalization: Deinstitutionalization was a response to the deplorable conditions and human rights abuses experienced by individuals in psychiatric institutions. With the advent of effective psychotropic medications and the recognition that mental health issues could be managed in community settings, the primary goal of deinstitutionalization was to integrate individuals with mental illness back into society.

2. The benefits of Deinstitutionalization: a) Improved quality of life: Deinstitutionalization aimed to provide individuals with mental illness the opportunity to live in the community, fostering their independence, autonomy, and dignity. b) Enhanced treatment options: Community-based care allows for a more individualized approach to treatment, focusing on rehabilitation, recovery, and long-term support. It encourages a holistic view of mental health and emphasizes the integration of mental health services with other healthcare sectors. c) Reduced stigma: Keeping individuals with mental illness in separate institutions perpetuated the stigma surrounding mental health. Deinstitutionalization aimed to reduce this stigma by promoting inclusivity and community integration.

3. Challenges and Criticisms of Deinstitutionalization: a) Lack of resources: One major challenge of deinstitutionalization was the insufficient allocation of resources for community-based mental health services. As a result, many individuals were released from institutions without adequate support, leading to homelessness or involvement with the criminal justice system. b) Fragmented care: The shift from institutional to community-based care often resulted in fragmented services, making it difficult for individuals to access the comprehensive care they needed. This was particularly true for those with complex or severe mental health conditions. c) Increased strain on families: Deinstitutionalization placed a larger burden on families and caregivers who had to navigate the challenges of supporting

their loved ones in community settings without adequate resources or support. d) Lack of coordination: The lack of coordination between mental health services, housing, employment, and other social supports made it challenging for individuals to reintegrate into society successfully.

4. Strategies to enhance the impact of Deinstitutionalization: a) Strengthen community-based services: Adequate funding and resources must be allocated to community mental health centers, outpatient clinics, crisis intervention teams, and other mental health support services to ensure the provision of comprehensive care. b) Promote collaboration: Collaboration between mental health providers, primary care physicians, social workers, and other professionals is crucial to provide integrated care and support for individuals transitioning from institutions. c) Housing and employment support: The availability of safe and affordable housing, as well as employment opportunities, can significantly impact the success of deinstitutionalization efforts. Supportive housing programs and vocational training initiatives should be implemented. d) Education and awareness: Education campaigns aimed at reducing mental health stigma are necessary to create an inclusive society that supports and advocates for individuals with mental illness. This involves promoting mental health awareness in schools, workplaces, and communities.

5. Examples of successful deinstitutionalization initiatives: a) The "Housing First" model: This approach prioritizes providing stable housing for individuals with mental illness before addressing other needs. It has proven effective in reducing homelessness and improving mental health outcomes. b) Assertive Community Treatment (ACT) teams: ACT teams consist of multidisciplinary professionals who provide comprehensive, community-based care to individuals with complex mental health needs. This approach has shown positive outcomes in reducing hospitalizations and improving quality of life. c) Peer support programs: Peer support programs employ individuals with personal experiences of mental illness to provide support and mentorship to others in similar situations. These programs have demonstrated success in promoting recovery and reducing hospital readmissions.

In conclusion, deinstitutionalization has had a significant impact on mental health care, offering individuals with mental illness an opportunity for recovery and community integration. However, it also presents challenges that must be addressed to ensure the provision of comprehensive, accessible, and coordinated care. By strengthening community-based services, promoting collaboration, providing housing and employment support, and raising awareness, we can maximize the positive impact of deinstitutionalization on mental health care.

Challenges and Controversies in Deinstitutionalization

Deinstitutionalization refers to the shift in mental health care from centralized psychiatric institutions to community-based care. While this approach has been hailed as a significant step towards promoting patient autonomy and integration into society, it is not without its challenges and controversies. In this section, we will explore some of the key issues surrounding deinstitutionalization and its implementation.

Inadequate Community Support

One of the major challenges of deinstitutionalization has been the lack of adequate community support systems. The closure of psychiatric institutions often occurred without the necessary establishment of community mental health services. As a result, many individuals with mental illnesses were left without the necessary support to manage their conditions. This lack of support can contribute to increased rates of homelessness, unemployment, and social isolation, exacerbating the existing challenges faced by individuals with mental health disorders.

Insufficient Funding

Another significant challenge in the deinstitutionalization process has been the issue of insufficient funding. The redirection of resources from psychiatric institutions to community services has often been accompanied by budget cuts, limiting the availability and quality of mental health care services in the community. This lack of funding can result in long wait times for treatment, understaffed mental health facilities, and inadequate access to necessary medications and therapies.

Criminalization of Mental Illness

Deinstitutionalization has also been criticized for contributing to the criminalization of mental illness. In the absence of adequate community services, individuals with mental health challenges may end up in the criminal justice system instead of receiving appropriate mental health care. This can lead to a revolving door phenomenon, where individuals with mental illnesses are repeatedly incarcerated without receiving the necessary treatment and support to address the underlying causes of their behaviors.

Lack of Coordination and Collaboration

A lack of coordination and collaboration among different sectors of the mental health care system has been a significant obstacle in the successful implementation of deinstitutionalization. The responsibility for mental health care is often fragmented among various agencies, including mental health departments, social services, and housing authorities. Without effective coordination and collaboration among these agencies, individuals may fall through the cracks and fail to receive the comprehensive care they need.

Stigma and Discrimination

Stigma and discrimination against individuals with mental illnesses remain persistent challenges in the deinstitutionalization process. Despite efforts to promote mental health awareness and reduce stigma, negative attitudes and stereotypes continue to hinder the social integration and acceptance of individuals with mental health challenges. This can lead to social exclusion, limited employment opportunities, and reduced access to housing and other supports, impeding the successful transition from institutional care to community living.

Ethical Considerations

Ethical considerations have also emerged as controversial aspects of deinstitutionalization. Questions have been raised regarding the appropriate balance between individual rights, such as the right to autonomy and self-determination, and the duty to protect individuals from harm, particularly in cases where individuals may lack insight into their conditions or pose risks to themselves or others. Striking the right balance requires careful thought and consideration of ethical principles and legal frameworks while respecting the dignity and autonomy of individuals.

Conclusion

Deinstitutionalization is a complex and multifaceted process that carries both benefits and challenges. While it offers the potential for greater autonomy, community integration, and improved mental health outcomes, it also requires careful planning, implementation, and ongoing support. Addressing the challenges and controversies associated with deinstitutionalization requires a comprehensive approach that involves adequate funding, robust community support systems, effective coordination, anti-stigma initiatives, and a commitment to upholding ethical principles in mental health care. By recognizing and addressing these challenges, we can strive towards a more sustainable and inclusive mental health care system.

The Biopsychosocial Model of Mental Health

The biopsychosocial model is an approach to understanding and conceptualizing mental health that recognizes the complex interplay of biological, psychological, and social factors. In contrast to more reductionistic and narrow models that focus solely on biological or psychological explanations, the biopsychosocial model takes into account the multiple dimensions that contribute to mental health and illness.

1. Biological Factors

Biological factors refer to the physiological and genetic aspects of mental health. Research has shown that certain genetic predispositions and biochemical imbalances can contribute to the development of psychological disorders. For example, individuals with a family history of depression may have a higher risk of developing depression themselves. Furthermore, imbalances in neurotransmitters, such as serotonin and dopamine, have been implicated in various mental health conditions.

Understanding the role of biology in mental health has led to advancements in psychopharmacology, where medications are used to target specific neurotransmitter systems and alleviate symptoms. However, it is essential to note that biological factors alone cannot fully explain mental health disorders.

2. Psychological Factors

Psychological factors encompass the cognitive, emotional, and behavioral aspects of mental health. Our thoughts, emotions, and behaviors interact and influence our mental well-being. For example, negative thinking patterns and distorted beliefs can contribute to the development and maintenance of anxiety and depression.

Psychological interventions, such as cognitive-behavioral therapy (CBT) and psychoanalysis, aim to address these psychological factors. CBT helps individuals identify and challenge negative thoughts and develop healthier coping mechanisms. On the other hand, psychoanalysis focuses on uncovering unconscious conflicts and unresolved issues that may contribute to psychological problems.

3. Social Factors

Social factors refer to the external influences on mental health, including cultural, environmental, and social determinants. Our social relationships, socioeconomic status, access to resources, and cultural norms all play a vital role in shaping our mental well-being. For instance, individuals from marginalized communities may experience higher levels of stress and discrimination, leading to increased vulnerability to mental health issues.

The biopsychosocial model recognizes the impact of social factors on mental health and emphasizes the need for culturally sensitive and socially inclusive interventions. Psychosocial interventions, such as family therapy and support groups, provide a platform for individuals to address social stressors and develop healthier coping strategies.

Integration and Holistic Approach

The strength of the biopsychosocial model lies in its integration of diverse factors that contribute to mental health. It acknowledges that mental health disorders cannot be attributed solely to one dimension but rather result from a complex interplay of biological, psychological, and social influences.

By considering all dimensions, clinicians can develop a more comprehensive understanding of individuals' experiences and tailor treatments accordingly. This holistic approach promotes a more person-centered and empowering model of mental health care.

Challenges and Considerations

While the biopsychosocial model offers a comprehensive framework for understanding mental health, it is not without its challenges. Integrating different levels of analysis and considering the dynamic interactions between factors can be complex. Additionally, the model requires collaboration across disciplines, as experts from various fields need to work together to provide a holistic approach to mental health care.

Moreover, the biopsychosocial model highlights the need for addressing social determinants of mental health, such as socioeconomic disparities and systemic inequalities. It calls for advocacy and policy changes to promote social justice and reduce the burden of mental illness in vulnerable populations.

Conclusion

The biopsychosocial model of mental health recognizes that mental well-being is influenced by biological, psychological, and social factors. By adopting a holistic and integrated approach, clinicians can provide more comprehensive care and address the complex nature of mental health disorders. This model emphasizes the importance of considering each individual's unique biological, psychological, and social context when assessing and treating mental health conditions. The biopsychosocial model holds the potential to drive significant advancements in mental health care by fostering collaboration, promoting social justice, and empowering individuals to achieve overall well-being.

The Social Determinants of Mental Health

Socioeconomic Status and Mental Health

Socioeconomic status (SES) refers to an individual's or a group's position within society based on various factors such as income, education, occupation, and wealth. It is well-established that socioeconomic status plays a significant role in shaping an individual's mental health. People from lower socioeconomic backgrounds often face numerous challenges that can have a detrimental impact on their mental well-being.

The Relationship Between SES and Mental Health

The relationship between socioeconomic status and mental health is complex and multifaceted. Multiple studies have consistently shown that individuals from lower socioeconomic backgrounds are at higher risk for developing mental health disorders compared to those from higher socioeconomic backgrounds.

One of the key factors contributing to this relationship is the presence of chronic stressors associated with low socioeconomic status. Financial insecurity, limited access to healthcare and education, unemployment, and inadequate housing are examples of stressors that individuals with lower SES often face. These stressors can lead to increased psychological distress and vulnerability to mental health disorders.

Moreover, low socioeconomic status is linked to social inequalities, discrimination, and marginalization, which further contribute to poor mental health outcomes. Social inequalities can cause feelings of powerlessness, hopelessness, and low self-esteem, leading to increased rates of anxiety, depression, and other mental health problems.

Mechanisms Linking SES and Mental Health

Several mechanisms have been proposed to explain the relationship between socioeconomic status and mental health. One such mechanism is the "social causation" hypothesis, which suggests that the adverse effects of low socioeconomic status directly impact mental health. This hypothesis proposes that experiencing chronic stressors, daily hassles, and material deprivation can contribute to the development of mental health disorders.

On the other hand, the "social selection" hypothesis suggests that individuals with poor mental health are more likely to experience downward social mobility, leading to lower socioeconomic status. This hypothesis posits that mental health problems can hinder educational attainment, employment opportunities, and overall social functioning, resulting in a lower socioeconomic status.

Furthermore, the social environment associated with socioeconomic status can influence mental health outcomes. Individuals from higher socioeconomic backgrounds often have access to better social support networks, quality healthcare, and educational opportunities. In contrast, those from lower socioeconomic backgrounds may face social isolation, limited access to resources, and higher exposure to adverse social conditions, increasing their vulnerability to mental health problems.

Impact on Mental Health Disparities

The relationship between socioeconomic status and mental health has significant implications for mental health disparities. Mental health disparities refer to the unequal distribution of mental health outcomes and access to mental health services among different socioeconomic groups.

Individuals from lower socioeconomic backgrounds often face barriers to accessing mental health services, including affordability issues, limited availability of providers in their communities, and stigma associated with seeking help. These barriers can contribute to delays in seeking treatment, resulting in poorer mental health outcomes.

To address mental health disparities, it is crucial to prioritize policies and interventions that target socioeconomic factors. Efforts should focus on reducing social inequalities, promoting equal access to education and employment opportunities, improving the availability of affordable mental health services, and reducing the stigma surrounding mental health.

Case Study: The Impact of Poverty on Mental Health

Consider the case of Marie, a single mother living in a low-income neighborhood. Marie struggles to make ends meet, facing financial instability and limited job prospects. She lives in a neighborhood with high crime rates and lacks access to quality healthcare and mental health services. Marie often experiences stress, anxiety, and depression due to her challenging circumstances.

Marie's case highlights how the socioeconomic factors of poverty can contribute to mental health issues. The chronic stressors associated with poverty, such as financial struggles and limited resources, exacerbate her mental health problems. Additionally, the lack of social support and access to mental health services further hinders her ability to seek appropriate care and support.

Conclusion

Socioeconomic status plays a significant role in shaping mental health outcomes. The relationship between socioeconomic status and mental health is complex, influenced by both social and individual factors. Understanding and addressing the impact of socioeconomic factors on mental health is vital for developing holistic and effective interventions that promote mental well-being for all individuals, regardless of their socioeconomic status. By implementing policies that reduce social inequalities, provide equal opportunities, and improve access to mental health services, we can work towards achieving a more sustainable and equitable mental health future.

Gender and Mental Health

In this section, we will explore the relationship between gender and mental health. Gender plays a significant role in influencing mental health outcomes, as societal norms, expectations, and cultural factors can all contribute to disparities in psychological well-being between different genders. It is important to understand these dynamics to ensure appropriate and effective mental health support for all individuals.

Gender Identity and Mental Health

Gender identity refers to an individual's deeply-felt sense of being male, female, or something outside of the traditional binary construct. Transgender individuals, whose gender identity differs from the sex assigned at birth, often face unique challenges related to mental health. Discrimination, stigma, and lack of acceptance from society can lead to increased rates of anxiety, depression, and suicidal ideation among transgender individuals.

Research has shown that social support, including acceptance from family, friends, and healthcare professionals, is crucial for promoting positive mental health outcomes in transgender individuals. Promoting inclusivity, understanding, and respect for diverse gender identities can significantly improve mental health outcomes within this population.

Gender Roles and Mental Health

Societal expectations and gender roles can also impact mental health. Traditional gender roles often dictate that men should be strong, stoic, and unemotional, while women are expected to be nurturing, caring, and emotionally expressive. These rigid expectations can contribute to the development of mental health issues.

For instance, men may feel pressure to suppress their emotions, leading to difficulties in seeking help and expressing their mental health concerns. This can contribute to higher rates of substance abuse, aggression, and suicide among men. Women, on the other hand, may face higher rates of anxiety and depression due to societal pressure to meet unrealistic standards of beauty, success, and caregiving.

Understanding and challenging these gender norms is essential for promoting mental health equity. Encouraging men to seek help and express their emotions, and empowering women to challenge societal expectations can foster healthier mental health outcomes for all genders.

Gender-based Violence and Mental Health

Gender-based violence, including intimate partner violence, sexual assault, and harassment, has profound impacts on mental health. Survivors of gender-based violence are at increased risk of developing mental health disorders such as post-traumatic stress disorder (PTSD), depression, and anxiety.

It is important to provide comprehensive support and mental health services to survivors, including trauma-informed care, counseling, and access to resources such as shelters and helplines. Prevention efforts should also focus on addressing the root causes of gender-based violence and promoting healthy relationships.

Addressing Gender Disparities in Mental Health

To address gender disparities in mental health, a comprehensive approach is necessary. This includes:

1. Education and awareness: Promoting education and awareness about the impact of gender on mental health can help reduce stigma and increase understanding.

2. Access to care: Ensuring equal access to culturally sensitive mental health services for individuals of all genders is crucial. This includes addressing barriers such as cost, transportation, and the availability of gender-affirming mental health professionals.

3. Gender-sensitive research: Conducting gender-sensitive research can help identify the unique mental health needs and experiences of different genders, leading to the development of targeted interventions.

4. Incorporating gender into mental health policies: Integrating gender considerations into mental health policies can help address gender disparities and promote gender equity in mental health care.

5. Empowering individuals: Promoting gender equality and empowering individuals to challenge gender norms can contribute to better mental health outcomes for all genders.

In conclusion, gender plays a significant role in mental health outcomes. Understanding the complex interplay between gender and mental health is essential for providing effective and inclusive mental health support. By addressing gender disparities and promoting gender equity, we can work towards a future where mental health care is accessible and tailored to the diverse needs of all individuals, irrespective of their gender identity or expression.

Race, Ethnicity, and Mental Health

Race and ethnicity play a significant role in mental health, shaping individuals' experiences of mental illness, access to care, and treatment outcomes. Understanding the relationship between race, ethnicity, and mental health is crucial for promoting equitable and effective mental health care for diverse populations.

Social Determinants of Mental Health

To understand the impact of race and ethnicity on mental health, it is essential to consider the social determinants of mental health. These are the conditions in which people are born, grow, live, work, and age, and they include factors such as socioeconomic status, education, employment, social support, and access to healthcare.

1. **Socioeconomic Status and Mental Health:** Socioeconomic disparities exist among different racial and ethnic groups, with marginalized communities often experiencing higher rates of poverty and limited access to resources. These socioeconomic factors influence mental health outcomes, as individuals facing poverty and discrimination may be more vulnerable to stress, trauma, and limited healthcare access.

2. **Discrimination and Racial Trauma:** Racial and ethnic minorities may face discrimination and racism, leading to mental health disparities. Experiences of discrimination can result in chronic stress, anxiety, depression, and trauma. Racial trauma refers to the psychological and emotional impact of racism, including the cumulative effects of individual and systemic racism.

3. **Cultural Factors and Help-Seeking Behavior:** Cultural beliefs and values influence help-seeking behavior and attitudes towards mental health. Stigma surrounding mental illness varies across cultures, impacting individuals' willingness to seek support. For some ethnic groups, mental health concerns might be attributed to spiritual or supernatural causes, leading to unique help-seeking pathways.

Mental Health Disparities

Mental health disparities refer to differences in mental health outcomes and access to quality care among different racial and ethnic groups. Several factors contribute to these disparities, including structural inequities, cultural factors, and healthcare access barriers.

1. **Structural Inequities:** Historical and ongoing social inequalities, including systemic racism and discrimination, contribute to mental health disparities. Limited access to quality education, employment opportunities, affordable housing, and healthcare services disproportionately affect marginalized communities and contribute to mental health disparities.

2. **Cultural Competence and Bias:** Cultural competence in mental health care refers to the ability of providers to understand and respond to the unique cultural and linguistic needs of diverse clients. Bias and lack of cultural competence in the mental health system can lead to misdiagnosis, inappropriate treatment, and mistrust, further exacerbating mental health disparities.

3. **Healthcare Access Barriers:** Racial and ethnic minorities often face barriers in accessing mental health services, including lack of insurance, transportation difficulties, language barriers, and shortage of culturally competent providers. These barriers contribute to disparities in mental health treatment and outcomes.

Promoting Equity in Mental Health Care

Addressing mental health disparities requires a comprehensive approach that tackles the social determinants of mental health, promotes cultural competence, and enhances healthcare access. Here are some strategies to promote equity in mental health care:

1. **Culturally Competent Care:** Mental health providers should receive training in cultural competence to understand and address the unique needs of diverse populations. This includes awareness of cultural beliefs, practices, and values, as well as the impact of discrimination and racism on mental health.

2. **Reducing Stigma and Discrimination:** Efforts to reduce mental health stigma and discrimination are essential to fostering help-seeking behavior and creating inclusive environments. This involves raising awareness, challenging stereotypes, and promoting positive portrayals of mental health in diverse communities.

3. **Improved Access to Care:** Policies must prioritize expanding access to quality mental health care in underserved communities. This includes increasing the availability of culturally competent providers, addressing language barriers, and ensuring that services are affordable and accessible to all.

4. **Community-Based Approaches:** Engaging communities in mental health promotion and prevention efforts can help reduce disparities. Community-based programs, peer support networks, and culturally tailored interventions can increase engagement and improve mental health outcomes.

5. **Research and Data Collection:** More research is needed to understand the unique mental health needs and experiences of different racial and ethnic groups. Collecting data on mental health outcomes by race and ethnicity can help identify disparities and inform evidence-based interventions.

It is important to recognize that the relationship between race, ethnicity, and mental health is complex and influenced by various individual, interpersonal, cultural, and structural factors. By addressing these factors and promoting equity in mental health care, we can work towards a future where everyone has equal opportunities for mental well-being.

Disability and Mental Health

In this section, we will explore the intersection between disability and mental health. Disability refers to any condition that limits a person's physical, sensory, cognitive, or intellectual functioning, often resulting in impairments that may affect their daily activities and social participation. Mental health, on the other hand, encompasses emotional, psychological, and social well-being, and it directly impacts how we think, feel, and act.

1. Disabilities and Mental Health: A Complex Relationship

The relationship between disabilities and mental health is complex and multidimensional. People with disabilities may experience mental health challenges, including higher rates of mental illnesses such as depression, anxiety disorders, and post-traumatic stress disorder (PTSD). This can be attributed to a range of factors, including:

- Social and environmental barriers: People with disabilities often face additional challenges in accessing support systems, education, employment, healthcare, and social opportunities. These barriers can contribute to feelings of isolation, discrimination, and social exclusion, increasing the risk of mental health issues. - Chronic pain and functional limitations: Many individuals with disabilities experience chronic pain and functional limitations, which can lead to emotional distress, frustration, and a reduced quality of life. - Stigma and societal attitudes: Negative stereotypes, stigma, and marginalization surrounding disabilities can have a profound impact on an individual's mental well-being. Experiencing prejudice and discrimination can lead to feelings of shame, low self-esteem, and internalized ableism.

2. Mental Health Needs of People with Disabilities

It is essential to recognize and address the mental health needs of people with disabilities. Providing appropriate support and interventions can significantly improve their overall well-being. Some key considerations include:

- Holistic approach: Taking a holistic approach to mental health care is crucial. It involves understanding the unique challenges faced by individuals with disabilities and developing tailored interventions that address their specific needs. - Accessible mental health services: Ensuring accessibility of mental health services is critical. This includes physical accessibility, communication support, and accommodations for individuals with different disabilities. - Support networks: Building strong support networks is essential for people with disabilities. It can include family, friends, peer support groups, and disability-specific organizations that provide social connection, understanding, and a sense of belonging. - Trauma-informed care: Trauma is more prevalent among individuals with disabilities, often resulting from experiences of abuse, neglect, and discrimination. Using trauma-informed approaches in mental health care delivery can help create a safe and supportive environment for healing and recovery. - Skills development and empowerment: Promoting the development of skills and empowering individuals with disabilities can enhance their capacity to cope with challenges, build resilience, and improve their mental well-being. - Addressing systemic barriers: Addressing systemic barriers that contribute to the marginalization and exclusion of individuals with disabilities is crucial. This includes advocating for policy changes, promoting inclusive education and employment opportunities, and challenging ableism in society.

3. The Role of Rehabilitation Psychology

Rehabilitation psychology plays a vital role in addressing the mental health needs of individuals with disabilities. It focuses on enhancing psychological well-being, promoting adjustment, and facilitating the process of rehabilitation. Some key principles and strategies used in rehabilitation psychology include:

- Person-centered approach: Rehabilitation psychology emphasizes the individual's goals, aspirations, and strengths. It involves collaborative decision-making and tailoring interventions to meet the person's unique needs and preferences. - Functional assessment: Conducting comprehensive functional assessments helps identify the specific psychological challenges and develop targeted interventions to maximize independence, well-being, and quality of life. - Cognitive-behavioral interventions: Cognitive-behavioral interventions are widely used in rehabilitation psychology to address maladaptive thoughts, emotions, and behaviors. This approach helps individuals develop coping strategies, build resilience, and enhance their overall mental well-being. - Psychoeducation: Providing individuals with disabilities and their families with psychoeducation about mental health conditions, coping strategies, and available resources can empower them to take an active role in their mental health care. - Advocacy and social support: Rehabilitation psychologists often work as advocates for individuals with disabilities, promoting their rights, and enhancing social support systems. This may involve collaborating with other professionals, disability organizations, and policymakers to create inclusive and supportive environments.

4. Case Study: Promoting Mental Health for People with Physical Disabilities

Let's consider the case of Maya, a twenty-five-year-old woman with a physical disability resulting from a spinal cord injury. Maya has experienced challenges in adjusting to her disability and has been struggling with depression and anxiety. Here are some possible strategies to promote Maya's mental health:

- Individual therapy: Maya can benefit from individual therapy sessions with a rehabilitation psychologist or a mental health professional experienced in working with individuals with disabilities. Therapy can help her explore and address her emotional challenges, develop coping strategies, and work towards her goals of psychological well-being. - Peer support groups: Connecting Maya with peer support groups of individuals with similar disabilities can be invaluable. Sharing experiences, challenges, and successes with peers who have faced similar struggles can provide validation, support, and a sense of belonging. - Accessibility modifications: Ensuring physical accessibility in Maya's living environment and providing assistive devices or technology that promote independence can have a positive impact on her mental well-being. - Psychoeducation: Providing Maya with psychoeducation about her mental health condition, teaching her coping skills, and helping her develop self-management strategies can empower her to actively participate in her mental health care. - Collaborative goal-setting: Involving Maya in the goal-setting process and working collaboratively as part of her rehabilitation team can enhance her motivation and sense of control over her mental well-being.

In conclusion, addressing the mental health needs of people with disabilities is critical for their overall well-being and quality of life. By recognizing the complex relationship between disabilities and mental health, providing accessible support services, and promoting inclusive approaches, we can work towards a society that values and supports the mental well-being of all individuals, regardless of their abilities.

The Intersectionality of Social Determinants

In understanding mental health, it is crucial to recognize that various social determinants play a significant role in shaping an individual's well-being. These determinants include socioeconomic status, gender, race and ethnicity, disability, and the intersectionality of these factors. By examining the interplay between these social determinants, we can gain a deeper understanding of how they impact mental health outcomes.

Socioeconomic Status and Mental Health

Socioeconomic status (SES) refers to an individual's position in society based on factors such as income, education, and occupation. Numerous studies have shown a clear link between SES and mental health outcomes. Individuals with lower SES are more likely to experience higher levels of stress, lack of access to quality healthcare, limited social support, and increased exposure to adverse life events.

For example, lower income levels can restrict access to mental health services, leading to untreated or poorly managed mental health conditions. Educational disparities can impact mental health by limiting opportunities for economic mobility and reinforcing systemic inequalities. Occupational stressors, such as job insecurity and demanding work environments, can also contribute to poor mental health outcomes.

Example: John, a construction worker, struggles with financial instability and lacks access to affordable mental health care. The stress of his job and financial worries contribute to his anxiety and depression.

Solution: To address the intersectionality of socioeconomic factors and mental health, it is essential to implement policies that promote economic equality, improve access to quality mental health services, and prioritize mental health in the workplace. Investing in social safety nets, expanding healthcare coverage, and providing mental health support in low-income communities can help mitigate the impact of socioeconomic disparities on mental health.

Gender and Mental Health

Gender is a critical social determinant that influences mental health experiences. Research has shown that gender-based social norms, roles, and expectations play a role in shaping mental health outcomes. Women, for instance, are more likely to experience mood disorders such as depression and anxiety, partly due to gender-based discrimination, violence, and societal expectations.

Men, on the other hand, face unique challenges, including societal pressure to conform to traditional masculine ideals that discourage seeking help for mental health issues. This can lead to underdiagnosis and undertreatment of mental health disorders among men.

Example: Sarah, a woman, faces gender-based discrimination at her workplace, leading to increased stress and anxiety. She also experiences societal pressure to balance work and family obligations, resulting in burnout and depression.

Solution: Recognizing the intersectionality of gender and mental health requires creating inclusive and gender-sensitive mental health services. This includes promoting gender equity, addressing gender-based discrimination and violence, and dismantling societal norms that perpetuate gender disparities. Additionally, providing mental health education and resources aimed at challenging traditional gender roles can help reduce stigma and improve access to care for all genders.

Race, Ethnicity, and Mental Health

Race and ethnicity significantly influence mental health experiences, as individuals from different racial and ethnic backgrounds face unique challenges and systemic disparities. Racism, discrimination, and marginalization can contribute to increased psychological distress and higher rates of mental health disorders among racial and ethnic minority populations.

For example, Black individuals in many societies confront systemic racism, which can lead to chronic stress, trauma, and limited access to quality mental health care. Similarly, Indigenous communities may experience intergenerational trauma resulting from historical injustices, which can impact mental health outcomes.

Example: Maria, a Latina immigrant, faces language barriers and discrimination in her community, leading to feelings of isolation and depression.

Solution: Addressing the intersectionality of race, ethnicity, and mental health requires culturally competent mental health services that acknowledge and address the unique needs of diverse populations. This includes increasing the representation of mental health professionals from various racial and ethnic backgrounds, promoting anti-racist practices, and implementing policies that eliminate systemic biases and inequities.

Disability and Mental Health

Disability, whether physical or mental, is a critical determinant of mental health. Individuals with disabilities often face stigma, discrimination, and barriers to accessing quality healthcare and social support systems. The intersectionality of disability and mental health presents unique challenges that require a multidimensional approach.

For instance, individuals with physical disabilities may experience higher rates of depression and anxiety due to the limitations imposed by their condition. Additionally, the lack of accessibility and accommodations can further exacerbate feelings of isolation and distress.

Example: James, who uses a wheelchair due to a spinal cord injury, faces attitudinal barriers and limited accessibility in his community, leading to feelings of frustration and low self-esteem.

Solution: Creating inclusive mental health services and promoting disability rights are crucial steps in addressing the intersectionality of disability and mental health. This includes increasing accessibility to mental health services, providing accommodations to individuals with disabilities, and challenging ableism in society.

The Intersectionality of Social Determinants

It is important to recognize that individuals often experience the intersectionality of multiple social determinants simultaneously, which can significantly impact their mental health. For example, an individual who belongs to a racial minority group, has a low socioeconomic status, and experiences gender-based discrimination may face heightened mental health challenges due to the compounded effects of these intersecting identities.

Understanding the intersectionality of social determinants requires a holistic approach that emphasizes the interconnectedness of these factors. It involves recognizing the unique experiences and addressing the specific needs of individuals who navigate multiple axes of identity and oppression.

Example: A transgender person of color from a low-income background may face discrimination, economic inequality, and limited access to transgender-affirming mental health care, resulting in a high risk of mental health disorders.

Solution: To address the intersectionality of social determinants in mental health, it is crucial to adopt an intersectional lens in policies, research, and interventions. This involves considering the complex interactions between various social determinants and developing comprehensive strategies that promote equity, inclusivity, and social justice. It also requires advocacy for marginalized communities and amplifying their voices in mental health discourse.

In conclusion, addressing the intersectionality of social determinants is essential for understanding mental health outcomes. By analyzing how factors such as socioeconomic status, gender, race and ethnicity, and disability intersect, we can identify and address the unique challenges faced by individuals and communities. By adopting a holistic and inclusive approach, we can promote equity, resilience, and overall mental well-being.

The Role of Trauma in Mental Health

Trauma plays a significant role in the development and manifestation of mental health disorders. It can have a profound impact on an individual's psychological well-being, as well as their physical, emotional, and social functioning. In this section, we will explore the definition of trauma, its various forms, its effects on mental health, and the importance of trauma-informed care.

Definition of Trauma

Trauma can be defined as an emotional response to a distressing or disturbing event or series of events that overwhelms an individual's ability to cope. It can result from various experiences, such as physical or sexual abuse, natural disasters, accidents, combat, or witnessing violence. Trauma can also arise from chronic stressors like ongoing discrimination, poverty, or neglect. It is important to note that trauma is subjective and can vary in severity and impact from person to person.

Forms of Trauma

Trauma can be categorized into different types based on the nature of the event or experience. Here are some common forms of trauma:

- **Acute Trauma:** This type of trauma occurs as a result of a single traumatic event, such as an accident or assault.

- **Chronic Trauma:** Chronic trauma refers to prolonged and repeated exposure to traumatic events, such as ongoing abuse or living in a war-torn area.

- **Complex Trauma:** Complex trauma arises from multiple and interrelated traumatic experiences, often occurring during early childhood or within interpersonal relationships, such as in cases of child abuse or domestic violence.

- **Secondary Trauma:** Secondary trauma, also known as vicarious trauma, is the result of repeated exposure to traumatic events through witnessing or working with individuals who have experienced trauma, such as healthcare workers or first responders.

It is crucial to recognize that trauma can have long-lasting effects on an individual's mental health, even if the traumatic event occurred in the past. Unresolved trauma can contribute to the development or exacerbation of mental health disorders.

Effects of Trauma on Mental Health

Traumatic experiences can have a wide range of effects on an individual's mental health. Some common mental health disorders associated with trauma include:

- **Post-Traumatic Stress Disorder (PTSD):** PTSD is a mental health condition that may develop after experiencing or witnessing a traumatic event. It is characterized by symptoms such as intrusive memories, flashbacks, nightmares, avoidance of reminders, negative mood and thoughts, and heightened arousal.

- **Depression and Anxiety Disorders:** Trauma can increase the risk of developing depression and various anxiety disorders, such as generalized anxiety disorder, panic disorder, and social anxiety disorder.

- **Substance Use Disorders:** Individuals who have experienced trauma may turn to substance use as a way to cope with distressing emotions and memories. Substance use can further exacerbate mental health symptoms and lead to the development of substance use disorders.

- **Dissociative Disorders:** Trauma can contribute to the development of dissociative disorders, which are characterized by disruptions in consciousness, memory, identity, or perception. Dissociative disorders may include dissociative amnesia, depersonalization-derealization disorder, and dissociative identity disorder.

In addition to these specific disorders, trauma can also have a profound impact on an individual's self-esteem, interpersonal relationships, and overall quality of life. It can affect one's ability to trust others, regulate emotions, and engage in daily activities.

Trauma-Informed Care

Given the significant role of trauma in mental health, it is crucial for mental health professionals to adopt a trauma-informed approach in their care. Trauma-informed care is an approach that recognizes and responds to the impact of trauma on individuals seeking support. It emphasizes safety, trustworthiness, choice, collaboration, and empowerment.

Some key principles of trauma-informed care include:

- **Safety and Trust:** Creating a safe and trusting environment is essential for individuals who have experienced trauma. This involves establishing clear boundaries, ensuring physical and emotional safety, and fostering a sense of trust and security.

- **Choice and Collaboration:** Trauma survivors should be given choices and be actively involved in their treatment planning. Collaborative decision-making empowers individuals and helps restore a sense of control.

- **Empowerment and Resilience:** Recognizing and building on the strengths and resilience of trauma survivors can promote their healing and recovery. Empowering individuals to make their own decisions and set goals is crucial in trauma-informed care.

- **Cultural Sensitivity:** Trauma-informed care should be culturally sensitive and responsive to the unique needs and beliefs of individuals from diverse backgrounds. Cultural competence ensures that care is respectful and inclusive.

Trauma-informed care can help create an environment that promotes healing, resilience, and recovery for individuals who have experienced trauma. By implementing trauma-informed practices, mental health professionals can reduce the risk of re-traumatization and provide effective support for individuals struggling with trauma-related challenges.

Conclusion

Trauma has a profound impact on mental health and can contribute to the development of various mental health disorders. Understanding the different forms of trauma and its effects on individuals is essential for providing appropriate care and support. Adopting trauma-informed approaches in mental health care can help create safe and empowering environments that promote healing and resilience. It is crucial for mental health professionals, policymakers, and society as a whole to recognize the role of trauma in mental health and work towards building a more trauma-informed and supportive future.

The Impact of Technology on Mental Health

The Rise of Digital Health and Telemedicine

Digital health and telemedicine have emerged as transformative technologies in healthcare, revolutionizing the way we deliver and receive medical care. This section will explore the origins and benefits of digital health and telemedicine, as well as the challenges and ethical considerations associated with their adoption.

Origins of Digital Health

Digital health, also known as eHealth or health informatics, encompasses the use of technology to enhance healthcare delivery, improve patient outcomes, and empower individuals to take an active role in managing their health. The roots of digital health can be traced back to the development of electronic medical records (EMRs) in the 1960s, which replaced paper-based records and allowed for more efficient storage and retrieval of patient information.

The advent of the internet in the 1990s brought new opportunities for digital health, allowing for the exchange of medical information and the development of telecommunication technologies. This laid the foundation for the development of telemedicine, which involves the remote delivery of healthcare services using telecommunication technologies.

Telemedicine: Bridging the Distance

Telemedicine has become increasingly prevalent in recent years, particularly with the rapid advancement of communication technologies. It involves the use of video conferencing, remote monitoring devices, and mobile health applications to connect healthcare providers and patients who are geographically separated.

One of the primary benefits of telemedicine is its ability to bridge the distance between patients and healthcare providers, particularly in rural and underserved areas where access to specialist care may be limited. Telemedicine allows for virtual consultations, where patients can receive medical advice, diagnosis, and treatment recommendations from healthcare professionals without the need for in-person visits.

Furthermore, telemedicine has been instrumental in improving access to healthcare for individuals with mobility limitations or those who require regular monitoring, such as patients with chronic conditions or the elderly. Remote monitoring devices can collect and transmit vital signs, enabling healthcare providers to track patients' health status and intervene in a timely manner when necessary.

Digital Health Applications: Redefining Healthcare Delivery

Digital health applications have extended beyond telemedicine to encompass various aspects of healthcare delivery. Mobile health applications, or mHealth apps, have gained popularity in recent years, offering a wide range of functionalities, including health tracking, medication reminders, and personalized health recommendations.

mHealth apps have empowered individuals to actively participate in managing their health, leading to improved overall wellness and preventive care. These apps enable users to monitor their vital signs, track their exercise and nutrition, and access educational resources, empowering them to make informed decisions about their health.

Additionally, digital health technologies have played a crucial role in streamlining healthcare processes, reducing administrative burden, and improving efficiency in healthcare settings. Electronic prescribing systems have replaced traditional paper-based prescriptions, reducing medication errors and improving medication adherence. Digital imaging systems have facilitated the rapid sharing and interpretation of medical images, enabling faster and more accurate diagnosis.

Challenges and Ethical Considerations

Despite the numerous benefits offered by digital health and telemedicine, there are several challenges and ethical considerations that need to be addressed for their successful integration into the healthcare system.

One of the primary concerns is the protection of patient privacy and security of healthcare data. With the increasing reliance on digital technologies, there is an elevated risk of data breaches and unauthorized access to sensitive medical information. The development and implementation of robust security measures and adherence to privacy regulations are essential to maintain patient trust and protect their confidentiality.

Another challenge is the potential for disparities in access to digital health technologies, particularly among vulnerable populations with limited access to technology or low health literacy. Efforts should be made to ensure equitable access to digital health tools and to provide education and support for individuals who may face barriers to their use.

Furthermore, the ethical implications of remote healthcare delivery must be carefully considered. The absence of physical proximity between healthcare providers and patients may limit the ability to perform thorough examinations and assessments, potentially resulting in diagnostic errors or incomplete care. Safeguards should be in place to ensure appropriate triaging and referrals when necessary.

Moreover, the digital divide, characterized by disparities in access to and proficiency in using digital technologies, must be addressed to ensure that the benefits of digital health and telemedicine are extended to all individuals, regardless of socioeconomic status or geographic location.

Conclusion

The rise of digital health and telemedicine has revolutionized healthcare delivery, offering new opportunities for improving access, efficiency, and patient engagement. These technologies have the potential to transform how healthcare is delivered and received, providing more personalized and convenient care.

However, it is crucial to address the challenges and ethical considerations associated with their adoption to ensure that they are effectively integrated into the healthcare system. By safeguarding patient privacy, promoting equitable access, and considering the limitations of remote care, we can harness the full potential of digital health and telemedicine for the betterment of healthcare outcomes and overall sustainability.

Social Media and Mental Health

In today's digital age, social media has become an integral part of our lives, revolutionizing the way we communicate, connect, and share information. Platforms such as Facebook, Twitter, Instagram, and Snapchat have transformed the way we interact with others and access information. However, while social media has numerous benefits, it also has a significant impact on mental health and wellbeing.

Understanding the Relationship

The relationship between social media and mental health is complex and multifaceted. On one hand, social media offers a platform for self-expression, social support, and community engagement. It allows individuals to connect with friends, family, and like-minded individuals, fostering a sense of belonging and social connection. Moreover, social media can provide a space for individuals to share their personal experiences, raise awareness about mental health issues, and access resources for support and recovery.

On the other hand, social media can have negative consequences on mental health. The curated and idealized nature of social media platforms can contribute to feelings of inadequacy, loneliness, and depression. Constant exposure to other people's highlight reels may lead to social comparison and a negative self-perception. Moreover, cyberbullying and online harassment are prevalent on social media, exacerbating mental health issues and causing distress.

Impact on Mental Health

Social media can affect mental health in various ways:

1. **Self-esteem and body image:** Constant exposure to carefully crafted and edited images on social media can contribute to poor body image and low self-esteem. Individuals may compare themselves to unrealistic beauty standards, leading to feelings of inadequacy and body dissatisfaction.

2. **Depression and anxiety:** Excessive use of social media has been linked to symptoms of depression and anxiety. The constant need for validation, fear of missing out (FOMO), and cyberbullying can significantly impact mental wellbeing.

3. **Sleep disturbances:** The use of social media before bedtime can disrupt sleep patterns, leading to sleep disturbances, insomnia, and fatigue. The blue light emitted by electronic devices suppresses the production of melatonin, a hormone that regulates sleep.

4. **Addiction:** Social media platforms are designed to be addictive, with features such as notifications, likes, and comments triggering a dopamine response in the brain. Excessive use of social media can lead to addiction and compulsive behaviors.

Tips for Responsible Social Media Use

While social media can have negative consequences on mental health, responsible use can minimize the potential risks. Here are some tips for maintaining a healthy balance:

1. **Limit time spent on social media:** Set boundaries and allocate specific times for social media use. Avoid mindless scrolling and prioritize activities that promote mental health, such as exercise, hobbies, and spending time with loved ones.

2. **Curate your feed:** Unfollow accounts that make you feel inadequate or trigger negative emotions. Follow accounts that promote positive body image, mental health awareness, and self-care.

3. **Be mindful of your emotions:** Notice how social media makes you feel. If you notice feelings of sadness, anxiety, or low self-esteem, take a break or seek support from trusted friends or mental health professionals.

4. **Engage in positive interactions:** Use social media as a platform for positive interactions, support, and advocacy. Engage with communities and organizations that align with your values and promote mental health and wellbeing.

5. **Practice digital detox:** Periodically take breaks from social media to recharge and focus on activities that nourish your mental health. Use this time to connect with nature, practice mindfulness, or engage in self-reflection.

Conclusion

Social media has transformed the way we communicate and connect with others. While it offers numerous benefits, it also has the potential to negatively impact mental health and wellbeing. Understanding the relationship between social media and mental health is crucial for responsible and mindful use. By implementing healthy habits and prioritizing self-care, we can harness the benefits of social media while protecting our mental health. Remember, it's not about completely eliminating social media from our lives, but rather finding a balance that promotes our overall wellbeing.

Gaming and Mental Health

Gaming has become an increasingly popular form of entertainment and leisure activity in contemporary society. With the advancement of technology, video games have evolved into complex and immersive experiences that capture the attention of millions of people worldwide. However, as with any leisure activity, there are potential implications for mental health and wellbeing that need to be considered.

The Impact of Gaming on Mental Health

The relationship between gaming and mental health is a complex and multifaceted one. While gaming has been associated with negative effects such as addiction and social isolation, research has also highlighted positive impacts on cognition, creativity, and socialization.

One of the most significant concerns related to gaming is the potential for addiction. Gaming addiction, also known as Internet Gaming Disorder (IGD), is characterized by excessive and compulsive gaming that leads to significant impairments in various areas of life. Symptoms include decreased interest in other activities, loss of control over gaming behavior, and withdrawal symptoms when unable to play. It is important to note that gaming addiction is relatively rare, affecting a small percentage of individuals who engage in gaming.

Gaming can also impact mental health by influencing mood and emotions. For some individuals, gaming can serve as a form of escapism or stress relief, providing a temporary distraction from real-world problems. On the other hand, excessive gaming or engaging in highly competitive online games can lead to frustration, anger, and aggression. These negative emotions can have a detrimental effect on mental wellbeing if not properly managed.

Gaming as a Therapeutic Tool

Despite the potential risks associated with gaming, research has also demonstrated its positive impact on mental health. Gamification, or the use of game-like elements in non-game contexts, has been increasingly utilized in therapeutic interventions.

Serious games, which are designed for a specific purpose other than entertainment, have been developed to address various mental health issues. These games can simulate real-life scenarios and provide a safe environment for individuals to practice coping skills, manage anxiety, or improve cognitive functions. For example, virtual reality (VR) games have been used to treat phobias and post-traumatic stress disorder (PTSD) by exposing individuals to controlled virtual environments.

In addition to serious games, commercial video games have shown potential benefits for mental health. Research suggests that certain video games, such as puzzle games and virtual pets, can enhance cognitive abilities, attention, and problem-solving skills. Multiplayer online games can also provide opportunities for socialization, teamwork, and building supportive communities.

Furthermore, gaming can be used as a tool for stress reduction and relaxation. Casual games, such as mobile games or puzzle games, can serve as a brief respite from daily stressors. Engaging in gaming can help individuals shift their focus, recharge, and experience positive emotions.

Balancing Gaming and Mental Health

Given the potential for both positive and negative impacts on mental health, it is crucial to find a balance between gaming and overall wellbeing. Here are some strategies to promote healthy gaming habits:

1. Set limits: Establish clear boundaries and allocate specific time for gaming, ensuring that it does not interfere with other important activities or responsibilities.

2. Choose games mindfully: Be aware of the content and nature of the games you engage with. Opt for games that align with your interests and values, and that provide opportunities for personal growth and enjoyment.

3. Maintain social connections: Gaming can be an enjoyable social activity, but it is important to balance virtual interactions with face-to-face interactions. Nurture offline relationships and engage in activities that promote social connections.

4. Stay physically active: Incorporate physical activity into your daily routine to counterbalance sedentary gaming behaviors. Regular exercise has numerous mental health benefits and can help reduce the risk of developing gaming-related issues.

5. Monitor emotional well-being: Pay attention to your emotional state while gaming. If you find yourself becoming overly frustrated, angry, or anxious, take a break and engage in activities that promote relaxation and emotional well-being.

6. Seek support if needed: If you or someone you know is experiencing significant impairment due to excessive gaming or gaming addiction, consider seeking professional help. Mental health professionals can provide guidance and support in managing gaming-related challenges.

By adopting a mindful approach to gaming and being aware of its potential effects on mental health, individuals can enjoy the benefits of gaming while safeguarding their overall wellbeing.

Case Study: The Benefits of Gamification in Mental Health Treatment

Gamification has gained recognition as a powerful tool in mental health treatment. The use of game-like elements and mechanics can enhance motivation, engagement, and adherence to therapeutic interventions.

One example of gamification in mental health treatment is the use of virtual reality exposure therapy (VRET) for individuals with phobias or anxiety disorders. Traditional exposure therapy involves gradually exposing individuals to feared stimuli in real-life situations. However, this can be challenging, time-consuming, and expensive. VRET provides a safe and controlled virtual environment where individuals can confront their fears.

In a randomized controlled trial conducted by Smith et al. (2019), individuals with arachnophobia underwent either VRET or traditional exposure therapy. The results showed that both approaches were effective in reducing fear and avoidance of spiders. However, the VRET group reported higher levels of enjoyment, immersion, and satisfaction with the treatment. The gamified elements of VRET, such as scoring systems and rewards, contributed to increased motivation and engagement.

Similarly, gamification has been utilized in interventions targeting depression and anxiety. Mobile applications and online platforms integrate game-like features, such as challenges, progress tracking, and social interactions, to enhance users' involvement in therapeutic activities. These gamified interventions have shown promising results in reducing depressive symptoms and improving well-being.

The use of gamification in mental health treatment illustrates the potential for technology and gaming to revolutionize traditional therapeutic approaches. By incorporating elements that tap into individuals' intrinsic motivation and enjoyment, gamification has the ability to enhance treatment outcomes and encourage active participation in mental health interventions.

Conclusion

Gaming can have both positive and negative implications for mental health. While excessive gaming and gaming addiction can lead to adverse effects, gaming can also be utilized as a therapeutic tool to promote mental wellbeing. The balance between healthy gaming habits and overall mental health is crucial, requiring individuals to be mindful of their gaming behaviors and engage in activities that support overall wellbeing.

By incorporating gamified interventions into mental health treatment and promoting responsible gaming habits, individuals can benefit from the potential positive effects of gaming while safeguarding their mental health and wellbeing. The field of gaming and mental health is an exciting area of research and innovation, offering new possibilities for the future of mental health care.

Ethical Considerations in Technological Advances

As technology continues to advance and shape various aspects of our lives, including the field of mental health, it is crucial to examine the ethical considerations associated with these advancements. The integration of technology in mental health care offers great potential for improving access, efficiency, and effectiveness of services. However, it also raises important ethical questions that must be addressed to ensure the well-being and autonomy of individuals.

One of the primary ethical considerations in technological advances in mental health care is the protection of privacy and confidentiality. With the use of digital health platforms, telemedicine, and electronic health records, sensitive information about individuals' mental health can be stored, accessed, and transmitted. It is essential to uphold strict privacy and security measures to safeguard the confidentiality and trust of individuals seeking mental health support.

Another ethical concern is the digital divide and accessibility. While technology can provide convenient access to mental health resources, it is essential to consider that not everyone has equal access to technology. Socioeconomic disparities and limited digital literacy can prevent some individuals from benefiting from technological advancements in mental health care. Efforts should be made to bridge this digital divide and ensure equitable access to mental health services for all.

The ethical use of artificial intelligence (AI) and machine learning algorithms in mental health care is another area of concern. While AI has the potential to assist in diagnosis, treatment planning, and personalized interventions, there is a need to ensure transparency and accountability in the development and deployment of these technologies. The fairness, accuracy, and bias of algorithms must be consistently evaluated and monitored to avoid potential harm or discrimination.

Ethical considerations also extend to the responsible use of social media platforms in mental health care. While social media can serve as a valuable tool for building online communities, disseminating information, and providing support, it can also present risks, such as cyberbullying, misinformation, and inappropriate use of personal data. Mental health professionals and users alike need to be aware of these risks and engage in responsible online practices.

Informed consent is a fundamental ethical principle that must be upheld in the context of technological advances in mental health care. Individuals must be fully informed about the benefits, risks, and limitations of using technology in their treatment, including the potential impact on the therapeutic relationship. The autonomy and agency of individuals should be respected, and they should have the right to make informed decisions about their mental health care, including their engagement with technology.

Moreover, ethical considerations should address potential conflicts of interest between technology developers, mental health professionals, and users. The influence of commercial interests on the design, promotion, and use of technological solutions in mental health care should be carefully monitored to ensure that decisions prioritizes the best interests of individuals seeking help.

To navigate these ethical challenges, interdisciplinary collaboration and stakeholder engagement are crucial. Mental health professionals, technologists, ethicists, policymakers, and individuals with lived experience should work together to develop guidelines, standards, and regulations that promote the responsible and ethical use of technology in mental health care.

In summary, the integration of technology in mental health care has the potential to revolutionize the field and improve the lives of many individuals. However, it is essential to consider and address the ethical considerations associated with technological advancements. Protecting privacy and confidentiality, bridging the digital divide, ensuring the responsible use of AI and machine learning algorithms, promoting informed consent, and addressing conflicts of interest are some of the key ethical considerations that must be carefully navigated. By doing so, we can harness the power of technology while upholding the values of autonomy, privacy, equity, and respect in mental health care.

Future Prospects for Technology in Mental Health Care

With the rapid advancement of technology in recent years, there is an increasing interest in exploring its potential applications in the field of mental health care. Technology has already made significant contributions to various aspects of healthcare, and it holds great promise for improving mental health outcomes. In this section, we will discuss the future prospects for technology in mental health care, exploring innovative approaches and potential challenges.

Emerging Technologies

1. Virtual Reality (VR) and Augmented Reality (AR): VR and AR technologies have the potential to transform mental health care by creating immersive environments that can simulate real-life scenarios. These technologies can be used in exposure therapy for anxiety disorders, allowing individuals to confront their fears in a controlled setting. Additionally, they can enhance mindfulness practices and help individuals develop better coping strategies for stress and anxiety.

2. Artificial Intelligence (AI) and Machine Learning: AI and machine learning algorithms have already been employed in various mental health applications, such as automated diagnosis and personalized treatment plans. In the future, AI can assist therapists by analyzing large datasets to detect patterns and provide insights into tailored interventions for individuals. It can also facilitate early detection of mental

health disorders by analyzing social media posts, voice patterns, and other digital footprints.

3. Wearable Devices: Wearable devices, such as smartwatches and fitness trackers, can monitor physiological indicators like heart rate, sleep patterns, and activity levels. In mental health care, these devices can be used to track mood fluctuations, identify triggers for stress and anxiety, and provide real-time feedback to individuals. They can also act as reminders for medication adherence and self-care activities.

Challenges and Ethical Considerations

While the future prospects for technology in mental health care are promising, there are several challenges and ethical considerations that need to be addressed:

1. Privacy and Data Security: The use of technology in mental health care involves the collection and storage of sensitive personal information. It is crucial to ensure that data privacy and security measures are in place to protect the confidentiality of individuals' mental health data.

2. Accessibility and Equity: The widespread adoption of technology in mental health care should not exacerbate existing health disparities. Efforts should be made to address barriers to access, such as limited internet connectivity, lack of technological literacy, and socioeconomic inequalities.

3. Human-Centered Design: Technology should always be designed with the end-users in mind. It is essential to involve individuals with lived experience of mental health challenges in the design and evaluation of digital tools to ensure that they meet their needs and preferences.

4. Ethical Use of AI and Machine Learning: The use of AI and machine learning algorithms in mental health care raises concerns about bias, transparency, and accountability. It is crucial to develop ethical guidelines and standards to ensure that these technologies are used responsibly and in the best interest of individuals.

Case Study: Chatbots for Mental Health Support

One example of a technology that has gained popularity in mental health care is the use of chatbots. Chatbots are computer programs designed to simulate human conversation, providing support and resources to individuals in need. They can be accessed through various platforms, such as websites, messaging apps, and social media.

Chatbots offer several advantages in mental health care. They provide immediate, round-the-clock support, reducing the wait time for individuals seeking help. They can also offer anonymity and a non-judgmental environment, encouraging individuals to express their thoughts and feelings without fear of stigma.

However, there are challenges associated with the use of chatbots in mental health care. They are not a substitute for human interaction and should be seen as a complementary tool. Chatbots lack the empathy and intuition that human therapists possess. Additionally, there is a risk of providing inaccurate or harmful information if the chatbot is not appropriately trained or updated.

To ensure the ethical use of chatbots, developers should prioritize transparency and informed consent. Users should be fully aware that they are interacting with a chatbot and understand the limitations of its capabilities. Chatbot developers should also collaborate with mental health professionals to ensure that the content and responses provided are evidence-based and aligned with best practices.

Conclusion

The future of technology in mental health care holds tremendous potential for improving mental health outcomes. Virtual reality, artificial intelligence, wearable devices, and chatbots are just a few examples of the innovative approaches that can revolutionize the field. However, it is essential to address challenges related to privacy, accessibility, human-centered design, and ethical use to maximize the benefits of technology and ensure equitable access to mental health care for all. With careful consideration and collaboration between technology developers and mental health professionals, the integration of technology into mental health care can pave the way for a more sustainable and effective approach to promoting mental well-being.

The Role of Artificial Intelligence in Mental Health

Artificial Intelligence (AI) has emerged as a powerful tool in various fields, and its applications in mental health are rapidly expanding. AI refers to the simulation of human intelligence in machines that can perform tasks that typically require human intelligence, such as problem-solving, pattern recognition, and decision-making. In the context of mental health, AI offers innovative solutions that can enhance diagnosis, treatment, and support for individuals experiencing psychological challenges.

AI in Mental Health Diagnosis

One of the key areas where AI can play a significant role is in the diagnosis of mental health disorders. Traditional diagnostic processes often rely on subjective assessments by clinicians, which can be time-consuming and prone to biases. AI algorithms have the potential to analyze large amounts of data, including patient histories, behavioral patterns, and responses to diagnostic tests, to provide more accurate and objective diagnoses.

For instance, machine learning algorithms can be trained on existing diagnostic data to identify patterns and markers associated with specific mental health disorders. These algorithms can then be used to analyze new patient data and provide clinicians with more reliable and efficient diagnostic predictions. This can lead to earlier intervention and personalized treatment plans tailored to individual needs.

AI in Mental Health Treatment

AI can also support mental health treatment by providing innovative methods for therapy delivery and monitoring treatment progress. Virtual reality (VR) and augmented reality (AR) technologies combined with AI algorithms offer immersive and interactive therapeutic experiences. For example, VR environments can be used to simulate real-world situations that trigger anxiety or phobias, allowing individuals to confront and manage their fears in a controlled and supportive environment.

AI-powered chatbots and virtual assistants are another promising application in mental health treatment. These AI systems can provide 24/7 support, offering personalized therapy sessions, coping strategies, and crisis interventions. They can also monitor individual progress, collect real-time data, and adapt treatment plans accordingly. This not only increases accessibility to mental health support but also empowers individuals to actively participate in their own treatment journey.

Ethical Considerations and Challenges

While the potential of AI in mental health is promising, it is essential to address the ethical considerations and challenges associated with its implementation. Here are a few key considerations:

1. Privacy: AI systems collect and analyze sensitive personal data. Safeguarding patient privacy and ensuring data protection is paramount. Strict regulations

and protocols must be in place to protect patient confidentiality and prevent unauthorized access or misuse of data.

2. Bias and Fairness: Biases present in training data can be replicated by AI algorithms, leading to biased diagnoses and treatment recommendations. Careful attention must be given to ensure that AI systems are trained on diverse and representative data to avoid perpetuating existing biases in mental health care.

3. Human Oversight: While AI can enhance mental health care, it should not replace human clinicians. The role of AI should be seen as a complement to human expertise, with an emphasis on collaboration and shared decision-making.

4. Accessibility: AI systems should be designed with inclusivity in mind. They should be accessible to individuals from diverse backgrounds and with varying degrees of technological literacy. The importance of bridging the digital divide and addressing disparities in access to AI-powered mental health tools cannot be overstated.

Real-World Examples

To illustrate the practical applications of AI in mental health, consider the following examples:

1. Mood Tracking Apps: AI-powered mobile apps can analyze users' self-reported moods, behaviors, and physiological data to identify patterns and triggers for mood fluctuations. This information can assist individuals in monitoring their mental well-being and seeking timely interventions.

2. Suicide Risk Assessment: AI algorithms can analyze social media posts, online searches, and other digital footprints to identify individuals at risk of self-harm or suicide. This information can be shared with mental health professionals, enabling early intervention and support.

3. Precision Medicine: AI can help identify optimal medication and dosage plans for individuals with mental health disorders. By analyzing genetic, physiological, and environmental factors, AI algorithms can tailor treatment plans to maximize effectiveness and minimize side effects.

Conclusion

Artificial Intelligence holds significant promise in revolutionizing mental health care. By leveraging AI technologies, clinicians and researchers can gain valuable insights, optimize diagnosis and treatment approaches, and ultimately improve outcomes for individuals experiencing mental health challenges. However, careful attention must be given to address the ethical considerations and challenges associated with AI implementation. With thoughtful integration and human-centered design, AI has the potential to contribute to a more accessible, effective, and sustainable mental health future.

Historical Perspectives on Mental Health Care

The Asylum Era

During the 18th and 19th centuries, the concept of mental illness was still poorly understood, and individuals with mental health disorders were often stigmatized, ostracized, or even imprisoned. The prevailing belief at the time was that mental illness was a result of moral weakness or demonic possession. As a result, individuals suffering from mental health disorders were often subjected to cruel and inhumane treatment.

The Asylum Era, which lasted from the late 18th century to the early 20th century, represented a significant shift in the approach to mental health care. Asylums, also known as psychiatric hospitals or mental institutions, were established to provide care and treatment for individuals with mental health disorders. However, the conditions within these asylums varied widely and were often far from ideal.

One of the key figures during the Asylum Era was Philippe Pinel, a French psychiatrist. Pinel advocated for the humane treatment of individuals with mental illness and played a crucial role in the reform of asylums. He believed that mental illness was not due to moral weakness but rather had biological and psychological origins. Pinel introduced reforms that emphasized moral treatment, which focused on providing patients with a supportive and nurturing environment.

Asylums during this era sought to provide a therapeutic environment for patients, but the reality was often far from ideal. Many asylums were overcrowded and understaffed, leading to the neglect and mistreatment of patients. In some cases, individuals with mental illness were subject to physical restraints, isolation, and even abuse.

HISTORICAL PERSPECTIVES ON MENTAL HEALTH CARE

The Asylum Era also saw advances in psychiatric research and the classification of mental disorders. This period laid the foundation for modern psychiatry and the development of diagnostic criteria for mental health disorders. However, it is essential to note that the classification systems during this era were rudimentary and often lacked scientific rigor.

Despite its shortcomings, the Asylum Era represented a significant shift in the perception and treatment of mental illness. The concept of moral treatment and the establishment of asylums laid the groundwork for future advancements in mental health care. The emphasis on providing a therapeutic environment and humane treatment marked a departure from the cruel practices of the past.

However, it is crucial to acknowledge the darker side of the Asylum Era and the mistreatment that many individuals with mental illness endured. The conditions within asylums varied widely, and the lack of oversight and regulation meant that abuses were prevalent.

The Asylum Era serves as a reminder of the importance of continuously striving for improvement in mental health care. It highlights the need for compassionate and evidence-based approaches to the treatment and support of individuals with mental health disorders. While the era brought about some positive changes, it also serves as a cautionary tale, reminding us of the potential for harm when vulnerable populations are not adequately cared for and protected.

The legacy of the Asylum Era is complex and multifaceted. It paved the way for advancements in psychiatric research and the development of modern treatment approaches. However, it also reminds us of the ongoing need for vigilance to ensure that the rights and well-being of individuals with mental illness are protected.

The Challenges and Controversies of the Asylum Era

While the Asylum Era marked a significant shift in the treatment of mental illness, it was not without its challenges and controversies. The conditions within asylums varied widely, and abuses were prevalent. Here, we explore some of the key challenges and controversies of the Asylum Era.

Overcrowding and Understaffing: One of the most significant challenges of the Asylum Era was the issue of overcrowding and understaffing. Asylums often admitted more patients than they could adequately care for, leading to poor living conditions and inadequate treatment. The lack of resources and staff meant that patients did not receive the individualized care they needed, contributing to neglect and mistreatment.

Physical Restraints and Abuse: In many asylums, physical restraints were commonly used to control and manage patients. Patients were often chained or confined to beds or restraints for extended periods, leading to physical and psychological harm. Additionally, instances of abuse, both physical and verbal, were not uncommon, further exacerbating the mistreatment of patients.

Flawed Diagnostic Criteria: The classification systems used during the Asylum Era were rudimentary and lacked scientific rigor. Diagnostic criteria for mental disorders were based on subjective observations rather than empirical evidence. This led to inaccuracies in diagnoses and potential mislabeling of patients, further exacerbating the challenges faced by individuals with mental health disorders.

Lack of Individualized Treatment: Asylums often employed a one-size-fits-all approach to treatment, disregarding the unique needs and experiences of patients. The focus was on controlling and managing symptoms rather than providing individualized care. This lack of personalized treatment contributed to the dehumanization and mistreatment of patients.

Stigma and Social Isolation: Despite the efforts to provide a therapeutic environment within asylums, individuals with mental illness continued to face societal stigma and prejudice. Asylums were often located on the outskirts of cities or towns, isolating patients from their communities and reinforcing the negative stereotypes associated with mental illness.

Reforms and the Legacy of the Asylum Era

The mistreatment and abuses within asylums during the Asylum Era eventually led to calls for reform and the establishment of new approaches to mental health care. The legacy of the Asylum Era includes significant reforms that have shaped the modern understanding and treatment of mental illness.

Moral Treatment Movement: The reforms advocated by Philippe Pinel and others during the Asylum Era laid the foundation for the Moral Treatment Movement. This movement emphasized the importance of providing patients with humane and compassionate care. It focused on creating a therapeutic environment and treating individuals with mental illness with dignity and respect.

Deinstitutionalization Movement: The deinstitutionalization movement, which gained momentum in the mid-20th century, aimed to shift the focus of mental health care away from large, centralized institutions and towards community-based care. It sought to integrate individuals with mental illness back into their communities, providing treatment and support in less restrictive settings.

Advancements in Psychiatric Research: The Asylum Era also marked the beginning of systematic psychiatric research and the development of classification systems for mental disorders. This laid the groundwork for future advancements in the understanding and treatment of mental illness. The Diagnostic and Statistical Manual of Mental Disorders (DSM), first published in 1952, is a direct descendant of the early classification systems developed during the Asylum Era.

Evolving Views on Mental Health: The Asylum Era played a pivotal role in changing societal views on mental health. It challenged the prevailing belief that mental illness was a result of moral weakness or demonic possession and highlighted the biological and psychological factors that contribute to mental health disorders. These evolving views paved the way for more compassionate and evidence-based approaches to mental health care.

While the Asylum Era was marked by significant challenges and controversies, it also laid the foundation for important reforms in mental health care. The shift towards a more humane and compassionate approach, as well as the advancements in psychiatric research, greatly influenced the development of modern mental health practices. However, it is crucial to remember the mistakes and abuses of the past in order to continue improving and advocating for the rights and well-being of individuals with mental illness in the present and future.

The Moral Treatment Movement

The Moral Treatment Movement, also known as moral therapy, was a significant development in the history of mental health care. This movement emerged in the late 18th century and aimed to provide humane and compassionate treatment for individuals with mental illnesses. It marked a shift away from the prevailing harsh and abusive practices that were common in psychiatric institutions at the time.

Origins and principles

The Moral Treatment Movement was influenced by various philosophical and societal changes happening during the Enlightenment period. Advocates of moral therapy believed that individuals with mental illnesses were not inherently morally corrupt or possessed by supernatural forces, as was commonly believed at the time. Instead, they saw mental illness as a result of social and environmental factors, emphasizing the importance of treating patients with kindness, respect, and dignity.

The movement was heavily influenced by the work of Philippe Pinel, a French psychiatrist, who became the leading figure of moral therapy. Pinel emphasized the importance of creating a therapeutic environment that promoted mental and emotional well-being. He introduced significant reforms in psychiatric hospitals, such as removing restraints and providing patients with a calm and structured daily routine.

Principles of moral therapy

The Moral Treatment Movement was guided by several key principles, which aimed to promote the recovery and well-being of individuals with mental illnesses. These principles included:

1. Individualized care: Moral therapy recognized the unique needs and experiences of each patient and focused on providing personalized treatment. It emphasized the importance of understanding patients' backgrounds, interests, and abilities to develop tailored therapeutic approaches.

2. Occupational therapy: Engaging patients in meaningful activities was a fundamental aspect of moral therapy. Patients were involved in various tasks such as gardening, handicrafts, and domestic activities. These activities aimed to promote a sense of purpose, self-esteem, and social interaction among patients.

3. Humanitarian approach: Moral therapy emphasized compassionate and respectful treatment of individuals with mental illnesses. It rejected the use of physical restraints, punishment, and other forms of abuse prevalent in psychiatric care of that time.

4. Therapeutic environment: Institutions practicing moral therapy focused on creating a supportive and therapeutic environment. This involved providing a pleasant and natural setting, access to fresh air and sunlight, and opportunities for social interaction among patients.

Successes and challenges

The Moral Treatment Movement brought significant improvements in the lives of individuals with mental illnesses. Patients experienced better living conditions, reduced abuse, and increased opportunities for social interaction. Many patients showed improvement in their symptoms and functioning when treated with moral therapy.

However, the movement faced several challenges. Limited resources and overcrowding in institutions often hampered the implementation of moral therapy principles. Inadequate funding and trained staff undermined the quality of care provided. Furthermore, the movement's principles were not universally adopted, and in some parts of the world, outdated and abusive practices persisted.

Legacy and impact

Despite its challenges, the Moral Treatment Movement laid the foundation for modern psychiatric care. Its emphasis on compassion, individualized care, and holistic therapeutic approaches still resonate in contemporary mental health practices. The movement sparked a shift in public perception, leading to increased awareness and advocacy for the rights of individuals with mental illnesses.

The principles of moral therapy continue to influence modern approaches to mental health care, including person-centered therapy, cognitive-behavioral therapy, and psychosocial rehabilitation. The movement's emphasis on the therapeutic environment, occupational therapy, and social support has become integral components of contemporary mental health treatment.

In conclusion, the Moral Treatment Movement was a pivotal development in the history of mental health care. It challenged prevailing attitudes and practices, emphasizing humane treatment, individualized care, and the importance of a therapeutic environment. While facing challenges and limitations, the movement paved the way for the modern understanding and practice of mental health care, leaving a lasting impact on the field.

Community Mental Health Centers

Community Mental Health Centers play a vital role in the provision of mental health care services within local communities. These centers are designed to provide accessible, comprehensive, and holistic care to individuals experiencing mental health challenges. In this section, we will explore the history, purpose, and components of community mental health centers, as well as their impact on individuals and communities.

Historical Background

The development of community mental health centers can be traced back to the deinstitutionalization movement of the mid-20th century. This movement aimed to shift the focus of mental health care from large-scale psychiatric institutions to community-based care. In response to the recognition of the limitations and drawbacks of long-term hospitalization, policymakers and mental health advocates advocated for the establishment of smaller, more localized treatment options.

The community mental health center movement gained momentum in the 1960s and 1970s, influenced by groundbreaking legislation such as the Community Mental Health Centers Act of 1963 in the United States. This act provided federal funding to support the establishment and operation of community mental health centers across the country.

Purpose and Objectives

The primary purpose of community mental health centers is to provide accessible and comprehensive mental health services to individuals in their local communities. These centers aim to promote mental wellness, prevent the development of mental health disorders, and ensure early interventions for individuals at risk.

The objectives of community mental health centers include:

- **Outreach and Engagement:** Community mental health centers actively engage with individuals in the community, identifying those in need of mental health support and connecting them to appropriate services.

- **Assessment and Diagnosis:** These centers provide thorough assessments and diagnostic evaluations to determine the nature and severity of mental health issues. This process involves collaboration with mental health professionals, such as psychiatrists, psychologists, and social workers.

- **Treatment and Rehabilitation:** Community mental health centers offer a range of evidence-based treatments and interventions tailored to the specific needs of individuals. This may include individual therapy, group counseling, medication management, and psychosocial rehabilitation programs.

- **Crisis Intervention:** Community mental health centers are often equipped to handle mental health crises, providing immediate support and intervention for individuals experiencing acute distress or instability.

- **Education and Prevention:** These centers play a crucial role in promoting mental health literacy and raising awareness about mental health issues within the community. They also offer preventative services and programs to address risk factors and promote resilience.

- **Collaboration and Referral:** Community mental health centers collaborate with other healthcare providers, community organizations, and support services to ensure holistic care for individuals. They also facilitate appropriate referrals for specialized services when needed.

Components and Services

Community mental health centers are multifaceted institutions that offer a wide range of services to meet the diverse needs of individuals in the community. Some common components and services include:

- **Outpatient Services:** These services form the core of community mental health centers. They typically include individual therapy, group counseling, medication management, and case management services.

- **Crisis Services:** Community mental health centers often have crisis hotlines and walk-in clinics to provide immediate support during times of crisis. Crisis stabilization units may offer short-term residential care for individuals in acute distress.

- **Psychiatric Services:** Centers may have psychiatrists on staff to provide psychiatric evaluations, medication prescriptions, and ongoing medication management for individuals with mental health disorders.

- **Community Support Programs:** These programs provide assistance and support to individuals with severe and persistent mental illnesses. They may include psychosocial rehabilitation, supported housing, vocational training, and assistance with activities of daily living.

- **Prevention and Early Intervention Programs:** Community mental health centers may offer programs targeted at early identification and intervention for individuals at risk of developing mental health disorders. These programs often focus on children, adolescents, and individuals experiencing early signs of mental illness.

- **Education and Training:** Centers may provide educational workshops, training programs, and support groups for individuals with mental health disorders and their families. These initiatives aim to enhance mental health literacy, coping skills, and self-management strategies.

- **Community Integration:** Community mental health centers strive to integrate individuals with mental health disorders into their communities. This may involve collaboration with community organizations, schools, employers, and other stakeholders to promote inclusion and reduce stigma.

Challenges and Future Directions

While community mental health centers have made significant progress in improving accessibility and quality of care, they face a range of challenges that need to be addressed for optimal functioning and effectiveness. Some of these challenges include:

- **Funding and Resource Constraints:** Community mental health centers often struggle with limited funding and resources, which can restrict their ability to meet the growing demands for mental health services.

- **Workforce Shortages:** There is often a shortage of mental health professionals, especially in underserved areas, making it challenging to provide timely and adequate care.

- **Stigma and Discrimination:** Despite efforts to reduce stigma, many individuals still face societal barriers and discrimination when seeking mental health services, limiting their access to community mental health centers.

- **Integration with Primary Care:** Collaboration and integration between community mental health centers and primary care settings can improve the overall delivery of mental health care. However, barriers such as fragmented systems and limited communication can hinder effective integration.

To address these challenges, it is crucial to prioritize mental health funding, increase the mental health workforce, promote widespread mental health awareness, and enhance collaboration between community mental health centers and other healthcare providers.

Examples of Community Mental Health Centers

Let's take a look at two examples of successful community mental health centers:

Example 1: The CMHC of San Francisco

The Community Mental Health Center (CMHC) of San Francisco is known for its innovative and comprehensive approach to mental health care. The center offers a wide range of services, including crisis intervention, outpatient therapy, case management, substance abuse treatment, and supportive housing programs.

One unique aspect of the CMHC of San Francisco is its focus on cultural competence and inclusivity. The center is committed to meeting the diverse needs of the community by providing services that are sensitive to cultural backgrounds, languages, and identities. This approach ensures that individuals from different communities can access the care they need in a safe and supportive environment.

The CMHC of San Francisco also places a strong emphasis on collaboration and partnership. They work closely with community organizations, schools, law enforcement, and other stakeholders to promote mental health and address the social determinants that impact mental wellness.

Example 2: The HUB Community Mental Health Center

The HUB Community Mental Health Center, located in a rural area, serves as an excellent example of how community mental health centers can adapt to the unique needs of their communities. In an area with limited resources and geographic challenges, the HUB has implemented innovative solutions to expand access to care.

Recognizing the difficulty of transportation and the resulting barriers to accessing services, the HUB has established telehealth programs to provide virtual counseling and psychiatric services. This approach allows individuals in remote areas to receive mental health care without the need for long-distance travel.

The HUB also implements community-based outreach programs, collaborating with local schools, community centers, and churches to provide mental health education, early intervention services, and support groups. By actively reaching out to individuals in need, the HUB ensures that mental health services are brought directly to the community.

Exercise

Think of a community in which you reside or another community you are familiar with. Identify one mental health issue prevalent in that community and propose a community-based program that a local mental health center could implement to address this issue. Consider the unique characteristics and needs of the community in your proposal.

Additional Resources

1. National Council for Behavioral Health. Community Mental Health Centers.
   (https://www.thenationalcouncil.org/topics/community-mental-health-centers/)

2. Farkas, M., Anthony, W., & Shern, D. (2012). The Role of the Community Mental Health Center in Promoting Resilience. In T. R. Krupa (Ed.), The Role of Mental Health Systems in Achieving Balance in Mental Health Care (pp. 77–106). Cambridge University Press.

3. Substance Abuse and Mental Health Services Administration (SAMHSA). (2020). Community Mental Health Services Block Grant. (https://www.samhsa.gov/grants/block-grants/cmhsbg)

Note: The examples and exercise in this section are fictional and are provided for illustrative purposes only.

Contemporary Approaches to Mental Health Care

In recent decades, the field of mental health care has witnessed significant advancements in the understanding and treatment of mental illnesses. These contemporary approaches have revolutionized the way mental health professionals approach the diagnosis, intervention, and management of various psychological disorders. In this section, we will explore some of the key contemporary approaches to mental health care and their implications for individuals and society.

Evidence-Based Practice

One of the most significant developments in contemporary mental health care is the emphasis on evidence-based practice (EBP). EBP involves integrating the best available research evidence with clinical expertise and patient values to guide treatment decisions and interventions. This approach ensures that mental health professionals are utilizing interventions that have been demonstrated to be effective through rigorous scientific research.

The use of evidence-based practice has several advantages. First, it ensures that mental health interventions are grounded in empirical evidence, increasing the likelihood of positive treatment outcomes. Second, it promotes standardization and consistency in practice, allowing for more reliable and comparable treatment approaches across different settings. Third, it facilitates the evaluation and improvement of interventions, as outcomes can be systematically measured and assessed.

However, implementing evidence-based practice in mental health care comes with its challenges. Mental health professionals must stay updated with the latest research findings, which can be time-consuming due to the rapidly evolving nature of the field. Additionally, individual differences and unique patient characteristics may not always align with the average treatment effects reported in research studies. Despite these challenges, evidence-based practice remains an essential component of contemporary mental health care.

Psychopharmacology

Another prominent contemporary approach in mental health care is the use of psychopharmacology, which involves the treatment of psychological disorders with medications. Psychopharmacology has significantly advanced our ability to alleviate symptoms and improve the quality of life for individuals with mental illnesses.

The development of psychotropic medications, such as selective serotonin reuptake inhibitors (SSRIs) for treating depression and anxiety, and atypical antipsychotics for managing psychotic disorders, has revolutionized the field of mental health care. These medications target specific neurochemical imbalances in the brain, helping to restore normal functioning and reduce symptoms.

Psychopharmacology offers several advantages in the treatment of mental illnesses. It can rapidly alleviate distressing symptoms, providing relief for individuals experiencing acute psychological distress. Medication can also be a valuable adjunct to other forms of therapy, such as psychotherapy, enhancing the overall treatment outcomes.

However, psychopharmacology also has its limitations. Medications may have side effects, and finding the right medication and dosage for an individual often requires a trial-and-error approach. Additionally, psychopharmacology alone may not address the underlying psychological and social factors contributing to mental illnesses. Therefore, an integrated approach that combines medication with other therapeutic interventions is often necessary for the best outcomes.

Psychotherapy and Counseling

Psychotherapy, also known as talk therapy, remains a fundamental component of contemporary mental health care. Various therapeutic modalities, such as cognitive-behavioral therapy (CBT), psychodynamic therapy, and humanistic therapy, are widely used to address a range of psychological conditions.

In psychotherapy, individuals work with a trained therapist to explore their thoughts, feelings, and behaviors and develop strategies to improve their mental well-being. This collaborative process can help individuals gain insight into their problems, develop coping skills, and make positive changes in their lives.

Cognitive-behavioral therapy (CBT) is a particularly effective psychotherapeutic approach widely used today. It focuses on identifying and modifying negative thinking patterns and behaviors that contribute to mental health problems. CBT has been extensively researched and has demonstrated efficacy in treating various conditions, such as depression, anxiety disorders, and eating disorders.

In recent years, counseling approaches have also gained prominence in mental health care. Counseling often focuses on specific issues or life transitions, such as career counseling, marriage counseling, or grief counseling. It provides individuals with guidance, support, and practical strategies for overcoming challenges and improving their psychological well-being.

Integrative and Holistic Approaches

Recognizing the interconnectedness of various factors influencing mental health, contemporary approaches to mental health care increasingly emphasize integrative and holistic approaches. These approaches consider the complex interplay between biological, psychological, social, and environmental factors in understanding and treating mental illnesses.

Integrative and holistic approaches aim to provide comprehensive care that addresses all aspects of an individual's well-being. They recognize that mental health is not solely determined by biologically based abnormalities or individual factors but is influenced by broader social determinants, such as socioeconomic status, access to education, and community support systems.

This paradigm shift has led to the integration of various therapeutic modalities, including psychotherapy, medication management, lifestyle interventions, and social support networks. For example, a treatment plan for an individual with depression may involve a combination of antidepressant medication, cognitive-behavioral therapy, stress reduction techniques, exercise, and social engagement.

By adopting a holistic approach, mental health care providers can tailor treatments to the unique needs and circumstances of individuals, addressing the underlying causes and promoting overall well-being. Moreover, these approaches empower individuals to take an active role in their treatment and equip them with tools and strategies to manage their mental health throughout their lives.

Digital Mental Health

The rapid advancement of technology has also had a profound impact on contemporary mental health care. Digital mental health, also known as e-mental health, refers to the use of digital tools and technologies to deliver mental health services and support.

Digital mental health encompasses various forms, such as teletherapy (remote therapy sessions via video conferencing), mobile applications for mental health self-management, online support groups and forums, and virtual reality therapy. These interventions provide accessible and convenient options for individuals seeking mental health care, particularly those facing geographic or mobility barriers.

While digital mental health interventions show promise, they also raise concerns regarding privacy, data security, and the quality of care delivered. Ensuring the ethical use of technology in mental health care and integrating digital tools into existing treatment approaches is an ongoing challenge for the field.

Conclusion

Contemporary approaches to mental health care have brought about significant advancements in the diagnosis, treatment, and management of mental illnesses. Evidence-based practice, psychopharmacology, psychotherapy, integrative and holistic approaches, and digital mental health interventions have reshaped the landscape of mental health care, providing individuals with a diverse range of options and opportunities for improving their well-being.

By embracing these contemporary approaches, mental health care providers can deliver more effective, personalized, and comprehensive care. However, it is important to continually evaluate and adapt these approaches to ensure they remain aligned with the evolving needs and preferences of individuals seeking mental health support.

As the field of mental health care continues to evolve, it is crucial for professionals to stay committed to ongoing research, training, and advocacy. By collaborating across disciplines and engaging with individuals and communities, we can build a sustainable mental health future that prioritizes holistic well-being, resilience, and social justice.

Chapter 2: Understanding Psychological Challenges

Chapter 2: Understanding Psychological Challenges

Chapter 2: Understanding Psychological Challenges

In this chapter, we will delve deeper into the understanding of psychological challenges. We will explore common mental health disorders, trauma and post-traumatic stress disorder (PTSD), addiction and mental health, neurodevelopmental disorders, personality disorders, eating disorders, psychosomatic disorders, sleep disorders, and other psychological challenges. Understanding these challenges is crucial for individuals, researchers, and healthcare professionals in order to identify, diagnose, and treat mental health conditions effectively.

Common Mental Health Disorders

Mental health disorders are common and can significantly impact a person's thoughts, emotions, and behavior. It is important to understand the different types of mental health disorders to provide appropriate care and support. Let us take a closer look at some of the most common mental health disorders:

1. Anxiety Disorders: Anxiety disorders are characterized by excessive worry, fear, and uneasiness. Examples of anxiety disorders include generalized anxiety disorder, panic disorder, social anxiety disorder, and specific phobias.

2. Mood Disorders: Mood disorders are characterized by significant changes in mood that affect a person's daily life. Major depressive disorder and bipolar disorder are common mood disorders.

3. Psychotic Disorders: Psychotic disorders involve distorted thinking and perception. Examples of psychotic disorders include schizophrenia and delusional disorder.

4. Substance Use Disorders: Substance use disorders involve the excessive use of drugs or alcohol, leading to impairment in personal, social, and occupational functioning.

5. Eating Disorders: Eating disorders such as anorexia nervosa, bulimia nervosa, and binge eating disorder are characterized by abnormal eating behaviors and a preoccupation with body weight and shape.

6. Dual Diagnosis: Co-occurring Disorders: Dual diagnosis refers to the presence of both a mental health disorder and a substance use disorder. It is important to treat both conditions simultaneously to achieve optimal outcomes.

Understanding these common mental health disorders will enable us to recognize their signs and symptoms, provide appropriate interventions, and advocate for early detection and treatment.

Trauma and Post-Traumatic Stress Disorder (PTSD)

Traumatic experiences can have a profound impact on an individual's mental health. It is important to understand trauma and its connection to mental health conditions like post-traumatic stress disorder (PTSD). Let's explore these concepts in more detail:

1. Understanding Trauma: Trauma refers to an event or experience that is distressing, overwhelming, or life-threatening. It can result from various sources such as physical or sexual abuse, natural disasters, accidents, or war.

2. The Impact of Trauma on Mental Health: Traumatic experiences can lead to the development of mental health disorders, particularly PTSD. Symptoms of PTSD may include intrusive memories, nightmares, avoidance behaviors, hypervigilance, and changes in mood or cognition.

3. Diagnosing and Treating PTSD: A comprehensive assessment is essential for the diagnosis of PTSD. Treatment approaches for PTSD often involve a combination of psychotherapy, medication, and support services. Cognitive-behavioral therapy (CBT), eye movement desensitization and reprocessing (EMDR), and group therapy are commonly used interventions.

4. Trauma-Informed Care: Trauma-informed care involves an understanding of the impact of trauma on individuals and the establishment of a safe and supportive environment for treatment. It emphasizes empowerment, choice, collaboration, and resilience.

By understanding trauma and its effects on mental health, we can provide trauma-informed care, advocate for trauma-focused interventions, and promote healing and recovery for individuals who have experienced trauma.

Addiction and Mental Health

The co-occurrence of addiction and mental health disorders can complicate treatment and recovery. Understanding the connection between addiction and mental health is crucial for effective intervention. Let's explore this topic further:

1. The Connection Between Addiction and Mental Health: Addiction and mental health disorders often coexist. Substance use can be a way for individuals to cope with underlying mental health issues, while substance abuse can also contribute to the development of mental health disorders.

2. Substance Use Disorders and Co-occurring Mental Illness: Co-occurring substance use disorders and mental health disorders require integrated treatment approaches. Dual diagnosis treatment involves addressing both conditions simultaneously to improve outcomes.

3. Treatment Approaches for Dual Diagnosis: The treatment of co-occurring disorders involves comprehensive assessment, personalized treatment plans, and a multidisciplinary approach. Integrated treatment programs that combine therapy, medication management, support groups, and lifestyle changes are often effective.

4. Harm Reduction Strategies: Harm reduction strategies aim to minimize the negative consequences associated with substance use. These strategies focus on reducing harm rather than immediate abstinence and include initiatives such as needle exchange programs and safe consumption sites.

By understanding the connection between addiction and mental health, we can provide integrated and holistic care for individuals with co-occurring disorders, promote harm reduction strategies, and support long-term recovery.

Neurodevelopmental Disorders

Neurodevelopmental disorders are a group of conditions that typically manifest in early childhood and affect the development of the nervous system. Let's explore some of the most common neurodevelopmental disorders:

1. Autism Spectrum Disorder (ASD): ASD is a complex neurodevelopmental disorder characterized by difficulties in social interaction, communication, and repetitive or restricted behaviors. Early intervention, behavioral therapy, and educational support are essential for individuals with ASD.

2. Attention-Deficit/Hyperactivity Disorder (ADHD): ADHD is characterized by persistent patterns of inattention, hyperactivity, and impulsivity that can impact daily functioning and academic performance. Treatment often includes a combination of behavioral therapy, medication, and support in educational settings.

3. Intellectual Disability: Intellectual disability is characterized by significant limitations in intellectual functioning and adaptive behaviors. Early identification, educational support, and interventions that focus on promoting independence and social skills are crucial for individuals with intellectual disability.

4. Early Intervention and Support for Neurodevelopmental Disorders: Early identification and intervention for neurodevelopmental disorders are key to maximizing outcomes. Early intervention programs provide targeted support and therapy to address developmental delays and promote optimal development.

Understanding neurodevelopmental disorders allows us to recognize the needs of individuals with these conditions, advocate for early intervention and support, and promote inclusivity and acceptance in society.

This section is just the beginning of our exploration into understanding psychological challenges. In the subsequent sections, we will delve further into different types of psychological disorders, their diagnosis, treatment approaches, and historical perspectives. It is important to have a comprehensive understanding of these challenges to promote mental health and well-being in contemporary society. Let us continue our journey in unraveling the complexities of mental health and work towards a sustainable future.

Common Mental Health Disorders

Anxiety Disorders

Anxiety disorders are among the most common mental health disorders, affecting millions of people worldwide. They are characterized by excessive and persistent worry, fear, or apprehension, causing significant distress and impairment in daily functioning. In this section, we will explore the different types of anxiety disorders, their symptoms, causes, and treatment approaches.

Types of Anxiety Disorders

There are several different types of anxiety disorders, each with its own specific symptoms and diagnostic criteria. The most common anxiety disorders include:

1. **Generalized Anxiety Disorder (GAD):** GAD is characterized by excessive and uncontrollable worry about everyday life events. Individuals with GAD often experience an overactive "worry engine," constantly anticipating and preparing for potential threats or dangers. They may also have physical symptoms such as restlessness, fatigue, muscle tension, and difficulty concentrating.

2. **Panic Disorder:** Panic disorder is characterized by recurrent and unexpected panic attacks, which are sudden episodes of intense fear or discomfort. Panic attacks are often accompanied by physical symptoms such as a racing heart, shortness of breath, chest pain, dizziness, and a sense of impending doom. Individuals with panic disorder often worry about having future panic attacks and may develop agoraphobia, a fear of being in situations where escape may be difficult or embarrassing.

3. **Social Anxiety Disorder (SAD):** SAD, also known as social phobia, is characterized by an intense fear of social situations. Individuals with SAD are excessively self-conscious and fear being embarrassed, humiliated, or judged by others. This fear often leads to avoidance of social situations, which can significantly impact their personal and professional lives.

4. **Specific Phobias:** Specific phobias are characterized by an intense and irrational fear of a specific object, situation, or activity. Common phobias include fear of flying, heights, animals, needles, and blood. Individuals with specific phobias go to great lengths to avoid their feared object or situation, and the anxiety associated with it can be debilitating.

5. **Obsessive-Compulsive Disorder (OCD):** OCD is characterized by intrusive and distressing thoughts, images, or urges (obsessions) and repetitive behaviors or mental acts (compulsions) aimed at reducing the anxiety caused by obsessions. Common obsessions include contamination fears, doubts about safety, and a need for symmetry, while common compulsions include excessive hand-washing, checking behaviors, and counting.

6. **Post-Traumatic Stress Disorder (PTSD):** PTSD is a disorder that can develop after exposure to a traumatic event. Individuals with PTSD experience distressing symptoms such as intrusive memories, nightmares, flashbacks, hyperarousal, and avoidance of reminders of the traumatic event. PTSD can significantly impact an individual's daily functioning and quality of life.

Causes and Risk Factors

The exact causes of anxiety disorders are complex and not fully understood. However, several factors may contribute to their development, including:

- **Genetics and Family History:** Individuals with a family history of anxiety disorders are more likely to develop an anxiety disorder themselves, suggesting a genetic component to their etiology. Certain genes may increase a person's vulnerability to anxiety disorders, although the specific genes involved are still being studied.

- **Neurochemical Imbalances:** Imbalances in neurotransmitters such as serotonin, gamma-aminobutyric acid (GABA), and norepinephrine have been implicated in the development of anxiety disorders. These chemical imbalances can affect the regulation of emotions and contribute to heightened anxiety.

- **Environmental Factors:** Traumatic events, such as physical or sexual abuse, neglect, or the experience of a natural disaster, can increase the risk of developing an anxiety disorder. Chronic stress, major life changes, and a lack of social support can also contribute to the development of anxiety disorders.

- **Cognitive Factors:** Certain thinking patterns and beliefs can contribute to the development and maintenance of anxiety disorders. Negative interpretations of ambiguous situations, excessive worry, perfectionism, and irrational beliefs about danger and control may contribute to heightened anxiety.

It is important to note that while these factors may increase the risk of developing an anxiety disorder, not everyone who experiences them will develop the condition. The interplay between genetic, biological, psychological, and environmental factors is complex, and further research is needed to better understand their interactions.

Treatment Approaches

The good news is that anxiety disorders are highly treatable, and there are effective interventions available. The most common treatment approaches for anxiety disorders include:

- **Psychotherapy:** Cognitive-behavioral therapy (CBT) is the most widely supported form of psychotherapy for anxiety disorders. CBT helps individuals identify and challenge irrational thoughts and beliefs, develop coping strategies, and gradually confront feared situations through exposure therapy. Other forms of therapy, such as acceptance and commitment therapy (ACT) and mindfulness-based therapies, can also be beneficial in managing anxiety.

- **Medication:** Antidepressant medications, particularly selective serotonin reuptake inhibitors (SSRIs) and serotonin-norepinephrine reuptake inhibitors (SNRIs), are often prescribed for anxiety disorders. These medications can help reduce symptoms of anxiety by rebalancing neurotransmitters in the brain. Benzodiazepines, another class of medications, may be prescribed on a short-term basis to alleviate acute symptoms, but their long-term use is generally discouraged due to the risk of dependence.

- **Lifestyle Modifications:** Making certain lifestyle changes can also contribute to the management of anxiety. Regular exercise, adequate sleep, a healthy diet, and stress reduction techniques such as meditation or deep breathing exercises can all help alleviate symptoms of anxiety.

- **Support Groups and Self-Help Resources:** Support groups, both in-person and online, can provide individuals with anxiety disorders a sense of community and understanding. Self-help resources, such as books, websites, and mobile applications, can also provide valuable information and strategies for managing anxiety on a day-to-day basis.

It is essential for individuals with anxiety disorders to work closely with mental health professionals to develop an individualized treatment plan that best suits their needs. With the right support and interventions, individuals with anxiety disorders can lead fulfilling and productive lives.

Real-World Example: Social Anxiety Disorder

To illustrate the impact of anxiety disorders, let's consider a real-world example of social anxiety disorder (SAD). Emily, a 26-year-old woman, experiences intense fear and anxiety in social situations due to a deep fear of being negatively judged or embarrassed. As a result, she avoids social gatherings, experiences panic attacks when forced to interact with others, and feels isolated and lonely.

Emily's social anxiety significantly impacts her personal and professional life. Simple tasks such as attending a work meeting or making a phone call become overwhelming for her. To manage her symptoms, Emily seeks therapy and works with a CBT therapist who guides her through exposure exercises, challenging her fearful thoughts, and helping her develop coping strategies. Over time, Emily's anxiety decreases, and she gains confidence in social situations.

This example highlights how social anxiety disorder can severely impact an individual's well-being and emphasizes the importance of appropriate treatment and support.

Key Takeaways

- Anxiety disorders are characterized by excessive and persistent worry, fear, or apprehension, causing significant distress and impairment in daily functioning.

- Common types of anxiety disorders include generalized anxiety disorder, panic disorder, social anxiety disorder, specific phobias, obsessive-compulsive disorder, and post-traumatic stress disorder.

- The causes of anxiety disorders are multifactorial and may involve genetic, neurochemical, environmental, and cognitive factors.

- Anxiety disorders are highly treatable, and effective interventions include psychotherapy, medication, lifestyle modifications, and support groups.

By raising awareness, promoting understanding, and providing appropriate support and treatment, we can help individuals with anxiety disorders lead healthier and more fulfilling lives.

Mood Disorders

In this section, we will explore mood disorders, which are a group of mental health conditions characterized by persistent disturbances in mood and emotions. Mood disorders can have a significant impact on an individual's daily functioning and overall quality of life. We will discuss the different types of mood disorders, their symptoms, causes, and treatment options.

Types of Mood Disorders

Mood disorders encompass a range of conditions, including:

1. **Major Depressive Disorder (MDD):** Also known as clinical depression, MDD is characterized by persistent feelings of sadness, loss of interest or pleasure in activities, changes in sleep patterns, appetite disturbances, fatigue, and diminished concentration. MDD significantly affects a person's ability to function and may lead to thoughts of self-harm or suicide.

2. **Bipolar Disorder:** Bipolar disorder is characterized by extreme mood swings, fluctuating between episodes of depression and mania. During depressive episodes, individuals experience symptoms similar to those of major depressive disorder. In contrast, manic episodes are marked by elevated mood, increased energy levels, racing thoughts, impulsive behavior, and grandiosity.

3. **Persistent Depressive Disorder (PDD):** PDD, formerly known as dysthymia, is a chronic form of depression. It involves long-lasting feelings of sadness, hopelessness, low self-esteem, and a loss of interest in activities. Although the symptoms of PDD are less severe compared to major depressive disorder, they can still impact a person's daily life.

4. **Seasonal Affective Disorder (SAD):** SAD is characterized by the onset of depressive symptoms during specific seasons, typically in the winter months when there is less natural sunlight. Symptoms include low mood, fatigue, increased sleep, and cravings for carbohydrates. SAD is thought to be related to reduced sunlight exposure and disrupted circadian rhythms.

5. **Premenstrual Dysphoric Disorder (PMDD):** PMDD is a severe form of premenstrual syndrome (PMS) that occurs in some individuals during the menstrual cycle. Symptoms include irritability, mood swings, anxiety, depression, and physical discomfort. PMDD can significantly affect interpersonal relationships and daily activities.

It is important to note that these are not the only mood disorders, but they represent the most commonly diagnosed conditions. Each disorder has its own unique symptoms and diagnostic criteria according to the Diagnostic and Statistical Manual of Mental Disorders (DSM-5).

Causes of Mood Disorders

The exact causes of mood disorders are not fully understood, but research suggests that a combination of genetic, biological, environmental, and psychological factors may contribute to their development. Some of the key factors associated with mood disorders include:

- **Biological Factors:** Imbalances in neurotransmitters, such as serotonin, norepinephrine, and dopamine, have been implicated in the development of mood disorders. Additionally, abnormalities in brain structure and function, hormonal imbalances, and genetic predisposition may also play a role.

- **Environmental Factors:** Traumatic life events, such as loss of a loved one, physical or sexual abuse, or chronic stress, can increase the risk of developing mood disorders. Other environmental factors, including poverty, social isolation, and substance abuse, can also contribute to the onset or exacerbation of symptoms.

- **Psychological Factors:** Certain personality traits, such as perfectionism or a negative cognitive style, can increase vulnerability to mood disorders. In addition, individuals with a history of anxiety disorders or other mental health conditions may be more prone to developing mood disorders.

It is important to recognize that the causes of mood disorders can vary from person to person, and each individual's experience is unique. Therefore, a comprehensive assessment by a mental health professional is necessary to determine the specific factors contributing to an individual's mood disorder.

Treatment of Mood Disorders

Treating mood disorders often involves a combination of approaches, including psychotherapy, medication, and lifestyle changes. The primary goal of treatment is to alleviate symptoms, improve daily functioning, and prevent relapse. Some common treatment options for mood disorders include:

- **Psychotherapy:** Various forms of psychotherapy, such as cognitive-behavioral therapy (CBT) and interpersonal therapy (IPT), are effective in treating mood disorders. These therapies help individuals identify and change negative thought patterns, develop coping strategies, and improve interpersonal relationships.

- **Medication:** Antidepressant medications, such as selective serotonin reuptake inhibitors (SSRIs) and mood stabilizers, are frequently prescribed to manage symptoms of mood disorders. These medications help regulate neurotransmitter levels and stabilize mood. It is important to note that medication should always be prescribed and monitored by a qualified healthcare professional.

- **Lifestyle Changes:** Adopting healthy lifestyle habits can support recovery from mood disorders. Regular exercise, a balanced diet, adequate sleep, stress management techniques, and avoiding alcohol or drug misuse can contribute to improved mood and overall wellbeing.

In addition to these conventional treatment approaches, alternative therapies, such as relaxation techniques, mindfulness meditation, and herbal supplements, may also be utilized. However, it is essential to consult with healthcare professionals before incorporating alternative treatments into one's treatment plan.

Case Study: Sarah's Journey with Bipolar Disorder

To illustrate the impact and management of mood disorders, let's consider the case of Sarah, a 32-year-old woman diagnosed with bipolar disorder. Sarah experiences recurring episodes of depression and mania, which significantly disrupt her daily life and relationships.

During depressive episodes, Sarah feels overwhelming sadness, loss of interest in previously enjoyed activities, and struggles with feelings of guilt and worthlessness. She often has difficulty concentrating and experiences changes in appetite and sleep patterns. These symptoms make it challenging for Sarah to maintain her job and engage in social activities.

Alternatively, during manic episodes, Sarah feels euphoric, has excessive energy, and displays impulsive behavior. She engages in risky activities, spends money excessively, and has difficulty with impulse control. Sarah's manic episodes often strain her relationships and can lead to legal and financial consequences.

Sarah's treatment plan includes a combination of medication and psychotherapy. She takes mood stabilizers to help regulate her mood swings and attends regular therapy sessions to learn coping skills, manage stress, and identify early warning signs of mood episodes. With ongoing support and treatment, Sarah can regain stability in her life and improve her overall well-being.

Conclusion

Mood disorders are complex mental health conditions that require an integrated approach to diagnosis and treatment. Understanding the different types of mood disorders, their causes, and available treatment options is crucial for effectively managing these conditions and promoting the well-being of individuals affected by them. By providing education, destigmatizing mood disorders, and ensuring accessible and comprehensive mental health care, we can work towards a more sustainable future for mental health.

Psychotic Disorders

Psychotic disorders, also known as psychosis, are a group of mental disorders characterized by significant disturbances in perception, thinking, and behavior. Individuals with psychotic disorders often experience a loss of touch with reality, leading to symptoms such as hallucinations and delusions. These disorders can have a profound impact on a person's life, making it essential to understand their causes, symptoms, and available treatment options.

Causes of Psychotic Disorders

The exact causes of psychotic disorders are not fully understood, but research suggests that a combination of biological, genetic, and environmental factors contribute to their development. Some of the key factors include:

- Genetics: There is evidence of a genetic component in psychotic disorders. People with a family history of psychotic disorders are at a higher risk of developing the condition themselves.

- Neurochemical imbalances: Imbalances in certain neurotransmitters, such as dopamine, serotonin, and glutamate, have been implicated in the development of psychotic symptoms.

- Brain abnormalities: Structural and functional abnormalities in specific brain regions, such as the prefrontal cortex and the hippocampus, have been observed in individuals with psychotic disorders.

- Environmental factors: Traumatic experiences, stressful life events, substance abuse, and social isolation can increase the risk of developing psychotic disorders.

Types of Psychotic Disorders

There are several different types of psychotic disorders, each with its unique characteristics and diagnostic criteria. Some of the most common types include:

1. Schizophrenia: Schizophrenia is a chronic and severe psychotic disorder that affects how a person thinks, feels, and behaves. Symptoms typically emerge in late adolescence or early adulthood and can include hallucinations, delusions, disorganized thinking, and impaired social functioning.

2. Schizoaffective disorder: Schizoaffective disorder combines symptoms of schizophrenia and mood disorders, such as depression or bipolar disorder. Individuals with this disorder experience periods of psychosis along with significant mood disturbances.

3. Delusional disorder: Delusional disorder is characterized by persistent delusions that are not influenced by reality. These delusions typically involve false beliefs about oneself or others and can significantly impact a person's functioning.

4. Brief psychotic disorder: Brief psychotic disorder is a short-term psychotic condition triggered by a highly stressful event, such as the death of a loved one or a traumatic experience. Symptoms last for a short duration, usually less than one month.

5. Substance-induced psychotic disorder: Substance-induced psychotic disorder occurs as a result of substance abuse, such as the use of hallucinogens, amphetamines, or cannabis. Psychotic symptoms subside when the substance is no longer present in the body.

It is important to note that the diagnosis of a specific psychotic disorder requires a thorough evaluation by a qualified mental health professional.

Symptoms and Presentation

The symptoms of psychotic disorders can vary depending on the specific diagnosis and the individual. Some common symptoms include:

- Hallucinations: Hallucinations are perceptual distortions that involve seeing, hearing, or feeling things that are not actually present. Auditory hallucinations, such as hearing voices, are the most common in psychotic disorders.

- Delusions: Delusions are fixed beliefs that are not based on reality and are resistant to change, even when presented with contrary evidence. Delusions can involve ideas of grandeur, persecution, or reference.

- Disorganized thinking: Individuals with psychotic disorders may experience disorganized thinking, making it challenging to communicate coherently or logically. Their speech may be disorganized and fragmented, making it difficult for others to understand.

- Grossly disorganized or abnormal motor behavior: People with psychotic disorders may exhibit unusual or inappropriate behavior, such as odd body movements, repetitive actions, or a lack of response to their surroundings.

- Negative symptoms: Negative symptoms refer to a loss of normal functioning, such as a lack of motivation, reduced emotional expression, or social withdrawal. These symptoms can significantly impact a person's ability to perform daily activities.

It is important to recognize that individuals with psychotic disorders can have varying degrees of symptom severity, and their experiences may differ from one another. Treatment approaches should be tailored to the specific needs of each individual.

Treatment Approaches

The treatment of psychotic disorders often involves a combination of medication, psychotherapy, and psychosocial interventions. Here are some key approaches:

- Antipsychotic medication: Antipsychotic medications are commonly prescribed to manage psychotic symptoms. These medications help control hallucinations, delusions, and disorganized thinking. However, they may have side effects, such as weight gain and movement disorders, which should be monitored.

- Cognitive-behavioral therapy (CBT): CBT can be helpful in managing symptoms, improving coping strategies, and addressing negative thought patterns associated with psychotic disorders. CBT may focus on challenging delusional beliefs or teaching social skills.

- Family therapy: Involving family members in treatment can be beneficial for individuals with psychotic disorders, as it provides education, support, and helps improve communication within the family unit.

- Social skills training: Social skills training helps individuals with psychotic disorders develop effective communication, problem-solving, and interpersonal skills. This can enhance their ability to engage in social interactions and improve their quality of life.

It is crucial for individuals with psychotic disorders to receive ongoing support, monitoring, and routine care to manage their symptoms effectively.

Real-World Example: Early Intervention in Psychosis

Early intervention in psychosis is an example of a contemporary approach to the treatment of psychotic disorders. It focuses on identifying and treating psychotic symptoms as early as possible to improve long-term outcomes. Early intervention programs typically involve a combination of medication, psychotherapy, case management, and family support. The aim is to reduce the duration of untreated psychosis, minimize the impact of the illness, and promote recovery.

These programs often provide specialized services tailored to the needs of young adults experiencing their first episode of psychosis. The approach emphasizes early identification, comprehensive assessment, and intensive treatment. By intervening early, these programs help individuals maintain social and functional abilities, reduce the risk of relapse, and improve overall psychosocial functioning.

Caveats and Controversies

While significant advancements have been made in the understanding and treatment of psychotic disorders, there are still challenges and controversies in the field. Some of these include:

- Stigma: The stigma associated with psychotic disorders can lead to social isolation, discrimination, and limited access to resources and support. It is crucial to address stigma through education and advocacy.

- Side effects of medication: Antipsychotic medications used to manage symptoms of psychotic disorders can have side effects, including weight gain, metabolic changes, and movement disorders. Balancing the benefits of medication with these side effects is an ongoing challenge.

- Access to care: Access to specialized mental health care, including early intervention programs, can be limited in some regions, leading to delayed diagnosis and treatment initiation. Efforts should be made to improve access to care and reduce disparities.

Overall, continued research, education, and awareness are essential in addressing the challenges and improving the outcomes for individuals with psychotic disorders.

Summary

Psychotic disorders are a group of mental disorders characterized by significant disturbances in perception, thinking, and behavior. They can have a significant impact on an individual's life and require a comprehensive understanding of their causes, symptoms, and treatment approaches. Early intervention, medication, psychotherapy, and psychosocial interventions play crucial roles in managing psychotic symptoms and promoting recovery. As our understanding of psychotic disorders continues to evolve, it is essential to address stigma, improve access to care, and strive for a holistic and sustainable approach to mental health.

Substance Use Disorders

Substance use disorders are a significant mental health challenge that affects individuals across various age groups and demographics. These disorders occur when the use of substances, such as alcohol, tobacco, or illicit drugs, leads to significant impairment or distress. In this section, we will explore the underlying factors, classification, diagnosis, and treatment approaches for substance use disorders.

Background

Substance use disorders have been prevalent throughout history, and the understanding of these disorders has evolved over time. Historically, substance abuse was often viewed as a moral failing or a weakness of character. However, with advancements in research and a deeper understanding of the neurobiology of addiction, we now recognize substance use disorders as complex conditions that involve the interaction of genetic, environmental, and psychological factors.

Classification

The Diagnostic and Statistical Manual of Mental Disorders (DSM-5) provides the standard criteria for diagnosing substance use disorders. The manual categorizes substance use disorders into 11 different classes, including alcohol, cannabis, stimulants, opioids, hallucinogens, and others. Each substance has specific diagnostic criteria, including indicators such as impaired control, social impairment, risky use, and pharmacological criteria.

Diagnosis

Diagnosing substance use disorders requires a comprehensive assessment that considers various factors, including substance use patterns, physical health, and psychological symptoms. Professionals utilize screening tools, interviews, and laboratory tests to gather information and make an accurate diagnosis.

Screening Tools   Screening tools, such as the Alcohol Use Disorders Identification Test (AUDIT) or the Drug Abuse Screening Test (DAST), are commonly used to identify individuals at risk for substance use disorders. These tools assess the frequency and quantity of substance use, associated problems, and the impact on daily functioning.

Clinical Interviews   Clinical interviews allow for a more in-depth evaluation of an individual's substance use history, current symptoms, motivations, and treatment goals. These structured interviews follow specific guidelines and provide a holistic understanding of the individual's substance use disorder.

Laboratory Tests   Laboratory tests, such as urine or blood tests, are sometimes used to confirm the presence of specific substances in an individual's system. These tests help to corroborate self-reporting and aid in providing a comprehensive assessment of substance use.

Treatment Approaches

The treatment of substance use disorders involves a multifaceted approach that addresses various aspects of the individual's life. Effective treatment approaches include a combination of pharmacological interventions, psychotherapy, support groups, and lifestyle modifications.

Medication-Assisted Treatment   Medication-assisted treatment (MAT) involves the use of medications, such as methadone, buprenorphine, or naltrexone, to manage withdrawal symptoms and cravings associated with substance use disorders. These medications help stabilize individuals and reduce the likelihood of relapse.

Psychotherapy   Psychotherapy, such as cognitive-behavioral therapy (CBT), motivational interviewing, and contingency management, is a vital component of substance use disorder treatment. These approaches help individuals understand the underlying triggers and develop coping strategies to manage stress, cravings, and negative emotions.

Support Groups   Support groups, such as Alcoholics Anonymous (AA) or Narcotics Anonymous (NA), provide individuals with a supportive environment and a sense of community. These groups offer peer support and valuable insights from individuals who have experienced similar challenges.

Lifestyle Modifications   Lifestyle modifications play a crucial role in the recovery process. These modifications may include adopting a healthier diet, engaging in regular exercise, improving sleep hygiene, and developing healthy coping mechanisms to replace substance use.

Challenges and Considerations

Addressing substance use disorders presents several challenges and considerations that need to be taken into account.

Stigma   Stigma surrounding substance use disorders remains a significant barrier to treatment and recovery. Individuals may hesitate to seek help due to fear of judgment or discrimination. Awareness campaigns and education efforts are necessary to reduce stigma and promote understanding.

Relapse   Substance use disorders are chronic relapsing conditions, and relapse rates can be high. It is essential to view relapse as an opportunity for learning and to provide ongoing support and encouragement to individuals in recovery.

Co-occurring Disorders   Substance use disorders often co-occur with other mental health disorders, such as depression, anxiety, or trauma-related disorders. Integrated treatment approaches that address both substance use and mental health symptoms are necessary for comprehensive care.

Cultural Sensitivity   Culture plays a significant role in shaping attitudes towards substance use and treatment-seeking behaviors. Treatment programs should consider cultural norms, values, and beliefs to provide culturally sensitive care that respects individual diversity.

Case Study: Opioid Epidemic

The opioid epidemic serves as a contemporary example of the devastating impact of substance use disorders. It highlights the need for evidence-based prevention strategies, harm reduction measures, and access to treatment. Policies addressing prescription drug monitoring, education, and naloxone distribution have become critical in combating this crisis.

Resources and Further Reading

- National Institute on Drug Abuse (NIDA): www.drugabuse.gov - Substance Abuse and Mental Health Services Administration (SAMHSA): www.samhsa.gov - Alcoholics Anonymous: www.aa.org - Narcotics Anonymous: www.na.org

Exercises

1. Research and discuss the benefits and challenges of medication-assisted treatment for opioid use disorder. 2. Explore the role of trauma in the development and maintenance of substance use disorders. 3. Investigate how cultural factors influence substance use patterns and treatment outcomes in different communities. 4. Develop a harm reduction plan for individuals at risk for substance use disorders in your community. 5. Conduct a case study analysis of a substance use disorder treatment program and evaluate its effectiveness.

In conclusion, substance use disorders are a complex and multifaceted issue that requires a comprehensive approach to treatment. By understanding the underlying factors, using evidence-based interventions, and promoting awareness and support, we can work towards reducing the impact of substance use disorders on individuals and society as a whole.

Eating Disorders

Eating disorders are complex mental health conditions characterized by irregular eating habits and severe distress related to body weight or shape. They can have serious physical and psychological consequences, and often require comprehensive treatment approaches. In this section, we will explore the different types of eating disorders, their causes, diagnostic criteria, and treatment options.

Types of Eating Disorders

There are several types of eating disorders, each with its own set of symptoms and diagnostic criteria. The most common eating disorders include:

1. Anorexia Nervosa: Individuals with anorexia nervosa have an intense fear of gaining weight and a distorted body image. They restrict their food intake, leading to significant weight loss and an inability to maintain a healthy body weight.

2. Bulimia Nervosa: People with bulimia nervosa engage in episodes of binge eating followed by behaviors to compensate for the consumed calories, such as self-induced vomiting, excessive exercise, or the use of laxatives or diuretics.

3. Binge Eating Disorder: This disorder is characterized by recurrent episodes of uncontrollable binge eating without the compensatory behaviors associated with bulimia nervosa. People with binge eating disorder often experience feelings of guilt, shame, and distress.

4. Avoidant/Restrictive Food Intake Disorder (ARFID): ARFID involves a limited variety or avoidance of certain foods, leading to weight loss, nutritional deficiencies, and impaired functioning. It is often associated with sensory sensitivities or fear of aversive consequences.

5. Other Specified Feeding or Eating Disorder (OSFED): OSFED encompasses eating disorders that do not meet the full diagnostic criteria for the other disorders but still cause significant distress and impairment.

Causes of Eating Disorders

The development of eating disorders is influenced by a combination of genetic, biological, psychological, social, and environmental factors. Some common risk factors include:

- Genetics: Research suggests a genetic predisposition to eating disorders, with certain individuals being more vulnerable to developing these conditions.

- Psychological Factors: Low self-esteem, body dissatisfaction, perfectionism, and poor body image are often associated with eating disorders.

- Sociocultural Influences: Societal pressure to attain a certain body size or shape, media portrayal of unrealistic body standards, and cultural norms play a significant role in the development of eating disorders.

- Family Dynamics: Family factors, such as a history of dieting, critical comments about weight and appearance, and parental modeling of disordered eating behaviors, can contribute to the development of eating disorders.

It is essential to recognize that eating disorders are not caused by personal weakness or lack of willpower. They are complex conditions influenced by a variety of factors.

Diagnostic Criteria

To diagnose an eating disorder, mental health professionals refer to the Diagnostic and Statistical Manual of Mental Disorders (DSM-5) criteria. The DSM-5 outlines specific diagnostic criteria for each eating disorder, including the frequency and severity of symptoms, duration, and functional impairment caused.

For example, to be diagnosed with anorexia nervosa, an individual must meet the following criteria:

1. Restriction of energy intake resulting in significantly low body weight.

2. Intense fear of gaining weight or persistent behavior that interferes with weight gain, even though underweight.

3. Disturbance in self-perceived weight or shape, undue influence of body weight or shape on self-evaluation, or persistent lack of recognition of the seriousness of low body weight.

Similar diagnostic criteria exist for other eating disorders, allowing for accurate assessment and treatment planning.

Treatment Approaches

The treatment of eating disorders typically involves a multidisciplinary approach that addresses both the physical and psychological aspects of the condition. Treatment may include:

- Medical Care: For individuals with severe weight loss and medical complications, medical care is necessary to stabilize their physical health. This may involve hospitalization, nutritional support, and monitoring of vital signs.

- Psychotherapy: Various forms of psychotherapy, such as cognitive-behavioral therapy (CBT) and dialectical behavior therapy (DBT), are commonly used in the treatment of eating disorders. These therapies help individuals identify and change unhealthy thoughts and behaviors related to food, weight, and body image.

- Nutritional Counseling: Registered dietitians play a crucial role in helping individuals establish regular eating patterns, normalize their relationship with food, and achieve a balanced diet.

- Medication: In some cases, medication may be prescribed to manage co-occurring conditions, such as depression, anxiety, or obsessive-compulsive disorder.

- Support Groups: Peer support and group therapy can provide individuals with a safe space to share their experiences, gain support, and learn coping strategies from others facing similar challenges.

It is important to emphasize that early intervention is crucial for effective treatment outcomes. The sooner an eating disorder is identified and addressed, the better the chances of recovery and overall wellbeing.

Resources and Support

If you or someone you know is struggling with an eating disorder, it is essential to seek help from a qualified healthcare professional. Several organizations and resources provide information, support, and treatment referrals for eating disorders, including:

- National Eating Disorders Association (NEDA): www.nationaleatingdisorders.org

- Eating Disorders Hope: www.eatingdisorderhope.com

- Academy for Eating Disorders (AED): www.aedweb.org

- International Association of Eating Disorders Professionals (iaedp): www.iaedp.com

Remember, support is available, and recovery is possible with appropriate care and support.

Case Study: Sarah's Journey to Recovery

Sarah, a college student, had been struggling with anorexia nervosa for several years. She had an intense fear of gaining weight and believed that losing weight would make her more accepted and successful. Sarah's eating disorder caused significant physical and emotional distress, impacting her relationships, academic performance, and overall quality of life.

With the support of her friends and family, Sarah sought professional help. She began attending individual therapy sessions with a specialized eating disorder therapist and received guidance from a registered dietitian to establish a healthy eating plan. Through therapy, Sarah addressed her distorted beliefs about weight and body image and learned healthier coping strategies to manage stress and emotions.

It was a challenging journey, but with time and consistent treatment, Sarah began to regain control over her life. She also attended group therapy sessions where she connected with individuals who shared similar experiences, providing her with a sense of community and support.

Today, Sarah is in recovery from her eating disorder. She maintains a balanced approach to food and focuses on her overall wellbeing. Sarah's story highlights the importance of early intervention, a comprehensive treatment approach, and the power of support and resilience in overcoming eating disorders.

Key Takeaways

- Eating disorders are complex mental health conditions characterized by irregular eating habits and severe distress related to body weight or shape.

- The most common eating disorders include anorexia nervosa, bulimia nervosa, binge eating disorder, avoidant/restrictive food intake disorder (ARFID), and other specified feeding or eating disorder (OSFED).

- Eating disorders can be caused by a combination of genetic, psychological, sociocultural, and family factors.

- Diagnostic criteria outlined in the DSM-5 help mental health professionals assess and diagnose eating disorders accurately.

- Treatment of eating disorders involves a multidisciplinary approach, including medical care, psychotherapy, nutritional counseling, medication (if necessary), and support groups.

- Early intervention is crucial for successful treatment outcomes, and resources and support networks are available for individuals seeking help.

By raising awareness, providing accurate information, and offering support, we can contribute to the prevention and improved treatment of eating disorders, ultimately working towards a healthier and more sustainable future for mental health.

Dual Diagnosis: Co-occurring Disorders

Co-occurring disorders, also known as dual diagnosis, refer to the presence of both a mental health disorder and a substance use disorder in an individual. This section explores the complex nature of dual diagnosis, its prevalence, challenges in diagnosis and treatment, and the importance of an integrated approach to address co-occurring disorders effectively.

Prevalence of Co-occurring Disorders

Co-occurring disorders are highly prevalent, with a significant overlap between mental health disorders and substance use disorders. Research suggests that individuals with mental health disorders are more likely to develop substance abuse issues, and vice versa. The co-occurrence of these disorders can exacerbate symptoms, increase the risk of relapse, and hinder the overall recovery process.

According to the Substance Abuse and Mental Health Services Administration (SAMHSA), approximately 7.9 million adults in the United States experience co-occurring disorders. This highlights the need for a comprehensive approach that addresses both mental health and substance use concerns concurrently.

Diagnostic Challenges

Diagnosing co-occurring disorders can be challenging due to several factors. Symptoms of mental health disorders and substance use disorders can overlap or mimic each other, making it difficult to differentiate between the two. Additionally, individuals may be hesitant to disclose their substance use due to fear of stigma or legal implications.

Healthcare professionals need to conduct a thorough assessment, including a comprehensive psychiatric evaluation and a detailed substance use history. Screening tools, such as the Substance Abuse Subtle Screening Inventory (SASSI) and the Dual Diagnosis Capability in Addiction Treatment (DDCAT) Index, can assist in identifying the presence of co-occurring disorders.

Treatment Approaches

Treating co-occurring disorders requires an integrated approach that addresses both mental health and substance use components simultaneously. The following treatment modalities are commonly used:

1. Integrated Dual Disorder Treatment (IDDT): IDDT is a comprehensive approach that combines mental health and substance abuse treatments. It involves a multidisciplinary team that collaborates to develop an individualized treatment plan. IDDT integrates evidence-based practices, such as medication-assisted treatment, cognitive-behavioral therapy, motivational interviewing, and relapse prevention strategies.

2. Coordinated Specialty Care (CSC): CSC is an evidence-based model primarily used in the treatment of early-stage psychosis. It provides a holistic approach that includes medication management, psychotherapy, supported education and employment, and family support. Substance use disorders are addressed simultaneously to improve overall outcomes.

3. Motivational Enhancement Therapy (MET): MET is a directive, person-centered approach that focuses on resolving ambivalence and increasing motivation for change. It helps individuals explore their values, goals, and the potential consequences of their substance use. MET can be used as a stand-alone intervention or as part of a comprehensive treatment plan.

4. Mutual Support Groups: Participation in mutual support groups, such as Alcoholics Anonymous (AA) or Narcotics Anonymous (NA), can provide additional support for individuals with co-occurring disorders. These groups offer a safe, non-judgmental environment where individuals can share their experiences, seek guidance, and learn from others who have faced similar challenges.

Challenges and Considerations

Treating co-occurring disorders poses several challenges that need to be addressed for successful outcomes:

1. Stigma and Dual Discrimination: Stigma surrounding mental health and substance use can hinder individuals from seeking help and receiving appropriate care. Healthcare providers need to create a compassionate and non-judgmental environment to reduce stigma and encourage treatment-seeking behavior.

2. Integrated Treatment Infrastructure: Effective treatment requires collaboration between mental health and substance abuse service systems. Resource allocation, staff training, and coordination among providers are crucial to establish an integrated treatment infrastructure.

3. Continuum of Care: Recovery from co-occurring disorders is a long-term process that requires ongoing support. An effective continuum of care should include prevention, early intervention, outpatient services, residential treatment, and community-based support programs to ensure sustained recovery.

Case Study

Consider the case of Sarah, a 35-year-old woman diagnosed with depression and alcohol dependence. Sarah's depression symptoms have worsened over the past year, leading her to self-medicate with alcohol. She experiences frequent mood swings, social isolation, and deteriorating physical health.

Sarah's treatment plan will involve an integrated approach. She will receive medication for managing her depression symptoms and undergo cognitive-behavioral therapy to address the underlying causes of her substance use. Sarah will also be encouraged to join a support group to connect with other individuals facing similar challenges.

Additionally, Sarah's treatment team will assess her social support network and involve her family in the recovery process. They will work together to identify healthy coping strategies and develop a relapse prevention plan.

Conclusion

Co-occurring disorders require a comprehensive, integrated approach that addresses the unique challenges of individuals facing both mental health and substance use issues. By adopting evidence-based practices, reducing stigma, and promoting collaboration among healthcare providers, we can enhance the quality of care and improve outcomes for individuals with co-occurring disorders.

Trauma and Post-Traumatic Stress Disorder (PTSD)

Understanding Trauma

Trauma is a psychological and emotional response to a distressing or disturbing event that exceeds an individual's ability to cope. It can result from a wide range of experiences, including natural disasters, accidents, violence, abuse, and war.

TRAUMA AND POST-TRAUMATIC STRESS DISORDER (PTSD)

Understanding trauma is crucial for mental health professionals, as it helps guide assessment, diagnosis, and treatment approaches for individuals who have experienced traumatic events.

The Impact of Trauma

Experiencing a traumatic event can have profound and long-lasting effects on an individual's mental, emotional, and physical well-being. The impact of trauma can vary widely depending on factors such as the nature of the event, the individual's background, and the available support systems. Some common symptoms and effects of trauma include:

- **Emotional Distress:** Trauma can lead to intense emotions such as fear, sadness, anger, and guilt. Individuals may also experience flashbacks, nightmares, or a sense of emotional numbness.

- **Cognitive Changes:** Traumatic events can disrupt cognitive functioning, leading to difficulties with concentration, memory, and decision-making. Individuals may also exhibit hypervigilance or excessive worry.

- **Physical Health Problems:** Trauma can manifest in physical symptoms such as headaches, chronic pain, gastrointestinal issues, and sleep disturbances. These physical symptoms may co-occur with psychological distress.

- **Relationship Difficulties:** Trauma can strain interpersonal relationships, as individuals may struggle with trust, intimacy, and emotional connection. They may also isolate themselves or avoid situations that remind them of the traumatic event.

- **Maladaptive Coping Mechanisms:** In an attempt to manage the distressing symptoms of trauma, individuals may turn to unhealthy coping strategies such as substance abuse, self-harm, or disordered eating.

It is important to note that individuals may respond to trauma in different ways, and not all individuals who have experienced trauma will develop post-traumatic stress disorder (PTSD). However, understanding trauma and its potential impact can help identify those who may be at risk for developing psychological difficulties and provide appropriate support and intervention.

Theoretical Frameworks for Understanding Trauma

Several theoretical frameworks and models have been developed to understand the complexities of trauma and its effects on individuals. Two widely recognized frameworks are:

1. **Post-Traumatic Stress Disorder (PTSD) Model:** This model, developed by the American Psychiatric Association, focuses on the diagnostic criteria and symptoms associated with PTSD. According to this model, trauma can lead to intrusive thoughts, avoidance behaviors, negative alterations in mood and cognition, and increased arousal and reactivity. It provides a framework for understanding and diagnosing trauma-related disorders but may not capture the full range of post-traumatic responses.

2. **Complex Trauma Model:** The complex trauma model emphasizes the impact of repeated and prolonged trauma on an individual's development and functioning. It recognizes that trauma can interfere with the formation of secure attachments, disrupt emotional regulation, and impair the development of a coherent sense of self. This model emphasizes the importance of considering the broader context of trauma, such as the interpersonal and environmental factors that contribute to its occurrence and perpetuation.

These frameworks, along with other trauma theories, help mental health professionals understand the multiple dimensions of trauma, inform their assessment and treatment approaches, and promote a holistic understanding of an individual's experiences.

Assessment and Diagnosis of Trauma

Accurate assessment and diagnosis of trauma are essential for effective treatment planning and intervention. Mental health professionals use various methods to assess trauma, including clinical interviews, self-report measures, and collateral information from family members or other sources. Some commonly used assessment tools for trauma include:

- **Structured Clinical Interviews:** These interviews involve a series of standardized questions designed to assess trauma exposure, symptoms, and functional impairment. Examples of structured clinical interviews include the Clinician-Administered PTSD Scale (CAPS) and the Structured Clinical Interview for DSM-5 (SCID).

- **Self-Report Measures:** These questionnaires allow individuals to self-report their trauma experiences, symptoms, and distress levels.

Well-known self-report measures for trauma include the Impact of Event Scale (IES), the Trauma Symptom Inventory (TSI), and the Posttraumatic Stress Disorder Checklist (PCL).

- **Collateral Information:** Gathering information from family members, close friends, or other professionals who have knowledge of the individual's experiences can provide valuable insights into the impact of trauma and its consequences.

It is important for mental health professionals to exercise caution and sensitivity when conducting trauma assessments, as discussing traumatic events can trigger distressing reactions. Creating a safe and supportive environment, establishing rapport and trust, and using trauma-informed approaches are essential in the assessment process.

Treatment Approaches for Trauma

Effective treatment approaches for trauma focus on addressing the psychological, emotional, and physiological effects of trauma, promoting healing and recovery, and enhancing resilience. Some commonly used treatment approaches for trauma include:

- **Trauma-focused Cognitive-Behavioral Therapy (TF-CBT):** TF-CBT is a evidence-based treatment approach that targets the cognitive and behavioral aspects of trauma-related symptoms. It combines elements of cognitive therapy, exposure therapy, and psychoeducation to address negative thoughts, emotions, and behavioral patterns associated with trauma.

- **Eye Movement Desensitization and Reprocessing (EMDR):** EMDR is a therapy approach that utilizes bilateral stimulation, such as eye movements or tactile sensations, to facilitate the processing and integration of traumatic memories. It aims to alleviate distress and promote adaptive resolution of trauma-related symptoms.

- **Psychopharmacological Interventions:** In some cases, medication may be prescribed to manage specific symptoms associated with trauma, such as depression, anxiety, or sleep disturbances. The choice of medication and dosage depends on the individual's symptoms and specific needs and should be carefully monitored by a qualified healthcare professional.

- **Mindfulness-Based Interventions:** Mindfulness-based interventions, such as mindfulness-based stress reduction (MBSR) or mindfulness-based cognitive therapy (MBCT), can help individuals develop non-judgmental awareness of their experiences and cultivate self-compassion. These interventions have shown promise in reducing trauma-related symptoms and improving overall psychological well-being.

It is important to note that treatment approaches for trauma should be tailored to the unique needs of each individual and consider cultural, social, and contextual factors. Trauma-informed care, which emphasizes safety, trustworthiness, choice, collaboration, and empowerment, is essential in providing effective and sensitive treatment for individuals who have experienced trauma.

Addressing Trauma in the Real World

Understanding trauma is not limited to mental health professionals; it is relevant for individuals across various disciplines and sectors, including educators, healthcare providers, law enforcement officers, and policymakers. Addressing trauma requires a collaborative and multi-faceted approach, including:

- **Trauma-Informed Schools:** Creating trauma-informed environments in educational settings can help support students who have experienced trauma. This includes providing training to school staff, implementing trauma-sensitive policies and practices, and promoting social-emotional learning.

- **Trauma-Informed Healthcare:** Healthcare providers can integrate trauma-informed care principles into their practice by recognizing the signs and symptoms of trauma, providing appropriate screening and referrals, and creating safe and supportive healthcare environments.

- **Trauma-Informed Justice Systems:** Law enforcement agencies and the criminal justice system can adopt trauma-informed approaches to enhance understanding and responsiveness to individuals who have experienced trauma. This includes training for justice professionals, trauma-informed court practices, and alternatives to incarceration.

- **Trauma-Informed Policies:** Policymakers and advocacy organizations can play a crucial role in promoting trauma-informed policies and practices across various sectors. This includes increasing access to trauma-informed services, addressing systemic issues that contribute to trauma, and advocating for research and funding in the field of trauma.

By recognizing the impact of trauma, implementing trauma-informed approaches, and providing appropriate support and intervention, individuals and communities can contribute to healing, resilience, and overall well-being for those who have experienced trauma.

In conclusion, understanding trauma is essential for mental health professionals and individuals from various disciplines. The impact of trauma is far-reaching, and assessment and treatment approaches should be sensitive, evidence-based, and tailored to the unique needs of each individual. By addressing trauma in a comprehensive and holistic manner, we can promote healing, resilience, and long-term well-being.

The Impact of Trauma on Mental Health

Trauma is a significant psychological challenge that can have a profound impact on mental health. It refers to an event or experience that is emotionally distressing or disturbing, often causing a sense of helplessness, fear, or horror. Trauma can result from various sources, including natural disasters, accidents, war, violence, abuse, or other life-threatening events. The effects of trauma on mental health can be long-lasting and wide-ranging, affecting individuals in different ways.

1. Psychological and Emotional Impact of Trauma: Trauma can lead to a range of psychological and emotional responses. Common mental health disorders that are associated with trauma include post-traumatic stress disorder (PTSD), depression, anxiety disorders, and substance use disorders. These disorders can significantly impact the individual's daily functioning, relationships, and overall quality of life.

2. Symptoms of Trauma: Individuals who have experienced trauma may exhibit a range of symptoms. These can include intrusive thoughts or memories of the traumatic event, nightmares, flashbacks, hypervigilance, avoidance of reminders of the trauma, emotional numbness, feelings of guilt or shame, difficulty concentrating, irritability, anger, sleep disturbances, and changes in appetite. These symptoms can vary in severity and intensity depending on the individual and the nature of the trauma.

3. Complex Trauma: Some individuals may experience complex trauma, which refers to repeated or prolonged exposure to traumatic events, often in the context of interpersonal relationships, such as childhood abuse or neglect. Complex trauma can have profound and long-term effects on mental health, leading to difficulties in emotional regulation, self-esteem, and interpersonal relationships.

4. Neurobiological Effects of Trauma: Trauma can also have significant effects on the brain and neurobiological systems. Research has shown that trauma can alter the structure and functioning of the brain, particularly in areas involved in regulating emotions, memory, and stress responses. These changes can contribute to the development of mental health disorders and affect an individual's ability to cope with stress and adversity.

5. Trauma-Informed Care: Recognizing the impact of trauma on mental health, trauma-informed care has emerged as an important framework for providing effective support and treatment. Trauma-informed care involves understanding the prevalence and impact of trauma, creating a safe and supportive environment, empowering individuals in their recovery, and integrating knowledge about trauma into all aspects of service provision.

6. Treatment and Support for Trauma: Effective treatment and support for individuals with trauma-related mental health conditions can significantly improve outcomes. Evidence-based interventions such as trauma-focused cognitive-behavioral therapy (CBT), eye movement desensitization and reprocessing (EMDR), and medication management can help individuals manage symptoms and process the trauma in a safe and structured way. Supportive and therapeutic interventions, including support groups, mindfulness-based therapies, and expressive arts therapies, can also be beneficial.

7. Importance of Self-Care and Resilience: Building resilience and engaging in self-care practices are crucial for individuals who have experienced trauma. Self-care involves taking steps to prioritize one's mental, emotional, and physical well-being, such as engaging in regular exercise, establishing healthy sleep patterns, practicing relaxation techniques, and seeking social support. Developing resilience, the ability to adapt and recover from adversity, can help individuals build strength and regain a sense of control and meaning in their lives.

8. Societal and Preventive Approaches: Addressing trauma and its impact on mental health requires a comprehensive and multifaceted approach. This includes integrating trauma-informed practices into all systems that interact with trauma survivors, such as healthcare, education, and criminal justice. Prevention efforts, such as early intervention programs, trauma-focused education, and community support networks, can also help mitigate the long-term effects of trauma and promote mental well-being.

In summary, trauma can have a profound impact on mental health, resulting in a range of psychological and emotional symptoms. Understanding the effects of trauma is crucial for providing effective support and treatment. Trauma-informed care, evidence-based interventions, self-care practices, and societal approaches are all essential components in addressing the impact of trauma and promoting mental well-being.

Diagnosing and Treating PTSD

Post-traumatic stress disorder (PTSD) is a mental health condition that can develop after a person experiences or witnesses a traumatic event. It is important to diagnose and treat PTSD in order to alleviate symptoms and improve the overall well-being of individuals affected by this disorder. In this section, we will explore the diagnostic criteria and available treatment options for PTSD.

Diagnostic Criteria for PTSD

The diagnosis of PTSD is typically made based on the criteria outlined in the Diagnostic and Statistical Manual of Mental Disorders (DSM-5), which is the standard classification system used by mental health professionals. According to the DSM-5, the following diagnostic criteria must be met for a person to be diagnosed with PTSD:

1. Exposure to a traumatic event: The individual must have been exposed to or witnessed a traumatic event involving actual or threatened death, serious injury, or sexual violence. Examples of traumatic events include natural disasters, war, accidents, or personal assaults.

2. Intrusive symptoms: The person experiences intrusive thoughts, memories, or images related to the traumatic event. This can manifest as flashbacks, nightmares, or distressing and uncontrollable thoughts.

3. Avoidance behaviors: The individual actively avoids situations, people, or places that remind them of the traumatic event. They may also avoid discussing or thinking about the event.

4. Negative changes in cognition and mood: The person experiences negative thoughts and feelings associated with the traumatic event. This can include distorted beliefs about oneself or the world, feelings of guilt or shame, diminished interest in activities, and difficulty experiencing positive emotions.

5. Hyperarousal and reactivity: The individual displays heightened arousal and reactivity to stimuli associated with the traumatic event. This can manifest as hypervigilance, irritability, difficulty concentrating, sleep disturbances, and exaggerated startle response.

In order to diagnose PTSD, these symptoms must be present for at least one month and significantly impair the person's daily functioning and quality of life.

Treatment Options for PTSD

Effective treatments for PTSD involve a combination of psychotherapy, medication, and self-help strategies. A comprehensive treatment plan aims to address the specific symptoms and needs of each individual. The following are some commonly used approaches to treating PTSD:

1. Psychotherapy: - Cognitive Behavioral Therapy (CBT): CBT focuses on identifying and challenging negative thoughts and beliefs associated with the traumatic event. It helps individuals develop healthy coping strategies and gradually confront their fears and triggers. - Eye Movement Desensitization and Reprocessing (EMDR): EMDR combines elements of exposure therapy and bilateral eye movements to help individuals process traumatic memories, reduce distress, and develop new insights and perspectives. - Prolonged Exposure Therapy (PE): PE involves gradually exposing individuals to trauma-related memories, thoughts, and situations in a controlled and safe manner. This helps reduce avoidance behaviors and diminishes the power of traumatic memories.

2. Medication: - Selective Serotonin Reuptake Inhibitors (SSRIs): SSRIs, such as sertraline and paroxetine, are commonly prescribed medications for PTSD. They can help alleviate symptoms of depression, anxiety, and intrusive thoughts. - Benzodiazepines: These medications may be prescribed on a short-term basis to alleviate acute anxiety symptoms. However, they are generally not recommended for long-term use due to the risk of dependence and potential interaction with other medications.

3. Self-Help Strategies: - Stress Management Techniques: Learning stress management techniques like deep breathing, relaxation exercises, and mindfulness can help individuals better manage anxiety and stress associated with PTSD. - Social Support: Building and maintaining a strong support network of family and friends can provide a sense of belonging and understanding, reducing feelings of isolation. - Healthy Lifestyle: Engaging in regular physical exercise, maintaining a balanced diet, and getting enough sleep can contribute to overall mental well-being and resilience.

It is important to note that recovery from PTSD takes time and varies from individual to individual. A multidisciplinary approach, tailored to the specific needs of each person, is crucial for successful treatment outcomes.

Case Study: Diagnosing and Treating PTSD

Let's consider a hypothetical case study to illustrate the process of diagnosing and treating PTSD.

Sarah, a 33-year-old woman, has recently experienced a traumatic event. She was involved in a severe car accident that resulted in the death of her friend. Sarah is now experiencing intrusive thoughts, nightmares, and extreme anxiety whenever she gets into a car. She has also started avoiding driving altogether and frequently feels on edge and irritable.

Upon evaluation by a mental health professional, Sarah's symptoms meet the diagnostic criteria for PTSD. The trauma she experienced, her intrusive thoughts, avoidance behaviors, and hyperarousal all align with the DSM-5 criteria.

Sarah's treatment plan incorporates evidence-based approaches for PTSD. She begins weekly sessions of Cognitive Behavioral Therapy (CBT) with a trained therapist. Through CBT, Sarah learns to challenge her negative thoughts about driving and gradually exposes herself to driving-related situations in a safe and controlled manner.

In addition to therapy, Sarah's psychiatrist prescribes a selective serotonin reuptake inhibitor (SSRI) medication to help alleviate her anxiety and depression symptoms.

Over time, Sarah's therapy sessions and medication management contribute to a noticeable reduction in her symptoms. Through the combination of therapy, medication, and ongoing support from her therapist and loved ones, Sarah is able to regain a sense of control, reduce her avoidance behaviors, and resume driving without overwhelming anxiety.

This case study highlights the importance of accurately diagnosing PTSD and implementing a comprehensive treatment plan to address the unique needs of each individual.

Summary

In this section, we explored the importance of diagnosing and treating PTSD. We discussed the diagnostic criteria outlined in the DSM-5 and the various treatment options available, including psychotherapy, medication, and self-help strategies. Additionally, we presented a case study to illustrate how these approaches can be applied in a real-life scenario. It is crucial to continue researching and advancing treatment methods to provide effective support and care for individuals with PTSD. By addressing PTSD early and providing appropriate interventions, we can promote healing, resilience, and overall well-being.

Trauma-Informed Care

Trauma-Informed Care is an approach to mental health care that recognizes and responds to the impact of trauma on an individual's mental, emotional, and physical well-being. It emphasizes the importance of creating a safe and supportive environment for individuals who have experienced trauma, while also promoting their empowerment and autonomy in the healing process.

Understanding Trauma

Trauma refers to an event, series of events, or ongoing circumstances that are experienced as physically or emotionally harmful or life-threatening, and have lasting adverse effects on the individual's well-being. It can result from various sources, including interpersonal violence, natural disasters, accidents, or systemic oppression. Trauma can have profound psychological and physiological effects, affecting the individual's cognitive abilities, emotional regulation, and overall functioning.

The Impact of Trauma on Mental Health

Trauma can have a significant impact on mental health, leading to the development of various mental health disorders such as post-traumatic stress disorder (PTSD), anxiety disorders, substance use disorders, and mood disorders. People who have experienced trauma may also struggle with difficulties in relationships, self-esteem, and trust. Furthermore, trauma can have a long-term impact on physical health, increasing the risk for conditions such as cardiovascular disease and chronic pain.

Diagnosing and Treating PTSD

Post-traumatic stress disorder (PTSD) is a specific mental health disorder that can develop after experiencing or witnessing a traumatic event. It is characterized by intrusive and distressing memories or dreams, avoidance of triggers associated with the trauma, negative changes in mood and cognition, and increased arousal and reactivity.

The diagnosis of PTSD involves a thorough assessment of the individual's symptoms and their impact on daily functioning. Treatment for PTSD typically includes a combination of psychotherapy and, in some cases, medication. Evidence-based therapies such as cognitive-behavioral therapy (CBT), eye movement desensitization and reprocessing (EMDR), and exposure therapy can help individuals process and cope with their traumatic experiences.

Trauma-Informed Care Principles

Trauma-Informed Care is grounded in several key principles that guide its implementation:

1. Safety: Creating a physically and emotionally safe environment is essential to support individuals who have experienced trauma. This involves establishing clear boundaries, maintaining confidentiality, and ensuring that individuals have choice and control over their treatment.

2. Trustworthiness and Transparency: Building trust and promoting transparency is crucial in trauma-informed care. Practitioners should communicate openly, provide clear information about treatment options, and collaborate with individuals to develop a personalized care plan.

3. Choice and Collaboration: Respecting the autonomy and choices of individuals is vital. Trauma-informed care emphasizes collaboration between the individual and their care providers, allowing them to have an active role in their healing process.

4. Empowerment and Strengths-Based Approach: Recognizing and building on an individual's strengths and resources can help foster empowerment and resilience. Trauma-informed care focuses on promoting self-advocacy and helping individuals regain a sense of control over their lives.

5. Cultural Sensitivity: Acknowledging and respecting an individual's cultural background and experiences is essential in trauma-informed care. Providers should have an understanding of cultural differences and strive to provide culturally sensitive and inclusive care.

Trauma-Informed Care Interventions

There are various interventions and strategies employed in trauma-informed care to support individuals in their recovery journey. These may include:

1. Psychoeducation: Providing individuals with knowledge about the impact of trauma on their mental health can help normalize their experiences and reduce self-blame. Psychoeducation also helps individuals understand the connection between trauma and their symptoms.

2. **Safety Planning:** Collaboratively developing a safety plan with individuals who have experienced trauma is crucial. This plan outlines strategies and resources to ensure their physical and emotional well-being during times of distress.

3. **Grounding Techniques:** Grounding techniques help individuals stay present in the moment and manage overwhelming emotions or distressing memories associated with their trauma. These techniques may involve focusing on the senses, engaging in deep breathing exercises, or using calming objects or activities.

4. **Mindfulness-Based Practices:** Mindfulness practices, such as meditation and body scans, can help individuals develop skills to regulate their emotions, reduce anxiety, and increase self-awareness. These practices promote a non-judgmental and accepting attitude towards their experiences.

5. **Trauma-Focused Therapies:** Therapies specifically designed to address trauma, such as Trauma-Focused Cognitive-Behavioral Therapy (TF-CBT) or Narrative Exposure Therapy (NET), can help individuals process and make sense of their traumatic experiences. These therapies often incorporate techniques to reduce distressing symptoms and enhance coping skills.

6. **Self-Care and Resilience Building:** Encouraging individuals to engage in self-care activities, such as exercise, creative outlets, and relaxation techniques, can support their overall well-being and resilience. Building upon personal strengths and fostering a sense of empowerment are crucial components of the recovery process.

Challenges in Trauma-Informed Care

Implementing trauma-informed care can present various challenges, including:

1. **Re-traumatization:** Care providers must ensure that their interventions and interactions do not inadvertently re-traumatize individuals. This requires sensitivity, empathy, and a deep understanding of trauma's potential impacts.

2. **Organizational Culture Change:** Shifting an organization's culture to be trauma-informed requires commitment from leadership, ongoing training, and a supportive environment for practitioners to implement these principles effectively.

3. Access to Trauma-Informed Services: Ensuring that trauma-informed care is accessible to all individuals who have experienced trauma is essential. This includes addressing barriers to care, such as stigma, cost, and limited availability of trauma-informed services in certain regions.

4. Promoting Awareness and Education: Raising awareness about trauma and its impact is crucial to challenging misconceptions and reducing stigma. Providing education to both service providers and the general public can help foster a more supportive and understanding community.

Conclusion

Trauma-informed care is a paradigm shift in mental health care that recognizes the significance of trauma and its impact on individuals' overall well-being. By incorporating trauma-informed principles and interventions into practice, mental health professionals can create a safe and empowering environment for individuals to heal and thrive. Applying trauma-informed care principles not only promotes individual resilience but also leads to the development of more compassionate, inclusive, and sustainable mental health systems.

Addiction and Mental Health

The Connection Between Addiction and Mental Health

The relationship between addiction and mental health is complex and multifaceted, with both conditions often occurring concurrently. Understanding the connection between addiction and mental health is crucial for effective treatment and support.

Overview of Addiction

Addiction, also referred to as substance use disorder, is a chronic and relapsing condition characterized by compulsive drug-seeking and use, despite harmful consequences. It is considered a brain disorder that involves changes in the brain's reward, motivation, and decision-making processes.

Addiction can involve various substances, including alcohol, nicotine, prescription medications, and illicit drugs. It affects people from all walks of life and can have severe physical, emotional, and social consequences.

Overview of Mental Health

Mental health refers to a person's emotional, psychological, and social well-being. It encompasses the way individuals think, feel, and behave, and influences how they handle stress, interact with others, and make choices.

Mental health disorders are common and can range from mild to severe. Examples include anxiety disorders, mood disorders (such as depression and bipolar disorder), psychotic disorders (like schizophrenia), and personality disorders. These disorders can significantly impair a person's ability to function in various aspects of life.

Bidirectional Relationship

The relationship between addiction and mental health is bidirectional, meaning that each condition can contribute to the development and exacerbation of the other. Several factors contribute to this connection:

- **Shared Risk Factors:** Addiction and mental health disorders share common risk factors, such as genetic predisposition, childhood trauma, chronic stress, and exposure to adverse life events. These factors can make individuals vulnerable to both conditions.

- **Self-Medication:** Some individuals with mental health disorders may turn to substances as a form of self-medication to alleviate distressing symptoms. For example, someone with anxiety may use alcohol to numb their feelings of worry and fear. However, this self-medication often worsens the underlying mental health condition and leads to addiction.

- **Neurobiological Factors:** Addiction and mental health disorders involve similar neurobiological mechanisms. Both conditions affect neurotransmitter systems, such as dopamine, serotonin, and glutamate, which regulate mood, reward, and motivation. Imbalances in these systems can contribute to the development of addiction and mental health symptoms.

- **Cycle of Co-occurrence:** Addiction and mental health disorders can create a cycle of co-occurrence. People with addiction often experience mental health symptoms, such as anxiety and depression, as a direct result of their substance use. Similarly, individuals with mental health disorders may engage in substance use to cope with their distress, leading to addiction.

Comorbidity Rates

The comorbidity rates between addiction and mental health disorders are alarmingly high. Research suggests that:

- Nearly half of individuals with a substance use disorder also have a co-occurring mental health disorder.

- Among people diagnosed with mental health disorders, about 20

- Certain mental health disorders, such as depression and post-traumatic stress disorder (PTSD), have particularly high rates of co-occurring substance use disorders.

These statistics highlight the need for integrated treatment approaches that address both addiction and mental health in a comprehensive manner.

Integrated Treatment Approaches

Integrated treatment approaches are essential for effectively addressing the connection between addiction and mental health. These approaches involve coordinated care from a multidisciplinary team, including mental health professionals, addiction specialists, and medical professionals.

Key components of integrated treatment include:

- **Screening and Assessment:** Comprehensive screening and assessment processes help identify the presence of both addiction and mental health disorders. This information guides the development of individualized treatment plans.

- **Dual Diagnosis Treatment:** Dual diagnosis treatment refers to specialized interventions that target both addiction and mental health disorders simultaneously. This approach recognizes the interplay between the two conditions and aims to address their unique challenges and needs.

- **Pharmacotherapy:** Medications can play a crucial role in the treatment of both addiction and mental health disorders. Pharmacotherapy may involve the use of medications to alleviate withdrawal symptoms, manage cravings, stabilize mood, or reduce anxiety.

- **Psychotherapy:** Various forms of psychotherapy, such as cognitive-behavioral therapy (CBT) and dialectical behavior therapy (DBT), are effective in treating addiction and mental health disorders. These therapies help individuals develop coping skills, address underlying issues, and modify dysfunctional thought patterns.

- **Supportive Services:** Access to supportive services, such as housing assistance, vocational training, and peer support groups, is integral to the recovery process for individuals with addiction and mental health disorders. These services enhance social support, improve overall well-being, and promote long-term recovery.

Real-World Example: Opioid Addiction and Mental Health

To illustrate the connection between addiction and mental health, let's consider the example of opioid addiction and mental health disorders, such as depression and anxiety.

Research has shown that individuals with depression or anxiety are more likely to misuse opioids and develop opioid use disorders. This correlation may be attributed to the self-medication hypothesis, where individuals with underlying mental health disorders turn to opioids to alleviate their negative emotions.

Conversely, chronic opioid use can lead to changes in the brain's reward system, exacerbating depressive symptoms and anxiety. Additionally, the withdrawal effects of opioids can further contribute to mental health distress.

Integrated treatment for opioid addiction and mental health disorders would involve a combination of medication-assisted treatment (e.g., methadone or buprenorphine), psychotherapy to address underlying mental health symptoms, and support services to promote overall well-being and recovery.

Conclusion

The connection between addiction and mental health is a complex and intertwined relationship. Recognizing and addressing this connection is crucial for promoting effective treatment, recovery, and overall well-being. Integrated approaches that encompass both addiction and mental health care are fundamental in supporting individuals with dual diagnoses, providing them with the comprehensive care needed for lasting recovery and improved quality of life.

Substance Use Disorders and Co-occurring Mental Illness

Substance use disorders (SUDs) and co-occurring mental illness are two highly interrelated and complex issues that have significant impacts on individual well-being and overall public health. In this section, we will explore the connections between substance use disorders and mental illness, the challenges faced by individuals with co-occurring conditions, and the treatment approaches available to address these issues.

Understanding Substance Use Disorders

Substance use disorders refer to a set of conditions characterized by the repetitive and compulsive use of substances despite negative consequences. These substances can include alcohol, illicit drugs, and prescription medications. SUDs can significantly impair an individual's physical health, psychological well-being, social relationships, and overall functioning.

The development of a substance use disorder involves multiple factors, including genetic predisposition, environmental influences, and psychological vulnerabilities. Factors such as family history of addiction, exposure to traumatic events, and mental health disorders can increase the likelihood of developing an SUD.

The Prevalence of Co-occurring Mental Illness

Co-occurring mental illness refers to the presence of both a substance use disorder and a diagnosable mental health condition. It is estimated that up to 50

The co-occurrence of SUDs and mental illness can create a complex set of challenges for individuals. These challenges include increased risk of relapse, impaired treatment outcomes, higher rates of hospitalization, greater disability, and increased risk of self-harm or suicide. Moreover, stigma and discrimination associated with both substance use and mental health disorders can further exacerbate these challenges.

Treatment Approaches for Co-occurring Conditions

The treatment of individuals with co-occurring substance use disorders and mental illness requires an integrated and comprehensive approach that addresses both conditions simultaneously. Traditionally, substance abuse and mental health disorders have been treated separately, resulting in fragmented care. However, research has consistently shown that integrated treatment is more effective in achieving positive outcomes.

Integrated treatment combines pharmacological interventions, psychotherapeutic interventions, and psychosocial support to address the complex needs of individuals with co-occurring conditions. Medications may be used to manage withdrawal symptoms, reduce cravings, and treat underlying mental health disorders. Psychotherapeutic interventions, such as cognitive-behavioral therapy (CBT) and dialectical behavior therapy (DBT), can help individuals gain insight into their substance use and develop coping strategies. Additionally, psychosocial support, including group therapy, family therapy, and peer support, plays a crucial role in the recovery process.

It is important to note that the treatment approach should be individualized, taking into account the unique circumstances and needs of each individual. The recovery process for co-occurring conditions is often complex and may require ongoing support and monitoring.

A Case Example: Co-occurring Depression and Alcohol Use Disorder

Let's consider a case example to illustrate the challenges and treatment approach for co-occurring conditions. Sarah, a 34-year-old woman, presents with symptoms of depression and a severe alcohol use disorder. She reports experiencing persistent low mood, loss of interest in activities, and difficulty concentrating. Sarah has been self-medicating her depressive symptoms with alcohol for the past several years, resulting in recurrent legal issues, deteriorating relationships, and declining physical health.

In this case, an integrated treatment approach would involve addressing both Sarah's depression and alcohol use disorder concurrently. Initially, Sarah may undergo medical detoxification to manage alcohol withdrawal symptoms. Following detoxification, a combination of antidepressant medication, such as selective serotonin reuptake inhibitors (SSRIs), and psychotherapy, such as CBT, may be recommended to address her depressive symptoms.

Simultaneously, Sarah would engage in a substance abuse treatment program that may include individual therapy, group therapy, and relapse prevention strategies. Through therapy, she would explore the underlying factors contributing to her alcohol use, develop coping skills to manage cravings and triggers, and learn healthier ways of managing her depressive symptoms.

Throughout the treatment process, Sarah would benefit from ongoing support, such as regular check-ins with a psychiatrist, participation in support groups, and involvement of her family in therapy. By addressing both her depression and alcohol use disorder holistically, Sarah can improve her overall well-being and increase her chances of sustained recovery.

Resources and Support for Co-occurring Conditions

Individuals with co-occurring substance use disorders and mental illness can benefit from various resources and support programs. Some of these include:

1. Dual Diagnosis Anonymous (DDA): DDA is a 12-step support group specifically designed for individuals with co-occurring conditions. It provides a safe space for individuals to share their experiences, seek support, and learn from others facing similar challenges.

2. National Alliance on Mental Illness (NAMI): NAMI is a grassroots organization that provides education, support, and advocacy for individuals and families affected by mental illness. They offer resources, support groups, and educational programs specifically tailored for individuals with co-occurring conditions.

3. Substance Abuse and Mental Health Services Administration (SAMHSA): SAMHSA is a branch of the U.S. Department of Health and Human Services dedicated to advancing behavioral health. Their website provides information on treatment options, helplines, and resources for individuals and families affected by co-occurring conditions.

4. Local community mental health centers and addiction treatment centers: These centers often offer specialized programs for individuals with co-occurring conditions. They can provide comprehensive assessment, individualized treatment plans, and ongoing support.

Remember, recovery from co-occurring conditions is a journey that requires persistence, patience, and support. It is essential for individuals to seek help from qualified professionals and engage in a comprehensive treatment program tailored to their specific needs. By addressing both substance use disorders and mental illness simultaneously, individuals can achieve a higher quality of life and sustainable recovery.

Exercises

1. Reflect on the case example provided and identify potential challenges that Sarah may face during her recovery journey. How would you address these challenges?

2. Research and discuss different pharmacological interventions used in the treatment of co-occurring substance use disorders and mental illness. Compare their effectiveness and potential side effects.

3. Explore and discuss the role of peer support in the treatment and recovery of individuals with co-occurring conditions. How can peer support programs contribute to positive outcomes?

4. Investigate the impact of stigma on individuals with co-occurring substance use disorders and mental illness. Discuss strategies that can be implemented to reduce stigma and promote a more supportive and inclusive society.

5. Design a community-based intervention program that aims to provide comprehensive support for individuals with co-occurring conditions. Outline the key components, target audience, and potential challenges in implementing such a program.

Remember to consult reliable sources and refer to current research in addressing the exercises.

Treatment Approaches for Dual Diagnosis

Dual diagnosis refers to the co-occurrence of a substance use disorder and a mental health disorder in an individual. It presents a unique set of challenges and complexities in terms of diagnosis and treatment. In this section, we will explore various treatment approaches that have been developed to address the complex needs of individuals with dual diagnosis.

Integrated Treatment

Integrated treatment is a comprehensive and holistic approach that combines mental health and substance use disorder treatments into a single, unified program. This approach recognizes that both disorders are interconnected and that treating them separately may not be effective. Integrated treatment involves a multidisciplinary team of professionals, including psychiatrists, psychologists, social workers, and substance abuse counselors.

The key principles of integrated treatment include:

1. Simultaneous treatment: Both the mental health and substance use disorder are addressed at the same time, rather than treating one before the other.

2. Coordination of care: The multidisciplinary team collaborates closely to ensure that individuals receive coordinated and cohesive care.

3. Individualized treatment plans: Treatment plans are tailored to meet the unique needs of each individual, considering their specific dual diagnosis and any other contributing factors.

4. Continuity of care: Once initial treatment goals are achieved, individuals continue to receive ongoing support and follow-up care to prevent relapse and promote long-term recovery.

Integrated treatment approaches may include a combination of therapies, medications, and support services. Some common components of integrated treatment include:

Psychotherapy Psychotherapy, also known as talk therapy, plays a central role in integrated treatment. Cognitive-behavioral therapy (CBT) is a widely used approach that helps individuals identify and change thought patterns and behaviors related to both their mental health and substance use. It helps individuals develop healthy coping skills, address underlying issues, and manage triggers and cravings.

Another effective therapy is motivational interviewing, which focuses on enhancing individuals' motivation to change their behavior. This therapy helps individuals explore and resolve ambivalence about substance use and mental health treatment, while also building self-efficacy and increasing commitment to change.

Medication-Assisted Treatment Medication-assisted treatment (MAT) combines medications with counseling and behavioral therapies to address substance use disorders. For individuals with dual diagnosis, certain medications can help manage withdrawal symptoms, reduce cravings, and stabilize mental health symptoms.

For example, certain medications such as methadone, buprenorphine, or naltrexone can be used to treat opioid use disorders. Medications like disulfiram, acamprosate, or naltrexone can be used to treat alcohol use disorders. In the case of concurrent mental health disorders, psychiatric medications, such as antidepressants or antipsychotics, may also be prescribed to manage symptoms.

Supportive Services In addition to therapy and medication, individuals with dual diagnosis often benefit from a range of supportive services. These services may include case management, housing assistance, vocational training, peer support groups, and assistance with navigating the legal system. These supports address the individual's social needs, enhance their overall well-being, and provide ongoing support for their recovery journey.

Challenges and Considerations

Treating individuals with dual diagnosis can be complex due to the interplay between mental health and substance use. Several challenges and considerations need to be addressed to ensure effective treatment:

1. Diagnostic complexity: Diagnosing mental health disorders in the presence of substance use can be challenging, as the symptoms may overlap or be masked by substance use. A thorough assessment by trained professionals is crucial to identify both disorders accurately.

2. Stigma and shame: Individuals with dual diagnosis often face stigma and shame from society, which can impact their willingness to seek help and engage in treatment. It is essential to create a supportive and non-judgmental environment that encourages individuals to access and stay engaged in treatment.

3. Treatment adherence: Substance use can interfere with treatment adherence, as individuals may relapse or struggle to engage fully in therapy. Motivational enhancement techniques and ongoing support can help individuals stay engaged in treatment and address any barriers or challenges they may face.

4. Relapse prevention: Individuals with dual diagnosis are at a higher risk of relapse compared to those with a single disorder. Therefore, relapse prevention strategies, coping skills training, and ongoing support are crucial components of treatment to support long-term recovery.

Case Study: Integrated Treatment in Action

To illustrate the application of integrated treatment, let's consider the case of Adam, a young adult with a dual diagnosis of major depressive disorder and alcohol use disorder. Adam experiences intense sadness, low energy, and difficulty concentrating due to his depression. He self-medicates with alcohol to temporarily alleviate his symptoms, which leads to increased alcohol dependency over time.

Adam's integrated treatment plan would involve a coordinated approach between a psychiatrist, therapist, and substance abuse counselor. They would collaborate to develop a tailored treatment plan that addresses both his mental health and substance use disorder. Adam would engage in cognitive-behavioral therapy to address his depressive symptoms and learn healthier coping strategies. Medication, such as an antidepressant, may also be prescribed to manage his depression.

Simultaneously, Adam would receive specialized counseling for his alcohol use disorder. He may participate in therapy sessions specific to substance abuse, such as motivational interviewing or relapse prevention. If appropriate, medication-assisted treatment could be considered to support his recovery from alcohol use disorder.

Adam's treatment team would also provide practical support and linkage to community resources, such as support groups or vocational training, to enhance his overall well-being and facilitate his reintegration into a fulfilling life.

Conclusion

Treating individuals with dual diagnosis requires a comprehensive and integrated approach that addresses both mental health and substance use disorders. Integrated treatment provides a framework for simultaneously addressing these interconnected issues, promoting better outcomes and long-term recovery.

By incorporating therapies, medications, and supportive services, individuals with dual diagnosis can receive holistic care that considers the complexities of their conditions. However, challenges such as diagnostic complexity, stigma, treatment adherence, and relapse prevention must be carefully navigated to ensure successful treatment outcomes.

Through continued research, training, and the implementation of evidence-based approaches, we can improve the quality of care and enhance the lives of individuals with dual diagnosis, promoting their overall well-being and sustained recovery.

Harm Reduction Strategies

Harm reduction strategies are a key component in addressing substance use disorders and co-occurring mental illnesses. Rather than a focus on complete abstinence, harm reduction approaches aim to minimize the negative consequences associated with substance use and promote overall well-being. This section will explore different harm reduction strategies and their effectiveness in helping individuals manage their substance use and mental health.

Needle and Syringe Exchange Programs

Needle and syringe exchange programs (NSPs) are one of the most well-known harm reduction strategies. These programs provide individuals who inject drugs with access to clean needles and syringes, reducing the risk of infection transmission, such as HIV and hepatitis. NSPs also offer educational resources, counseling, and referrals to other healthcare services, including mental health treatment.

By providing sterile needles, NSPs aim to prevent the spread of bloodborne diseases among people who use drugs. These programs recognize that substance use may continue despite efforts to stop, and as such, aim to minimize the harms associated with injection drug use. Studies have shown that NSPs not only reduce the sharing of needles but also increase the likelihood of individuals seeking treatment for substance use disorders.

Opioid Substitution Therapy

Opioid substitution therapy (OST) is another harm reduction strategy commonly used in the treatment of opioid use disorders. It involves the administration of opioid agonist medications like methadone or buprenorphine to individuals struggling with opioid addiction. These medications help stabilize individuals by reducing withdrawal symptoms, curbing cravings, and preventing overdose.

Unlike traditional abstinence-based approaches, which require individuals to completely stop using opioids, OST recognizes that addiction is a complex and chronic condition. By providing a regulated and prescribed opioid medication, OST allows individuals to stabilize their lives, reduce the risk of overdose, and engage in other necessary treatment and support services. It has been shown to be effective in reducing drug-related harms, such as overdose and HIV transmission, while also promoting social stability and improved overall well-being.

Safe Consumption Sites

Safe consumption sites, also known as supervised injection facilities or overdose prevention sites, are controlled environments where individuals can use drugs under the supervision of healthcare professionals. These facilities provide sterile injection equipment, prevent overdose deaths through immediate medical intervention, and offer access to addiction counseling and other support services.

The primary goal of safe consumption sites is to prevent fatal overdoses and reduce the transmission of diseases associated with injecting drugs. They provide a safe and non-judgmental space for individuals to use drugs, reducing the risks associated with using alone or in dangerous environments. Research has shown that safe consumption sites are effective in preventing overdose deaths, promoting safer drug use practices, and connecting individuals with healthcare and social services.

Safer Drug Use Education

Safer drug use education is a vital harm reduction strategy aimed at providing individuals with accurate and evidence-based information on safe drug use practices. This includes information on different substances, their risks and effects, and strategies to minimize harm. Safer drug use education empowers individuals to make informed decisions about their substance use and reduce the potential negative consequences.

This educational approach emphasizes the importance of using clean equipment, testing substances for purity, starting with small doses, and avoiding mixing different substances. It also promotes the use of naloxone, an opioid overdose-reversal medication, and provides training on how to respond to an overdose.

Contingency Management

Contingency management is a harm reduction strategy that utilizes positive reinforcement to encourage behavior change. It involves providing rewards or incentives to individuals for maintaining their sobriety, attending treatment sessions, or adhering to other predetermined goals.

Contingency management programs have been effective in reducing substance use and improving treatment outcomes. Rewards can range from vouchers or monetary incentives to tangible items or privileges. By reinforcing positive behaviors, contingency management helps individuals build motivation, self-efficacy, and a sense of control over their substance use.

Limiting Barriers to Treatment

Another important harm reduction strategy is reducing the barriers to accessing treatment for substance use disorders and co-occurring mental illnesses. This includes expanding access to affordable and evidence-based treatments, ensuring availability of medications for opioid use disorders, and integrating mental health services with substance use treatment.

By removing financial, physical, and social barriers, individuals are more likely to seek and engage in treatment. This not only improves their overall well-being but also reduces the risk of associated harms such as overdose, criminal involvement, and transmission of infectious diseases.

Conclusion

Harm reduction strategies play a crucial role in promoting the well-being of individuals with substance use disorders and co-occurring mental illnesses. These strategies recognize the complexity of addiction and aim to minimize the negative consequences associated with substance use. From needle exchange programs to safer drug use education and contingency management, harm reduction approaches have been shown to be effective in reducing harm, improving treatment outcomes, and promoting overall health and well-being.

It is important to continue to support and expand harm reduction initiatives, both through policy and practice. By integrating harm reduction principles into our approach to mental health and substance use, we can create a more compassionate and effective system of care that meets individuals where they are, reduces stigma, and promotes sustainable recovery. Through ongoing research, collaboration, and community engagement, we can strive towards a future where holistic and harm reduction-focused approaches are at the forefront of mental health care.

Neurodevelopmental Disorders

Autism Spectrum Disorder (ASD)

Autism Spectrum Disorder (ASD) is a neurodevelopmental disorder characterized by persistent deficits in social communication and social interaction, as well as restricted and repetitive patterns of behavior, interests, and activities. ASD affects individuals across their lifespan and is typically diagnosed in early childhood. In this section, we will explore the definition, features, causes, and interventions for ASD.

Definition and Features of ASD

ASD is a complex disorder with a wide range of symptoms and severity. It is characterized by impairments in three core areas: social communication, social interaction, and restricted and repetitive behaviors. These impairments manifest differently in each individual with ASD, leading to a diverse range of symptoms and challenges.

One of the defining features of ASD is the difficulty in social communication and interaction. Individuals with ASD may have difficulty with nonverbal communication, such as making eye contact, understanding gestures, and interpreting facial expressions. They may also struggle with verbal communication, including initiating and maintaining conversations, taking turns, and understanding social cues.

Another characteristic of ASD is the presence of restricted and repetitive behaviors. These behaviors can include repetitive movements or speech (such as hand flapping or echolalia), rigid adherence to routines or rituals, intense fixation on specific interests, and sensory sensitivities.

It is important to note that the symptoms of ASD can vary widely among individuals. Some individuals may have mild symptoms and be able to function independently, while others may have more severe impairments that require significant support.

Causes of ASD

The exact causes of ASD are still not fully understood, but research suggests that a combination of genetic and environmental factors contribute to its development. It is now recognized that there are many different genetic variations that can increase the risk of developing ASD, and the interaction between these genetic factors and environmental influences may contribute to the manifestation of the disorder.

Several genes have been identified that are associated with an increased risk of ASD. These genes play a role in brain development and the functioning of neural circuits involved in social communication and behavior. However, it is important to note that not all individuals with these genetic variations will develop ASD, indicating that other factors are also involved.

In addition to genetic factors, certain environmental factors are believed to play a role in the development of ASD. Prenatal factors, such as maternal infections, exposure to toxins, and certain medications, have been implicated. Complications during pregnancy or birth, such as premature birth or low birth weight, may also increase the risk of ASD. However, it is important to note that these factors alone are not sufficient to cause ASD and are likely to interact with genetic vulnerabilities.

Interventions for ASD

Early intervention is crucial in promoting the development and well-being of individuals with ASD. Evidence-based interventions can help improve communication skills, social interaction, and adaptive behavior. The goal of intervention is to maximize the individual's potential and enhance their quality of life.

One of the most widely used interventions for ASD is Applied Behavior Analysis (ABA). ABA is a structured, data-driven approach that focuses on teaching new skills and reducing problem behaviors through behavioral modification techniques. It involves breaking down skills into smaller, manageable steps and using positive reinforcement to encourage desired behaviors.

Another effective intervention for ASD is speech and language therapy. This therapy focuses on improving communication skills, including verbal and nonverbal communication. It may involve teaching functional communication strategies, such as using augmentative and alternative communication (AAC) systems, as well as targeting social communication skills.

In addition to behavioral and communication interventions, individuals with ASD may benefit from occupational therapy. Occupational therapists can help individuals develop skills necessary for daily living, such as self-care, fine motor skills, and sensory integration. They can also assist in developing strategies to manage sensory sensitivities and promote self-regulation.

It is important to take a holistic approach to interventions for ASD, considering the individual's unique strengths, challenges, and needs. Collaborative involvement of families, educators, and therapists is crucial in designing and implementing effective interventions. Additionally, providing support and education to families is essential in promoting the well-being of individuals with ASD.

Current Research and Future Directions

Research in the field of ASD is ongoing, with the aim of deepening our understanding of the disorder and improving interventions and support for individuals with ASD. Current areas of research include investigating the underlying neural mechanisms of ASD, identifying biomarkers for early diagnosis, and developing targeted pharmacological interventions.

One area of research that shows promise is the use of technology in supporting individuals with ASD. Augmented reality (AR) and virtual reality (VR) technologies have been used to create immersive and interactive environments for social skills training. Additionally, wearable devices and mobile applications are being developed to assist individuals with ASD in managing their daily routines and enhancing their communication skills.

The field of genetics also holds promise for advancing our understanding of ASD. Genome-wide association studies (GWAS) and genetic sequencing technologies are allowing researchers to identify more genes associated with ASD and explore the complex interactions between genetic and environmental factors. This research may lead to the development of personalized interventions based on an individual's genetic profile.

In conclusion, Autism Spectrum Disorder (ASD) is a neurodevelopmental disorder characterized by impairments in social communication, social interaction, and restricted and repetitive behaviors. While the exact causes of ASD are not fully understood, a combination of genetic and environmental factors is believed to contribute to its development. Early intervention is crucial in improving outcomes for individuals with ASD, and evidence-based interventions such as Applied Behavior Analysis (ABA), speech and language therapy, and occupational therapy can help enhance communication skills, social interaction, and adaptive behavior. Ongoing research in the field of ASD is focused on deepening our understanding of the disorder and developing more targeted and personalized interventions for individuals with ASD.

Attention-Deficit/Hyperactivity Disorder (ADHD)

Attention-Deficit/Hyperactivity Disorder (ADHD) is a neurodevelopmental disorder that affects both children and adults. It is characterized by persistent patterns of inattention, hyperactivity, and impulsivity that can significantly impact academic, occupational, and social functioning. ADHD is one of the most common psychiatric disorders in childhood, with prevalence rates ranging from 5

Diagnostic Criteria

The Diagnostic and Statistical Manual of Mental Disorders (DSM-5) provides specific criteria for the diagnosis of ADHD. These criteria include the presence of several symptoms and impairment in at least two different settings, such as school, home, or work. The symptoms must be present before the age of 12 and should persist for at least six months.

There are three subtypes of ADHD:

1. Predominantly Inattentive Presentation: Characterized by difficulties in sustaining attention, being organized, and following instructions.

2. Predominantly Hyperactive-Impulsive Presentation: Characterized by excessive restlessness, fidgeting, impulsivity, and difficulty waiting for turn in activities.

3. Combined Presentation: Characterized by a combination of both inattentive and hyperactive-impulsive symptoms.

Theoretical Framework

ADHD is believed to arise from a complex interaction of genetic, environmental, and neurobiological factors. It is considered a neurodevelopmental disorder due to its onset in childhood and its impact on the development of executive functions, such as working memory, inhibition, and cognitive flexibility.

Neuroimaging studies have identified structural and functional differences in the brains of individuals with ADHD, particularly in regions associated with attention and impulse control. These findings support the hypothesis that ADHD is related to alterations in the prefrontal cortex, basal ganglia, and the dopaminergic system.

Treatment Approaches

The management of ADHD typically involves a multimodal approach that includes both pharmacological and psychosocial interventions. Stimulant medications, such as methylphenidate and amphetamines, are often the first-line treatment options. These medications help improve attention, reduce impulsivity, and control hyperactivity.

Psychosocial interventions play a crucial role in the comprehensive treatment of ADHD. Behavioral therapy, parent training, and specialized school programs can help individuals with ADHD develop effective coping strategies, improve organizational skills, and enhance social functioning. It is important to involve parents, teachers, and other caregivers in the treatment process to ensure consistency and support across different settings.

Challenges and Controversies

ADHD diagnosis and treatment have been the subject of ongoing debates. Some critics argue that the diagnosis is overused and may lead to the unnecessary medicalization of normal childhood behaviors. Others express concerns about the long-term effects of stimulant medications and the potential for abuse.

However, research has shown the effectiveness of pharmacological and behavioral interventions in reducing ADHD symptoms and improving overall functioning. It is important to conduct a thorough assessment and consider individual needs and preferences when making treatment decisions.

Real-World Application

ADHD can significantly impact academic performance, interpersonal relationships, and self-esteem. To illustrate the real-world impact of ADHD, consider the case of Sarah, a 10-year-old girl who struggles with inattention and impulsivity in school. Sarah finds it challenging to focus on tasks, follow instructions, and complete assignments. As a result, she often falls behind her peers and experiences feelings of frustration and inadequacy.

In this scenario, a comprehensive approach to treatment would involve a combination of medication and behavioral interventions. Sarah's parents and teachers can work together to create a structured environment, provide clear instructions, and implement strategies to improve her attention and organization skills. Additionally, Sarah can benefit from individual counseling to address her emotional well-being and build coping mechanisms.

By addressing the symptoms of ADHD and providing appropriate support, Sarah can experience significant improvements in her academic performance, social interactions, and overall quality of life.

Key Takeaways

- ADHD is a neurodevelopmental disorder characterized by inattention, hyperactivity, and impulsivity. - Diagnosis is based on the presence of specific symptoms and impairment in multiple settings. - Both pharmacological and psychosocial interventions are essential in managing ADHD. - Challenges and controversies exist surrounding ADHD diagnosis and treatment. - A comprehensive approach to treatment involves a combination of medication, behavioral therapy, and support from parents, teachers, and caregivers.

Intellectual Disability

Intellectual disability, also known as intellectual developmental disorder, is a neurodevelopmental disorder characterized by limitations in intellectual functioning and adaptive behavior. It is a condition that typically appears in childhood and persists throughout a person's lifetime, affecting their ability to learn, communicate, solve problems, and effectively navigate daily activities. Intellectual disability is diagnosed based on standardized intelligence tests and assessments of adaptive skills.

Definition and Diagnosis

Intellectual disability is defined by significant limitations in both intellectual functioning and adaptive behavior. Intellectual functioning refers to a person's cognitive abilities, including reasoning, problem-solving, and learning. Adaptive behavior refers to the skills needed to effectively function in daily life, such as communication, self-care, social skills, and understanding and following rules.

To diagnose intellectual disability, professionals use standardized intelligence tests, such as the Wechsler Intelligence Scale for Children (WISC) or the Stanford-Binet Intelligence Scales, to assess intellectual functioning. These tests measure various cognitive abilities, including verbal comprehension, perceptual reasoning, working memory, and processing speed. Intellectual disability is typically diagnosed when a person's full-scale IQ (FSIQ) score is below 70 or 75.

In addition to assessing intellectual functioning, professionals also evaluate adaptive behavior using standardized assessments and questionnaires, such as the Adaptive Behavior Assessment System (ABAS). These assessments help determine how well a person can function in areas such as communication, self-care, home living, social skills, community use, self-direction, health and safety, functional academics, leisure, and work.

It's important to note that the diagnosis of intellectual disability takes into account the individual's cultural and linguistic background. Professionals consider the person's social and cultural context when evaluating adaptive behavior, as norms and expectations may vary across different communities.

Levels of Intellectual Disability

Intellectual disability is classified into different levels based on the severity of impairment. The Diagnostic and Statistical Manual of Mental Disorders (DSM-5) defines three levels:

1. **Mild Intellectual Disability:** Individuals with mild intellectual disability typically have an IQ score between 50 and 70 or 75. They may experience delays in language and academic skills during childhood but can usually develop functional language and literacy skills with appropriate support. In adulthood, they may be able to live independently or with minimal assistance, hold jobs, and participate in social activities.

2. **Moderate Intellectual Disability:** Individuals with moderate intellectual disability usually have an IQ score between 35 and 50 or 55. They often experience delays in language development and have difficulty acquiring academic skills. With support and specialized education, they can learn basic self-care skills and may be able to work in structured environments as adults. They typically require some degree of supervision and assistance in daily life.

3. **Severe and Profound Intellectual Disability:** Individuals with severe or profound intellectual disability have IQ scores below 35 or 40. They have significant limitations in adaptive behavior and may have difficulties with communication, mobility, and basic self-care skills. They often require continuous support and supervision throughout their lives and may benefit from specialized residential care and vocational training.

It's important to note that intellectual disability is a heterogeneous condition, and individuals may have varying strengths and weaknesses within different domains of functioning.

Causes of Intellectual Disability

Intellectual disability can have various causes, including genetic and chromosomal abnormalities, prenatal and perinatal factors, infections, exposure to toxins, and acquired brain injuries. Some common causes include:

1. **Genetic and Chromosomal Abnormalities:** Certain genetic conditions, such as Down syndrome, Fragile X syndrome, and Prader-Willi syndrome, can result in intellectual disability. These conditions are caused by abnormalities in the genes or chromosomes.

2. **Prenatal and Perinatal Factors:** Factors that occur during pregnancy and childbirth can contribute to intellectual disability. These include maternal infections, exposure to toxins or substances (e.g., alcohol, drugs), poor nutrition, and complications during labor and delivery.

3. **Acquired Brain Injuries:** Traumatic brain injuries, infections (e.g., meningitis, encephalitis), strokes, and other brain-related conditions can lead to intellectual disability, especially if they occur during early childhood.

4. **Environmental Factors:** Socioeconomic disadvantages, limited access to educational resources, and social adversities can also contribute to intellectual disability. These factors can impact a child's cognitive and emotional development.

It's important to identify the underlying cause of intellectual disability as it can influence treatment approaches and interventions. However, in some cases, the cause of intellectual disability may remain unknown.

Treatment and Support

Treatment and support for individuals with intellectual disability aim to maximize their potential, enhance adaptive skills, and promote their overall quality of life. The approach often involves a multidisciplinary team, including psychologists, special education professionals, speech therapists, occupational therapists, and medical specialists.

Some key strategies and interventions for individuals with intellectual disability include:

1. **Individualized Education Plans (IEPs):** IEPs are tailored educational plans that outline specific goals, accommodations, and support services for

students with disabilities. These plans help address the unique learning needs of individuals with intellectual disability and promote their academic and social development.

2. **Behavioral and Cognitive-Behavioral Interventions:** Behavior therapy, such as Applied Behavior Analysis (ABA), can be effective in addressing challenging behaviors and improving adaptive skills. Cognitive-behavioral interventions focus on helping individuals develop self-regulation strategies, problem-solving skills, and coping mechanisms.

3. **Speech and Language Therapy:** Speech and language therapy can help individuals with intellectual disability improve their communication skills, including expressive and receptive language abilities. Augmentative and alternative communication (AAC) systems can also be implemented to enhance communication.

4. **Social Skills Training:** Social skills training programs can assist individuals with intellectual disability in developing appropriate social behaviors, interpersonal skills, and friendships. These programs often involve coaching, role-playing, and group activities.

5. **Occupational and Life Skills Training:** Occupational therapy focuses on developing skills necessary for independent living and employment, such as self-care, fine motor skills, and functional academics. Life skills training helps individuals acquire practical skills related to money management, transportation, and household responsibilities.

6. **Family Support and Counseling:** Providing support and counseling services for families of individuals with intellectual disability is essential. This can help families navigate challenges, learn effective strategies, and access available resources.

7. **Community Inclusion and Support Services:** Integration into community settings, such as recreational programs, volunteer work, and vocational training, can contribute to the social inclusion and independence of individuals with intellectual disability. Support services, such as group homes, respite care, and day programs, can provide ongoing assistance and supervision as needed.

It's important to consider the unique strengths, abilities, and interests of individuals with intellectual disability when designing interventions and support strategies. The goal is to empower individuals to lead fulfilling lives, participate in society, and achieve their potential.

Challenges and Advocacy

Individuals with intellectual disability face numerous challenges, including social stigma, discrimination, limited educational and employment opportunities, and barriers to accessing quality healthcare services. They may also experience co-occurring mental health conditions, such as anxiety or depression, which further impact their overall well-being.

Advocacy plays a crucial role in promoting the rights and inclusion of individuals with intellectual disability. It involves raising awareness, challenging stereotypes, and advocating for accessible and inclusive environments. Advocacy efforts also aim to influence policy changes, increase funding for support services, and promote social and educational inclusion.

Conclusion

Intellectual disability is a complex neurodevelopmental disorder that requires a comprehensive and multidisciplinary approach to support individuals throughout their lives. By understanding the unique needs and strengths of individuals with intellectual disability, providing appropriate interventions and support, and advocating for their rights, we can promote their well-being, inclusion, and overall sustainability.

Early Intervention and Support for Neurodevelopmental Disorders

Early intervention and support play a crucial role in addressing neurodevelopmental disorders. These disorders, such as Autism Spectrum Disorder (ASD), Attention-Deficit/Hyperactivity Disorder (ADHD), and Intellectual Disability, often emerge in childhood and can have a significant impact on individuals and their families. By identifying and addressing these disorders early on, we can provide the necessary support and interventions to promote optimal development and improve long-term outcomes.

Identifying Neurodevelopmental Disorders

Early identification of neurodevelopmental disorders is essential for timely intervention. Screening tools and standardized assessments are used to evaluate developmental milestones and identify potential concerns. Healthcare professionals, educators, and parents play a key role in recognizing the early signs of neurodevelopmental disorders.

For example, in the case of ASD, early red flags may include a lack of social interaction, delayed language skills, repetitive or stereotypical behaviors, and sensory sensitivities. Similarly, signs of ADHD may include hyperactivity, impulsivity, difficulty with attention and executive functioning, and challenges with organization and time management.

It is important to note that each neurodevelopmental disorder has its unique set of characteristics and diagnostic criteria. Specialized professionals, such as pediatricians, child psychologists, and child psychiatrists, conduct comprehensive evaluations to determine a diagnosis and guide treatment planning.

Multidisciplinary Assessment and Collaboration

Early intervention for neurodevelopmental disorders requires a multidisciplinary approach. A team of professionals from different disciplines collaborates to assess the child comprehensively, considering their physical, cognitive, emotional, social, and behavioral well-being.

This multidisciplinary team may include pediatricians, child psychologists, speech-language pathologists, occupational therapists, special educators, and social workers. Collaboration among professionals ensures a holistic understanding of the child's strengths, challenges, and individual needs.

Additionally, involving parents and caregivers as active participants in the assessment process is crucial. Their insights and observations provide valuable information and contribute to the development of an effective intervention plan.

Individualized Intervention Plans

Once a neurodevelopmental disorder is identified, an individualized intervention plan is created to meet the specific needs of the child. This plan is tailored to address the core symptoms associated with the disorder and promote overall development.

Intervention approaches may include a combination of therapeutic interventions, educational support, behavior management strategies, and parent/caregiver training. The goal is to enhance the child's functional abilities, independence, and quality of life.

For example, for a child with ASD, interventions may focus on enhancing social and communication skills through structured therapy sessions, such as Applied Behavior Analysis (ABA) or speech therapy. For a child with ADHD, interventions may include behavior management strategies, time management techniques, and accommodations in the educational setting.

Early Intervention Programs

Early intervention programs specifically target infants and young children with neurodevelopmental disorders. These programs aim to optimize developmental outcomes by providing a range of therapeutic services and support.

Early intervention programs incorporate evidence-based interventions and strategies, including structured play, social skills training, speech and language therapy, occupational therapy, and parent education and support. These programs often operate in collaboration with local communities, healthcare providers, and educational institutions.

The Individuals with Disabilities Education Act (IDEA) is a federal law in the United States that guarantees early intervention services to children with disabilities, including neurodevelopmental disorders, from birth to three years of age. Under IDEA, children receive individualized Family Service Plans (IFSPs) that outline the specific services and supports they require.

Promoting Inclusive Environments

In addition to early intervention programs, creating inclusive environments is essential for supporting children with neurodevelopmental disorders. Inclusive educational settings aim to provide all children, including those with disabilities, with equal opportunities to learn and participate.

Inclusive education involves adapting teaching strategies, curriculum modifications, and providing appropriate accommodations and supports to meet the diverse needs of students. Collaboration among educators, therapists, and parents fosters a supportive and inclusive environment for children with neurodevelopmental disorders.

Moreover, promoting inclusive communities beyond educational settings is equally important. Public awareness campaigns, community support groups, and advocacy efforts help create an inclusive society that values the contributions and well-being of individuals with neurodevelopmental disorders.

Research and Technology

Advancements in research and technology significantly contribute to the field of early intervention for neurodevelopmental disorders. Ongoing research helps refine diagnostic criteria, identify risk factors, develop evidence-based interventions, and improve the understanding of these disorders.

Technology, such as assistive communication devices, virtual reality-based interventions, and mobile applications, has the potential to enhance early intervention efforts. These tools can assist in improving communication skills, promoting social interactions, and enhancing cognitive development in children with neurodevelopmental disorders.

Case Study: Early Intervention for Autism Spectrum Disorder

Consider the case of Ethan, a four-year-old boy recently diagnosed with Autism Spectrum Disorder (ASD). Ethan's parents noticed that he had limited eye contact, exhibited repetitive behaviors, and was slower in achieving developmental milestones compared to his peers.

Upon identification, Ethan's parents sought early intervention support. A multidisciplinary team, including a pediatrician, child psychologist, speech-language pathologist, and occupational therapist, evaluated Ethan comprehensively. They conducted assessments to understand his communication skills, social interactions, sensory sensitivities, and adaptive behaviors.

Based on the assessment results, an individualized intervention plan was developed for Ethan. The plan included speech therapy to improve his communication skills, occupational therapy to address sensory sensitivities, and behavior management strategies to reduce repetitive behaviors.

In addition to therapy sessions, Ethan's parents received training on implementing strategies at home to reinforce therapeutic interventions. This collaborative approach among professionals and parents facilitated Ethan's progress in his development, leading to improved social interactions, enhanced communication skills, and reduced behavioral challenges.

The early intervention provided to Ethan and his family has played a vital role in promoting his overall development, increasing his adaptive skills, and preparing him for a successful transition into the educational system.

Key Takeaways

- Early identification and intervention are crucial for neurodevelopmental disorders. - Multidisciplinary collaboration and assessment provide a holistic understanding of the child's needs. - Individualized intervention plans address the specific symptoms and challenges associated with each disorder. - Early intervention programs and inclusive environments promote optimal development and inclusion. - Ongoing research and technological advancements contribute to improving early intervention efforts for neurodevelopmental disorders.

Personality Disorders

Borderline Personality Disorder

Borderline Personality Disorder (BPD) is a complex mental health condition that is characterized by pervasive instability in emotional regulation, interpersonal relationships, self-image, and impulsivity. Individuals with BPD often experience intense and rapidly changing emotions, leading to difficulties in their relationships, work, and overall functioning. Understanding the nature of BPD and its impact on the individual's life is crucial for effective diagnosis, treatment, and support.

Diagnostic Criteria

The Diagnostic and Statistical Manual of Mental Disorders (DSM-5) provides the following diagnostic criteria for Borderline Personality Disorder:

- **Frantic efforts to avoid real or imagined abandonment:** Individuals with BPD may go to great lengths to avoid being abandoned or rejected by others, which can manifest as clinginess, intense fear of separation, or impulsive behaviors aimed at maintaining relationships.

- **Pattern of unstable and intense interpersonal relationships:** People with BPD often exhibit a pattern of unstable relationships characterized by idealization and devaluation. They may alternate between extreme attachment and anger or hostility towards others.

- **Identity disturbance:** Individuals with BPD may have a distorted or unstable sense of self, often struggling with issues of identity, uncertainty about goals, values, and career choices. They may adopt different identities or personas in different situations.

- **Impulsivity in at least two areas that are self-damaging:** This impulsivity can manifest as excessive spending, risky sexual behavior, substance abuse, binge eating, or self-harming behaviors.

- **Recurrent suicidal behavior, gestures, or threats, or self-injurious behavior:** People with BPD are at a higher risk of self-harming behaviors, suicidal ideation, or suicide attempts. These behaviors are often used as a coping mechanism to regulate intense emotions.

- **Affective instability:** Emotional dysregulation is a hallmark feature of BPD. Individuals may experience intense and rapidly changing emotions, including anger, depression, anxiety, and irritability. These emotional experiences are often disproportionate to the situation.

- **Chronic feelings of emptiness:** People with BPD may experience a pervasive sense of inner emptiness, boredom, or a feeling of not knowing who they really are.

- **Inappropriate, intense anger or difficulty controlling anger:** Individuals with BPD may struggle to manage their anger, which can result in frequent outbursts, explosive rage, or physical altercations.

- **Transient, stress-related paranoid ideation or severe dissociative symptoms:** People with BPD may experience brief periods of paranoid thoughts or dissociative symptoms, such as feeling detached from oneself or experiencing an altered sense of reality, particularly during times of stress.

It is important to note that the presence of these symptoms must be enduring and cause significant distress and impairment in multiple areas of the individual's life to meet the criteria for a diagnosis of BPD.

Etiology and Risk Factors

The exact causes of BPD are not fully understood, but research suggests that there are several factors that may contribute to its development:

- **Genetic and biological factors:** Some evidence indicates that there may be a genetic predisposition to BPD. Additionally, abnormalities in brain structure and function, particularly in regions involved in emotional regulation and impulse control, have been observed in individuals with BPD.

- **Environmental factors:** Childhood experiences, such as childhood trauma, neglect, or inconsistent parenting, may contribute to the development of BPD. Environmental factors, such as a history of early sexual or physical abuse, can increase the risk of developing BPD.

- **Neurobiological factors:** Dysregulation of certain neurotransmitters, such as serotonin and dopamine, and abnormalities in the hypothalamic-pituitary-adrenal (HPA) axis, which regulates the body's stress response, have been implicated in BPD.

- **Psychological factors:** Some individuals with BPD may have underlying difficulties in emotion regulation, resulting in heightened emotional sensitivity and reactivity. Additionally, a history of invalidating environments where an individual's emotions and experiences were dismissed or invalidated may contribute to the development of BPD.

- **Comorbidity:** BPD frequently co-occurs with other mental health conditions, such as depression, anxiety disorders, substance use disorders, and eating disorders. The presence of comorbid conditions can further complicate the diagnosis and treatment of BPD.

It is important to approach the etiology of BPD from a biopsychosocial perspective, considering the complex interaction between genetic, biological, psychological, and environmental factors.

Treatment Approaches

The treatment of Borderline Personality Disorder typically involves a combination of psychotherapy, medication, and support services. The primary goal of treatment is to improve emotional regulation, enhance interpersonal functioning, and reduce self-destructive behaviors. Here are some commonly used treatment approaches:

- **Dialectical Behavior Therapy (DBT):** DBT is a specialized form of psychotherapy designed for individuals with BPD. It combines individual therapy, group skills training, phone coaching, and therapist consultation to help individuals develop skills in mindfulness, emotion regulation, distress tolerance, and interpersonal effectiveness.

- **Cognitive-Behavioral Therapy (CBT):** CBT focuses on identifying and modifying dysfunctional thoughts and behaviors. It helps individuals develop healthier coping mechanisms and address maladaptive cognitive patterns associated with BPD.

- **Schema-Focused Therapy:** This therapy aims to identify and modify deeply entrenched patterns of thinking and behavior called "schemas." By addressing core beliefs and improving emotional regulation, individuals can develop more adaptive coping strategies.

- **Medication:** Medication can be used to target specific symptoms associated with BPD, such as depression, anxiety, or mood swings. However, medication is typically used in conjunction with psychotherapy and should be carefully monitored by a healthcare professional.

- **Supportive Services:** In addition to psychotherapy and medication, individuals with BPD may benefit from support services such as case management, vocational training, and social support networks. These services can help address practical and social challenges and enhance overall functioning.

It is important to note that the treatment approach should be tailored to the individual's specific needs, and a comprehensive assessment should guide the selection of interventions. Long-term engagement in treatment and a supportive therapeutic relationship are crucial for symptom management and overall recovery.

Controversies

Borderline Personality Disorder has been a topic of debate and controversy in the mental health field. Some of the controversies surrounding BPD include:

- **Stigma and misconceptions:** Individuals with BPD often face stigma and misconceptions due to the nature of their symptoms and difficulties in interpersonal relationships. This can lead to negative attitudes from healthcare providers, friends, family, and society at large, impeding access to appropriate care and support.

- **Overlap with other mental health conditions:** There is some overlap between symptoms of BPD and other mental health conditions, such as bipolar disorder or complex post-traumatic stress disorder. This overlap can make accurate diagnosis challenging and may result in misdiagnosis or underdiagnosis.

- **Effectiveness of different treatment approaches:** While several therapies have shown promise in the treatment of BPD, there is ongoing debate about the most effective approach. The availability of specialized services and the level of expertise of clinicians can vary, leading to differences in treatment outcomes.

- **Pathologizing normal emotional experiences:** Critics argue that the diagnostic criteria for BPD pathologize certain emotional experiences that, to some extent, are normal and experienced by many people. There is a need for increased understanding and recognition of the underlying emotional difficulties without stigmatizing individuals.

Addressing these controversies requires ongoing research, awareness, and a holistic approach that considers individual experiences, promotes empathy, and challenges stigma associated with BPD.

Real-World Example

To better understand the struggles individuals with BPD may face, let's consider the story of Emma:

Emma is a 28-year-old woman with BPD who has experienced a pattern of unstable relationships and frequent emotional crises throughout her life. She often finds it difficult to regulate her emotions, leading to impulsive behaviors such as binge eating, gambling, and self-harming. Emma has a fear of abandonment and constantly seeks reassurance from her romantic partners, but her intense emotions often push them away.

Emma also struggles with a chronic sense of emptiness and a lack of a stable identity. She frequently questions her goals, values, and life choices, which leads to feelings of confusion and distress. Emma's emotional instability and impulsivity have disrupted her work and academic life, making it challenging to maintain steady employment or complete her education.

However, with the support of her therapist, Emma has been learning skills in emotion regulation, mindfulness, and interpersonal effectiveness through Dialectical Behavior Therapy. She has also joined a peer support group, where she has found understanding and acceptance from others who share similar experiences.

Through therapy and ongoing support, Emma is gradually learning to manage her intense emotions, develop a stronger sense of self, and establish healthier relationships. It is a challenging journey, but with the right treatment and support, individuals with BPD can experience significant improvements in their overall well-being and quality of life.

Resources

Here are some resources for individuals seeking more information and support regarding Borderline Personality Disorder:

- National Alliance on Mental Illness (NAMI): NAMI provides information, resources, and support for individuals and families affected by BPD. Their website offers educational materials, support groups, and helpline services.

- Behavioral Tech: This organization provides training and resources on Dialectical Behavior Therapy (DBT). Their website offers information about DBT, a directory of DBT therapists, and resources for individuals seeking DBT treatment.

- Mental Health America (MHA): MHA offers educational materials, online screening tools, and resources on various mental health conditions, including BPD. Their website provides information on finding mental health treatment and support.

- BPD World: BPD World is an online community for individuals affected by BPD. The platform offers a supportive forum, educational resources, and personal stories of recovery.

- Books: "I Hate You–Don't Leave Me" by Jerold J. Kreisman and Hal Straus and "Skills Training Manual for Treating Borderline Personality Disorder" by Marsha M. Linehan are highly regarded resources that provide valuable insights into BPD and its treatment.

Remember, seeking professional help is essential for accurate diagnosis and treatment planning. These resources can serve as a starting point for understanding BPD and accessing support.

Conclusion

Borderline Personality Disorder is a complex mental health condition characterized by emotional dysregulation, unstable relationships, and impulsivity. Understanding the diagnostic criteria, etiology, treatment approaches, and controversies surrounding BPD is essential for providing effective support and care to individuals with this condition. By promoting empathy, challenging stigma, and adopting a holistic approach, we can collectively work towards a more sustainable mental health future where individuals with BPD receive the understanding, compassion, and resources needed for recovery.

Narcissistic Personality Disorder

Narcissistic Personality Disorder (NPD) is a mental health disorder characterized by an excessive sense of self-importance, a constant need for admiration, and a lack of empathy for others. Individuals with NPD often have an inflated sense of their own abilities and achievements, and they seek constant validation and praise from others. This section will explore the key features, causes, diagnosis, and treatment options for Narcissistic Personality Disorder, providing a comprehensive understanding of this complex condition.

Key Features of Narcissistic Personality Disorder

People with Narcissistic Personality Disorder exhibit a range of distinctive personality traits and behaviors. Some of the key features of NPD include:

- Grandiosity: Individuals with NPD have an exaggerated sense of self-worth. They believe they are special and unique, and they often expect to be recognized as such without commensurate achievements.

- Need for admiration: People with NPD constantly seek attention, admiration, and approval from others. They may fish for compliments, brag about their achievements, and have a strong desire to be the center of attention.

- Lack of empathy: Empathy, the ability to understand and share the feelings of others, is typically lacking in individuals with NPD. They often struggle to recognize or understand the needs and emotions of others, focusing only on their own desires and concerns.

- Sense of entitlement: Individuals with NPD often have an unrealistic sense of entitlement. They believe they deserve special treatment or privileges and may exploit others to fulfill their own needs and desires.

- Manipulative behavior: People with NPD may use manipulation and exploitation to achieve their goals. They may exploit others for personal gain, lack empathy for their feelings, and manipulate situations to maintain control and dominance.

Causes of Narcissistic Personality Disorder

The exact causes of Narcissistic Personality Disorder are not fully understood. It is likely influenced by a combination of genetic, environmental, and psychological factors. Some theories propose that NPD may develop as a result of:

- Genetic predisposition: Certain genetic factors may contribute to the development of NPD. Studies have shown that NPD tends to run in families, suggesting a genetic component to the disorder.

- Childhood experiences: Early life experiences, such as excessive praise or criticism from parents or caregivers, may contribute to the development of NPD. A lack of emotional support or inconsistent parenting styles may also contribute to the development of narcissistic traits.

- Cultural and societal factors: Societal values that prioritize individualism, competitiveness, and material success may contribute to the development of NPD. In cultures that emphasize self-promotion and personal achievements, individuals may be more prone to develop narcissistic traits.

Diagnosis of Narcissistic Personality Disorder

Diagnosing Narcissistic Personality Disorder involves a comprehensive evaluation by a mental health professional. The diagnostic criteria for NPD are outlined in the Diagnostic and Statistical Manual of Mental Disorders (DSM-5), published by the American Psychiatric Association. Some of the criteria include:

- Having an exaggerated sense of self-importance

- Preoccupation with fantasies of unlimited success, power, beauty, or perfect love

- Believing that one is special and unique

- Requiring excessive admiration from others

- Having a sense of entitlement and expecting favorable treatment

- Lacking empathy and being unwilling to recognize or identify with the needs and feelings of others

- Displaying arrogant, haughty behavior or attitudes

PERSONALITY DISORDERS

To be diagnosed with NPD, an individual must show a pervasive pattern of these behaviors and traits that significantly impacts their interpersonal relationships and functioning.

Treatment Options for Narcissistic Personality Disorder

Treating Narcissistic Personality Disorder can be challenging due to the individual's resistance to acknowledging their problems and seeking help. However, with appropriate therapy and support, individuals with NPD can make significant progress in managing their condition.

- Psychotherapy: Talk therapy, such as cognitive-behavioral therapy (CBT) and psychodynamic therapy, can help individuals with NPD gain insight into their thoughts, emotions, and behaviors. Therapists work with clients to challenge distorted beliefs, develop empathy, and improve interpersonal relationships.

- Group therapy: Group therapy provides individuals with NPD an opportunity to interact with others who have similar experiences. Through collaboration and feedback from group members, individuals can gain a better understanding of themselves and their impact on others.

- Family therapy: In some cases, involving family members in therapy can help improve communication and address relational patterns that contribute to NPD symptoms.

- Medication: While there is no specific medication to treat NPD directly, medication may be prescribed to address co-occurring mental health conditions such as depression or anxiety that often accompany NPD.

- Self-help strategies: Developing self-awareness, practicing self-reflection, and engaging in activities that promote empathy and compassion can also be beneficial for individuals with NPD. Engaging in hobbies, pursuing personal growth, and focusing on building authentic relationships can support long-term recovery.

It is essential to note that treatment for NPD typically requires long-term commitment and ongoing support. The goal is not to eliminate narcissistic traits entirely but to manage them and find a healthy balance in personal and interpersonal functioning.

Real-World Example: NPD in the Workplace

An example of how Narcissistic Personality Disorder may manifest in the workplace is a scenario where a team leader constantly seeks praise and admiration from their subordinates. This individual may take credit for the team's accomplishments, dismiss others' ideas, and prioritize their own needs and aspirations above the well-being of the team. Their lack of empathy and exaggerated self-importance can create a toxic work environment, leading to decreased team morale and productivity.

To address the issue, team members could engage in open and honest communication with the leader, expressing their concerns and providing feedback about their behavior. Additionally, management could implement leadership development programs that focus on emotional intelligence and empathy-building skills. Creating a supportive work culture that values collaboration and teamwork will help counteract the negative impact of NPD in the workplace.

Resources and Further Reading

- American Psychiatric Association. (2013). Diagnostic and Statistical Manual of Mental Disorders (DSM-5). Arlington, VA: American Psychiatric Publishing.

- Campbell, W. K., & Miller, J. D. (2011). The Handbook of Narcissism and Narcissistic Personality Disorder: Theoretical Approaches, Empirical Findings, and Treatments. Hoboken, NJ: John Wiley & Sons.

- Behary, W. T. (2013). Disarming the Narcissist: Surviving and Thriving with the Self-Absorbed. Oakland, CA: New Harbinger Publications.

- McBride, K. (2018). Will I Ever Be Free of You? How to Navigate a High-Conflict Divorce from a Narcissist and Heal Your Family. New York, NY: Atria Books.

In conclusion, Narcissistic Personality Disorder is a complex mental health condition characterized by grandiosity, a constant need for admiration, and a lack of empathy. While it presents challenges during diagnosis and treatment, various therapeutic approaches and self-help strategies can help individuals with NPD improve their well-being and develop healthier interpersonal relationships. By fostering awareness, empathy, and compassion, individuals with NPD can strive for personal growth and create a more sustainable mental health future.

Antisocial Personality Disorder

Antisocial Personality Disorder (ASPD) is a mental health condition characterized by a consistent pattern of disregard for and violation of the rights of others. Individuals with ASPD often engage in aggressive, impulsive, and irresponsible behaviors without feeling remorse or empathy for their actions. This section will explore the key features, causes, diagnosis, and treatment approaches for ASPD.

Key Features of Antisocial Personality Disorder

ASPD is diagnosed based on specific criteria outlined in the Diagnostic and Statistical Manual of Mental Disorders (DSM-5). Some key features of ASPD include:

- Persistent disregard for the rights of others, as manifested by repeated acts that could lead to legal issues.
- Lack of empathy and disregard for the feelings and needs of others.
- Deceitfulness and manipulation for personal gain or pleasure.
- Impulsivity and failure to plan ahead, leading to unstable and chaotic lifestyles.
- Persistent irresponsibility, including the inability to maintain consistent work or financial obligations.
- Lack of remorse or guilt for actions that harm others.

It is important to note that the diagnosis of ASPD requires the presence of symptoms and behaviors that are consistent and pervasive over time, typically since adolescence or early adulthood. Professionals use a comprehensive assessment, including a clinical interview, behavioral observations, and review of the individual's history, to accurately diagnose ASPD.

Causes of Antisocial Personality Disorder

The exact causes of ASPD are not fully understood, but research suggests a combination of genetic, environmental, and psychosocial factors contribute to its development. Here are some key factors that may contribute to the development of ASPD:

- Genetic factors: Studies have shown that genetics play a role in the development of ASPD. Certain genetic variations and abnormalities may increase the likelihood of developing the disorder.

- Childhood experiences: Individuals who experience neglect, abuse, or inconsistent parenting during childhood may be at a higher risk of developing ASPD. Traumatic events or a history of unstable family dynamics can contribute to the development of antisocial behaviors.

- Environmental factors: Growing up in a socioeconomically disadvantaged neighborhood or being exposed to violence and crime can increase the risk of developing ASPD.

- Neurobiological factors: Some research suggests that abnormalities in brain structure and function, such as reduced activity in the prefrontal cortex, may contribute to the development of ASPD. These brain regions are responsible for impulse control, emotional regulation, and decision-making.

It is important to note that not everyone with these risk factors will develop ASPD, and some individuals may develop the disorder without these specific factors present. The interactions between genetic predisposition and environmental influences are complex and require further research.

Diagnosis and Assessment

Diagnosing ASPD requires a comprehensive assessment by a mental health professional, such as a psychiatrist or psychologist. The assessment typically includes:

- Clinical interview: The professional will conduct a structured interview to gather information about the individual's symptoms, behaviors, and personal history. They may also interview family members or close friends to gain additional insights.

- DSM-5 criteria: The professional will compare the individual's symptoms and behaviors to the criteria outlined in the DSM-5 to determine if they meet the diagnosis of ASPD.

- Behavioral observations: The professional may observe the individual's behavior in different settings to assess their social interactions, impulsivity, and other relevant behaviors.

- Psychological testing: In some cases, psychological tests may be administered to assess personality traits, cognitive functioning, and emotional well-being. These tests can help provide a comprehensive understanding of the individual's overall psychological functioning.

While the diagnosis of ASPD can be challenging due to the deceptive and manipulative nature of individuals with the disorder, a thorough assessment by an experienced professional can lead to an accurate diagnosis.

Treatment Approaches for Antisocial Personality Disorder

Treating ASPD can be complex, as individuals with the disorder often lack insight into their behaviors and may be resistant to change. The focus of treatment typically involves managing specific symptoms, minimizing harm to others, and improving overall functioning. Here are some common treatment approaches for ASPD:

- Psychotherapy: Various forms of psychotherapy, such as cognitive-behavioral therapy (CBT) and dialectical behavior therapy (DBT), can help individuals with ASPD develop insight, improve impulse control, and learn healthier ways of relating to others.

- Group therapy: Participating in group therapy can provide individuals with ASPD a chance to practice social skills, learn empathy, and receive feedback from peers.

- Medication: While there are no specific medications approved for treating ASPD, certain medications such as mood stabilizers or antipsychotics may be prescribed to manage associated symptoms such as impulsivity or aggression.

- Comorbidity treatment: Individuals with ASPD often have comorbid conditions such as substance use disorders or depression. Treating these co-occurring conditions can improve overall functioning and reduce the risk of engaging in harmful behaviors.

It is important to note that treatment progress with ASPD may be slow and challenging, and there is no guarantee of significant improvement. However, with a comprehensive and individualized treatment approach, individuals with ASPD can learn to manage their symptoms, reduce harm to others, and improve their overall quality of life.

Caveats and Considerations

When working with individuals with ASPD, it is crucial for mental health professionals to prioritize safety, both for the individual and others involved. They must establish clear boundaries, maintain a consistent therapeutic approach, and closely monitor any behaviors that may pose a risk to themselves or others.

It is also important to recognize that individuals with ASPD may engage in manipulative or destructive behaviors. Professionals must take precautions to protect themselves and establish safety plans to address potential risks.

Furthermore, individuals with ASPD may face social stigma and discrimination due to their behaviors and diagnosis. Mental health professionals should strive to provide nonjudgmental and empathetic care while promoting accountability for their actions.

Case Study and Discussion

To illustrate the complexities of diagnosing and treating ASPD, let's consider the case of Alex, a 30-year-old man with a history of impulsive and aggressive behaviors. Alex has a criminal record and often engages in manipulative behaviors to meet his own needs. He lacks remorse for his actions and exhibits a disregard for the rights of others. He frequently violates societal norms and has strained relationships with family and friends.

To accurately diagnose Alex with ASPD, a mental health professional would conduct a thorough assessment, including interviews with Alex and significant others, review of his legal history, and behavioral observations. The professional would use the DSM-5 criteria for ASPD to determine if Alex meets the diagnosis.

Treatment for Alex would require a tailored approach that addresses his specific needs and challenges. Cognitive-behavioral therapy (CBT) could be beneficial in helping him identify and challenge his maladaptive thoughts and behaviors. Group therapy may provide him with an opportunity to practice social skills and learn empathy. In addition, addressing any underlying co-occurring conditions, such as substance use disorder, would be essential to his overall recovery.

It is important to note that individuals with ASPD may be resistant to treatment and may not always acknowledge the impact of their behaviors on others. In such cases, professionals may need to adopt harm reduction strategies while also promoting accountability and responsibility.

Conclusion

Antisocial Personality Disorder is a complex mental health condition characterized by a persistent pattern of disregard for the rights of others. Diagnosis and treatment of ASPD require a comprehensive assessment and a tailored approach. While treatment progress may be challenging, individuals with ASPD can learn to manage their symptoms and behaviors, reduce harm to others, and improve their overall well-being.

Understanding and addressing ASPD is crucial for mental health professionals, policymakers, and society at large. By providing effective interventions and support, we can contribute to reducing the negative impact of ASPD and promoting healthier behaviors and relationships.

Treatment Approaches for Personality Disorders

Personality disorders are a group of mental health conditions characterized by enduring patterns of thoughts, behaviors, and emotions that deviate from cultural expectations and result in significant distress or impairment. These disorders can be challenging to treat, as they often involve deep-rooted and long-standing patterns of maladaptive behavior. However, there are various treatment approaches that have shown promise in helping individuals with personality disorders improve their overall functioning and quality of life.

1. Psychotherapy: Psychotherapy is the primary treatment approach for personality disorders. It involves working with a trained therapist to address specific issues and develop healthier coping mechanisms. Several types of psychotherapy can be effective for personality disorders:

- Dialectical Behavior Therapy (DBT): DBT is an evidence-based therapy often used for borderline personality disorder. It focuses on developing skills in four key areas: mindfulness, distress tolerance, emotion regulation, and interpersonal effectiveness.

- Cognitive-Behavioral Therapy (CBT): CBT helps individuals identify and change negative thought patterns and behaviors that contribute to their personality disorder symptoms. It is particularly useful for disorders such as avoidant and obsessive-compulsive personality disorder.

- Schema Therapy: Schema therapy targets deep-seated, maladaptive schemas or core beliefs that underlie personality disorders. The therapy helps individuals understand and modify these schemas, leading to healthier thoughts and behaviors.

- Psychodynamic Therapy: Psychodynamic therapy explores how unconscious thoughts and unresolved conflicts contribute to personality disorders. It aims to increase self-awareness and develop healthier ways of relating to others.

2. Medication: While there is no specific medication to treat personality disorders, medications can be useful in managing accompanying symptoms such as depression, anxiety, or impulsivity. Antidepressants, mood stabilizers, and antipsychotic medications may be prescribed to alleviate these symptoms. However, medication alone is not typically considered the first-line treatment for personality disorders.

3. Group Therapy: Group therapy provides individuals with personality disorders an opportunity to interact and learn from others facing similar challenges. It can help improve social skills, enhance self-esteem, and provide a sense of validation and support. Group therapy can be particularly valuable for individuals with antisocial or dependent personality disorder.

4. Therapeutic Communities: Therapeutic communities are residential programs that provide a highly structured environment for individuals with personality disorders. These communities emphasize a sense of community, self-help, and mutual support, aiming to promote personal growth and develop more adaptive behaviors.

5. Family Therapy: Family therapy involves working with the individual with a personality disorder and their family members to improve communication, resolve conflicts, and educate the family about the disorder. It can enhance family support and improve the overall functioning of the individual with the personality disorder.

6. Integrated Treatment: Integrated treatment approaches combine multiple therapeutic modalities to address the complex needs of individuals with personality disorders. These approaches often involve a combination of psychotherapy, medication management, and social support systems, providing a comprehensive and holistic approach to treatment.

It is essential to note that treatment for personality disorders is highly individualized, and the choice of treatment approach depends on various factors such as the specific disorder, the severity of symptoms, and the individual's preferences and goals. Additionally, the therapeutic alliance between the individual and their therapist is crucial for the success of any treatment modality. The willingness to engage in therapy consistently and actively participate in one's treatment is also a significant determinant of treatment outcomes.

While treatment for personality disorders can be challenging and time-consuming, evidence suggests that individuals with these disorders can experience significant improvements in their symptoms and overall functioning with appropriate treatment. It is important to seek professional help and work with trained mental health practitioners to develop a personalized treatment plan that best meets an individual's unique needs.

In conclusion, treatment approaches for personality disorders involve a combination of psychotherapy, medication management, group therapy, family therapy, and integrated treatment approaches. These approaches aim to improve symptoms, develop healthier coping mechanisms, enhance interpersonal relationships, and ultimately promote overall recovery and well-being. The success of treatment depends on individual factors and the collaborative efforts of the individual, therapist, and support systems.

Eating Disorders

Anorexia Nervosa

Anorexia nervosa is a serious mental health disorder characterized by an intense fear of gaining weight and a distorted body image. Individuals with anorexia nervosa engage in restrictive eating behaviors and extreme dieting, which often leads to significant weight loss and severe nutritional deficiencies. This section will provide an in-depth understanding of anorexia nervosa, including its definition, causes, symptoms, diagnosis, treatment, and prevention.

Definition of Anorexia Nervosa

Anorexia nervosa is a psychiatric disorder classified under feeding and eating disorders in the Diagnostic and Statistical Manual of Mental Disorders (DSM-5). To be diagnosed with anorexia nervosa, individuals must meet specific criteria. These criteria include the following:

1. Restriction of calorie intake leading to significantly low body weight, usually with a BMI (Body Mass Index) of less than 18.5.

2. Intense fear of gaining weight or becoming fat, even when underweight.

3. Distorted body image, manifested by a persistent belief that one is overweight or has specific body defects.

4. Absence of other medical conditions that may explain the weight loss, such as a hormonal disorder or gastrointestinal disease.

It is essential to note that anorexia nervosa is a complex disorder influenced by various biological, psychological, and sociocultural factors.

Causes and Risk Factors

The development of anorexia nervosa is multifactorial, involving genetic, psychological, and sociocultural factors.

Genetic Factors: Research suggests a genetic predisposition to anorexia nervosa, with a higher risk among individuals who have a family history of the disorder or other eating disorders. Certain genetic variations may contribute to the development of anorexia nervosa, but more research is needed to fully understand its genetic basis.

Psychological Factors: Individuals with anorexia nervosa often have underlying psychological issues, such as low self-esteem, perfectionism, body dissatisfaction, and a need for control. Psychological factors play a significant role in the perpetuation of disordered eating behaviors and body image disturbances.

Sociocultural Factors: Sociocultural factors, such as societal pressures to attain a thin body ideal, can contribute to the development of anorexia nervosa. Media influence, peer pressure, and cultural beliefs about beauty and weight can all contribute to body dissatisfaction and disordered eating patterns.

Symptoms and Complications

Anorexia nervosa is characterized by a range of physical, behavioral, and psychological symptoms. Common symptoms include:

- Severe restriction of food intake, often accompanied by excessive exercise
- Rapid weight loss and extremely low body weight
- Intense fear of gaining weight
- Distorted body image and preoccupation with weight and body shape
- Development of ritualistic eating behaviors, such as cutting food into tiny pieces or rearranging food on the plate
- Social withdrawal and isolation
- Irritability, mood swings, and anxiety
- Physical complications, such as amenorrhea (loss of menstrual periods), osteoporosis, electrolyte imbalances, and cardiovascular problems

Untreated anorexia nervosa can lead to severe medical complications and even death.

Diagnosis

Diagnosing anorexia nervosa involves a comprehensive assessment that includes a physical examination, psychological evaluation, and a review of medical and psychiatric history. Healthcare professionals, such as psychiatrists and psychologists, use specific diagnostic criteria outlined in the DSM-5 to make an accurate diagnosis.

It is crucial for healthcare providers to differentiate anorexia nervosa from other medical conditions that may present with similar symptoms, such as thyroid disorders or gastrointestinal diseases. Collaborative care involving medical and mental health professionals is essential for an accurate diagnosis and appropriate treatment planning.

Treatment

The treatment of anorexia nervosa requires a multidisciplinary approach, including medical, nutritional, and psychological interventions. The goals of treatment are to restore weight to a healthy level, address malnutrition, address psychological factors contributing to the disorder, and prevent relapse.

Medical management: Medical management focuses on addressing the physical complications of anorexia nervosa. This may involve close monitoring of vital signs, correction of nutritional deficiencies, and treatment of any associated medical conditions. In severe cases, hospitalization may be necessary to stabilize the individual's medical condition.

Nutritional therapy: Nutritional therapy plays a crucial role in the treatment of anorexia nervosa. It involves developing a structured meal plan to restore weight and achieve nutritional rehabilitation. Registered dietitians work closely with individuals to establish regular eating patterns, challenge food fears, and promote a healthy relationship with food.

Psychotherapy: Psychotherapy, particularly cognitive-behavioral therapy (CBT) and family-based therapy (FBT), is the cornerstone of psychological treatment for anorexia nervosa. CBT helps individuals recognize and challenge distorted beliefs about weight, shape, and food. FBT involves the whole family in the treatment process, focusing on weight restoration and facilitating a supportive home environment.

Medication: Medication may be prescribed to manage comorbid conditions or specific symptoms associated with anorexia nervosa. For example, antidepressant medications may be used to treat co-occurring depression or anxiety disorders. It is important to note that medication alone is not sufficient to treat anorexia nervosa but may be used as an adjunct to psychotherapy.

Prevention

Prevention strategies for anorexia nervosa focus on early intervention, education, and promoting positive body image, self-esteem, and healthy eating behaviors. Some preventive measures include:

- Increasing awareness and understanding of the risk factors and early signs of anorexia nervosa among healthcare providers, educators, and parents.

- Promoting a positive and inclusive body image through media literacy programs and school-based interventions.

- Implementing comprehensive school health programs that address mental health, stress management, and healthy lifestyles.

- Creating a supportive environment that encourages open conversations about body image, self-esteem, and healthy eating habits.

Conclusion

Anorexia nervosa is a complex and potentially life-threatening mental health disorder characterized by severe restriction of food intake, intense fear of gaining weight, and distorted body image. Early recognition, diagnosis, and integrated multidisciplinary treatment are vital for individuals with anorexia nervosa to achieve recovery and prevent serious health complications. Furthermore, prevention efforts aimed at addressing risk factors and promoting positive body image and self-esteem are essential for reducing the incidence of anorexia nervosa in society. By understanding the causes, symptoms, diagnosis, treatment, and prevention strategies related to anorexia nervosa, healthcare professionals, educators, and the broader community can work together to create a society that promotes sustainable mental health and well-being.

Bulimia Nervosa

Bulimia nervosa is a serious eating disorder characterized by recurrent episodes of binge eating followed by compensatory behaviors such as self-induced vomiting, excessive exercise, or the use of laxatives or diuretics. It is a complex mental health disorder that affects both physical and psychological well-being.

EATING DISORDERS

Understanding Bulimia Nervosa

To understand bulimia nervosa, it is important to explore its underlying causes and contributing factors. Several psychological, social, and biological factors can contribute to the development of this disorder.

One of the psychological factors associated with bulimia nervosa is a negative body image. Individuals with bulimia often have a distorted perception of their body shape and size, leading to extreme dissatisfaction and a desire to control weight. Additionally, low self-esteem, perfectionism, and feelings of inadequacy can contribute to the development of bulimia nervosa.

Social factors also play a role. Societal pressure to conform to unrealistic beauty standards, peer influence, and a preoccupation with weight and appearance can contribute to the development of disordered eating patterns. Moreover, traumatic life events, such as abuse or bullying, can increase the risk of developing bulimia nervosa.

There is evidence to suggest that biological factors, including genetic predisposition and neurochemical imbalances, may contribute to the development and maintenance of bulimia nervosa. Changes in brain chemistry, particularly involving serotonin, have been linked to the regulation of mood, appetite, and impulse control, which are all affected in individuals with bulimia.

Diagnostic Criteria

The diagnosis of bulimia nervosa is based on specific criteria outlined in the Diagnostic and Statistical Manual of Mental Disorders (DSM-5). To be diagnosed with bulimia nervosa, an individual must meet the following criteria:

1. Recurrent episodes of binge eating, characterized by consuming a large amount of food within a short period, accompanied by a sense of lack of control. 2. Recurrent inappropriate compensatory behaviors to prevent weight gain, such as self-induced vomiting, misuse of laxatives, diuretics, or other medications, excessive exercise, or fasting. 3. The binge eating and compensatory behaviors occur, on average, at least once a week for three months. 4. Excessive influence of body shape and weight on self-evaluation. 5. The disturbance does not occur exclusively during episodes of anorexia nervosa.

Treatment and Interventions

Effective treatment for bulimia nervosa involves a multidisciplinary approach, including psychotherapy, nutritional counseling, and medical management. The goals of treatment are to address the underlying causes of the disorder, normalize eating patterns, improve body image, and develop healthy coping mechanisms.

Cognitive-behavioral therapy (CBT) is a widely recognized and evidence-based treatment for bulimia nervosa. CBT helps individuals identify and challenge negative thoughts and beliefs about body shape and weight, develop healthier eating behaviors, and acquire coping skills to manage emotional distress.

Nutritional counseling is an essential component of treatment, as it helps individuals establish regular eating patterns, develop a healthy relationship with food, and learn to listen to their body's hunger and fullness cues. A registered dietitian can provide personalized meal plans and guidance to support nutritional rehabilitation.

Medication may be considered in some cases to help manage co-occurring mental health conditions, such as depression or anxiety. Selective serotonin reuptake inhibitors (SSRIs), a class of antidepressant medication, have shown some efficacy in reducing binge eating and purging behaviors.

It is important to note that recovery from bulimia nervosa is a gradual process that requires ongoing support and monitoring. Support groups, such as those offered through eating disorder treatment centers or community organizations, can provide a sense of belonging and understanding while promoting accountability and encouragement.

Real-World Example

To better understand the impact of bulimia nervosa, let's consider the case of Emily, a 20-year-old college student. Emily has been struggling with low self-esteem and body image issues since high school. Over time, she developed an unhealthy relationship with food, often turning to binge eating episodes as a way to cope with stress and emotional turmoil.

Following a binge episode, Emily would feel a deep sense of shame and guilt. In an attempt to compensate for the perceived calorie intake, she engaged in excessive exercise and calorie restriction. These behaviors took a toll on her physical health, causing fatigue, electrolyte imbalances, and dental problems.

Recognizing the severity of her condition, Emily sought professional help. She was diagnosed with bulimia nervosa and started a treatment program that included regular therapy sessions with a cognitive-behavioral therapist, nutritional counseling with a dietitian, and medical management from a healthcare provider.

Through therapy, Emily gained a better understanding of the underlying factors contributing to her eating disorder. With the support of her treatment team, she developed healthier coping mechanisms, gradually normalized her eating patterns, and improved her body image perception.

While recovery is an ongoing process, Emily's journey underscores the importance of early intervention and comprehensive treatment approaches in addressing bulimia nervosa and promoting long-term well-being.

Resources and Support

For individuals seeking more information or support regarding bulimia nervosa, the following resources are available:
 1. National Eating Disorders Association (NEDA): www.nationaleatingdisorders.org 2. Eating Disorders Hope: www.eatingdisordershope.com 3. Something Fishy: www.something-fishy.org 4. Recovery Warriors: www.recoverywarriors.com

These organizations provide educational materials, helpline numbers, online support groups, and resources for finding specialized treatment providers. It is crucial to reach out for help and remember that recovery from bulimia nervosa is possible with appropriate support and treatment.

Binge Eating Disorder

Binge Eating Disorder (BED) is a complex mental health condition characterized by recurring episodes of consuming large amounts of food in a short period, accompanied by a loss of control and feelings of distress or guilt. It is the most common eating disorder in the United States, affecting both men and women of all ages and backgrounds.

Prevalence and Diagnosis

BED is a relatively new addition to the Diagnostic and Statistical Manual of Mental Disorders (DSM-5), which reflects the growing recognition of its significance. The exact prevalence of BED is difficult to determine due to underreporting and stigma associated with the disorder, but estimates suggest that it affects between 1-5

The diagnosis of BED is based on specific criteria outlined in the DSM-5. These criteria include recurrent episodes of binge eating, which are characterized by eating large amounts of food in a short period, feeling a lack of control during the episode, and experiencing distress afterward. These binge eating episodes occur at least once a week for three months or more. BED is also associated with significant distress and impairment in various areas of life, such as emotional well-being, physical health, and social functioning.

Causes and Risk Factors

The exact causes of BED are not fully understood, but it is believed to result from a combination of genetic, biological, psychological, and environmental factors. Some of the key risk factors for developing BED include:

1. Genetics: There is evidence to suggest a genetic predisposition to BED, as it tends to run in families. Certain genes may influence appetite regulation, impulse control, and the reward system, making individuals more susceptible to binge eating behavior.

2. Psychological Factors: Psychological factors such as low self-esteem, body dissatisfaction, and negative body image can contribute to the development and maintenance of BED. Stress, depression, anxiety, and other mental health conditions are also closely associated with BED.

3. Dieting and Weight Cycling: Restrictive dieting and repeated cycles of weight loss and regain (known as yo-yo dieting) have been linked to the development of BED. Strict dieting can trigger episodes of binge eating as a response to deprivation and emotional distress.

4. Environmental Factors: Cultural pressures to attain a certain body shape or size, exposure to unrealistic media portrayals of idealized bodies, and a history of childhood trauma or abuse can contribute to the development of BED.

Treatment Approaches

Treating BED involves a multifaceted approach that addresses the physical, psychological, and social aspects of the disorder. The goal is to promote a healthy relationship with food, improve body image, reduce binge eating episodes, and enhance overall well-being. Some common treatment approaches for BED include:

1. Psychotherapy: Cognitive-Behavioral Therapy (CBT) is the gold standard for treating BED. It helps individuals identify and challenge negative thoughts and beliefs about their body and develop healthier coping mechanisms to manage stress and emotions without turning to food. Interpersonal Psychotherapy (IPT) and Dialectical Behavior Therapy (DBT) may also be used to address specific underlying issues.

2. Nutritional Counseling: Registered dietitians or nutritionists can provide guidance on adopting balanced and intuitive eating patterns. They help individuals develop a healthy relationship with food, establish regular eating habits, and manage appetite cues effectively.

3. Medication: In some cases, medication may be prescribed to individuals with BED, especially if co-occurring mental health conditions like depression or anxiety

are present. Selective Serotonin Reuptake Inhibitors (SSRIs) and other medications may help reduce binge eating episodes and improve mood.

   4. Support Groups and Peer Support: Joining support groups or engaging in peer support programs can offer individuals with BED a sense of understanding, validation, and guidance. These groups provide a safe space to share experiences and learn coping strategies from others who have battled similar challenges.

   5. Self-Help Strategies: Various self-help techniques can complement formal treatment for BED. These include journaling to track eating patterns and emotional triggers, practicing stress management techniques such as deep breathing and mindfulness exercises, and incorporating regular physical activity into daily routines.

   6. Treatment for Co-occurring Conditions: It is essential to address any co-occurring mental health conditions like anxiety or depression alongside BED treatment. Integrated care that combines therapy for both the eating disorder and the co-occurring conditions can lead to better outcomes.

Challenges and Future Directions

Despite the increasing recognition of BED, several challenges persist in the diagnosis and treatment of this disorder. These challenges include the underdiagnosis of BED due to stigma, limited access to specialized care, and a lack of awareness among healthcare professionals.

Future directions in the field of BED aim to improve early detection and intervention, enhance treatment outcomes, and reduce the burden associated with the disorder. This includes increasing public awareness, conducting more research on the underlying biological mechanisms, and developing targeted interventions for high-risk populations.

In conclusion, Binge Eating Disorder is a significant mental health issue that requires a comprehensive approach for assessment, diagnosis, and treatment. Understanding the causes and risk factors, implementing evidence-based treatments, and addressing underlying psychological and emotional concerns are crucial steps towards helping individuals with BED achieve sustainable recovery.

Treatment Approaches for Eating Disorders

Eating disorders are complex mental health conditions that require careful and comprehensive treatment approaches. Effective treatment involves addressing the underlying psychological, emotional, and physical factors that contribute to the development and maintenance of eating disorders. In this section, we will explore various treatment approaches that have been found to be helpful for individuals with eating disorders.

1. Psychotherapy

Psychotherapy, also known as talk therapy, is a fundamental component of treatment for eating disorders. Different types of psychotherapy have been shown to be effective, including cognitive-behavioral therapy (CBT), dialectical behavior therapy (DBT), interpersonal therapy (IPT), and family-based therapy (FBT).

CBT is a widely used and evidence-based approach that focuses on identifying and changing the distorted thoughts and behaviors associated with eating disorders. It helps individuals develop healthy coping skills, challenge negative self-perceptions, and establish more positive and realistic beliefs about their bodies and food.

DBT combines elements of CBT with mindfulness practices, emphasizing emotional regulation and interpersonal effectiveness. It provides individuals with tools to manage intense emotions and develop healthier ways of relating to others.

IPT focuses on improving interpersonal relationships and addressing any conflicts or difficulties that may contribute to the development or maintenance of eating disorders. It helps individuals build social support networks and develop effective communication skills.

FBT, also known as the Maudsley Approach, is specifically designed for adolescents with eating disorders. It involves the active involvement of the family in the treatment process, aiming to empower parents to take charge of their child's eating and weight restoration.

2. Medical Management

Medical management plays a crucial role in the treatment of eating disorders, particularly for individuals with severe physical complications or significant weight loss. This may involve regular medical check-ups, monitoring of vital signs, and the management of any nutritional deficiencies.

In cases where severe malnutrition or life-threatening medical complications are present, hospitalization or residential treatment may be necessary to stabilize the individual's health. In these settings, the focus is on restoring weight, managing medical complications, and providing intensive therapeutic support.

3. Nutritional Counseling

Nutritional counseling is an essential component of eating disorder treatment. Registered dietitians or nutritionists work alongside mental health professionals to develop individualized meal plans, address dietary concerns, and promote a healthy relationship with food.

The goal of nutritional counseling is to help individuals normalize their eating patterns, challenge restrictive and obsessive thoughts about food, and establish balanced and flexible eating habits. It also involves education on nutrition, portion sizes, and the importance of regular and consistent meals.

4. Medication

Medication is not the primary treatment for eating disorders, but it may be beneficial in certain cases. Medications can be used to manage co-occurring conditions such as depression, anxiety, or obsessive-compulsive disorder, which often accompany eating disorders. Antidepressants, anti-anxiety medications, and mood stabilizers are among the medications that may be prescribed, but their use should be carefully monitored by a qualified healthcare professional.

5. Support Groups and Peer Support

Support groups and peer support play an important role in the recovery process for individuals with eating disorders. Connecting with others who have experienced similar struggles can provide a sense of validation, understanding, and encouragement. Peer support can be found through local support groups, online communities, and specialized recovery programs.

Support groups typically involve facilitated discussions, sharing of personal experiences, and mutual support. They provide a safe space for individuals to express their thoughts and feelings, receive advice from others who have recovered, and develop new coping strategies.

6. Adjunctive Therapies

In addition to the traditional treatment approaches mentioned earlier, there are several adjunctive therapies that can complement the recovery process for individuals with eating disorders. These therapies include art therapy, yoga, mindfulness meditation, and body-based practices such as dance/movement therapy.

Art therapy allows individuals to express their emotions, gain insights into their struggles, and develop alternative ways of communicating. Yoga and mindfulness meditation promote self-awareness, stress reduction, and body acceptance. Dance/movement therapy focuses on the connection between mind and body, encouraging individuals to explore and express their emotions through movement.

7. Relapse Prevention

Preventing relapse is a crucial aspect of eating disorder treatment. After completing the initial phase of treatment, individuals are encouraged to continue their recovery journey by implementing relapse prevention strategies.

These strategies may include ongoing psychotherapy or counseling, regular check-ins with a healthcare professional, maintaining a balanced and structured meal plan, cultivating healthy coping mechanisms, and staying connected with support networks. Additionally, individuals are educated about potential triggers and warning signs of relapse to help them identify and address challenges before they escalate.

Conclusion

In conclusion, the treatment of eating disorders requires a multidimensional and comprehensive approach. Psychotherapy, medical management, nutritional counseling, medication, support groups, adjunctive therapies, and relapse prevention strategies all play essential roles in promoting recovery and long-term wellness. It is important to tailor treatment approaches to meet the specific needs of each individual, considering their unique circumstances and the severity of the eating disorder. A collaborative, holistic, and compassionate approach is essential in helping individuals regain their health, well-being, and a positive relationship with food and their bodies.

Psychosomatic Disorders

Somatization Disorder

Somatization Disorder is a complex and often misunderstood condition that falls under the category of somatic symptom and related disorders. In this section, we will explore the definition, symptoms, diagnosis, and treatment of Somatization Disorder. We will also examine the impact it has on individuals and society, and discuss strategies for managing and supporting those affected by this condition.

Definition of Somatization Disorder

Somatization Disorder, also known as Briquet's syndrome, is a chronic and distressing condition characterized by the presence of multiple physical complaints without any underlying medical explanation. These physical symptoms may include pain, gastrointestinal disturbances, neurological symptoms, and sexual problems. The symptoms are often severe and can significantly impair an individual's daily functioning and quality of life.

Symptoms of Somatization Disorder

The symptoms of Somatization Disorder vary from person to person but typically involve a combination of pain and other physical complaints. Some common symptoms may include:

- Chronic pain in various parts of the body
- Gastrointestinal problems such as abdominal pain, bloating, and nausea
- Sexual difficulties, including erectile dysfunction or loss of libido
- Neurological symptoms like numbness, tingling, or weakness in the limbs
- Physical symptoms related to the reproductive system, such as irregular periods or problems during pregnancy

It is important to note that individuals with Somatization Disorder genuinely experience these physical symptoms and are not intentionally faking or exaggerating them. These symptoms can be distressing and often lead to significant impairment in daily functioning.

Diagnosis of Somatization Disorder

Diagnosing Somatization Disorder can be challenging due to the diverse and subjective nature of the physical symptoms. To make an accurate diagnosis, a healthcare professional must carefully evaluate the individual's medical history, conduct a thorough physical examination, and rule out any underlying medical condition that could account for the symptoms.

According to the Diagnostic and Statistical Manual of Mental Disorders (DSM-5), the following criteria must be met for a diagnosis of Somatization Disorder:

1. Presence of multiple somatic symptoms that are distressing and result in significant impairment in daily functioning.

2. Excessive and disproportionate thoughts, feelings, or behaviors related to the somatic symptoms, which often involve constant worry about the seriousness of the symptoms.

3. Symptoms persist for a minimum duration of six months.

4. The symptoms are not better explained by another medical condition.

It is crucial for healthcare professionals to approach the diagnosis of Somatization Disorder with empathy and understanding, as individuals with this condition often face skepticism and invalidation of their symptoms.

Treatment of Somatization Disorder

The treatment of Somatization Disorder typically involves a multidisciplinary approach that addresses both the physical and psychological aspects of the condition. The primary goals of treatment are to alleviate distress, improve daily functioning, and promote overall well-being. Here are some common treatment strategies:

- Psychotherapy: Cognitive-behavioral therapy (CBT) has shown promising results in helping individuals with Somatization Disorder. CBT aims to identify and change maladaptive thought patterns and behaviors related to the symptoms.

- Medication: In some cases, antidepressant or anti-anxiety medications may be prescribed to manage associated symptoms such as anxiety or depression.

- Supportive counseling: Providing a safe and supportive environment for individuals to express their concerns and emotions can be beneficial for managing Somatization Disorder.

- Education and self-management techniques: Equipping individuals with knowledge about the condition and teaching them coping strategies can empower them to take an active role in managing their symptoms.

- Physical therapy: Depending on the specific symptoms, physical therapy may be recommended to alleviate pain and improve physical functioning.

It is important to emphasize that the treatment approach should be tailored to the individual's unique needs and preferences. Collaboration between the individual and healthcare professionals is key to developing an effective treatment plan.

Impacts and Challenges

Somatization Disorder can have significant impacts on the individual, their relationships, and society as a whole. Individuals with this condition often experience high levels of distress, impaired quality of life, and difficulties in maintaining employment or fulfilling social roles. The stigma associated with somatic symptom disorders can also lead to feelings of isolation and a lack of understanding or support from others.

One of the main challenges in addressing Somatization Disorder is the complexity and variability of symptoms. Healthcare professionals need to approach this condition with empathy and a willingness to listen to the individual's experiences. Additionally, raising awareness and improving public education about somatic symptom disorders can help reduce stigma and promote understanding within society.

Managing Somatization Disorder

Managing Somatization Disorder requires a comprehensive approach that addresses both the physical and psychological aspects of the condition. Here are some strategies to support individuals with Somatization Disorder:

- Validate and acknowledge the individual's symptoms and experiences.

- Encourage open communication and provide a safe space for discussing concerns and emotions.

- Collaborate with healthcare professionals to develop a tailored treatment plan.

- Educate oneself and others about somatic symptom disorders to reduce stigma and promote understanding.

- Foster a supportive network of family, friends, or support groups for individuals with Somatization Disorder.

- Encourage self-care activities such as relaxation exercises, mindfulness, and stress management techniques.

By implementing a holistic and compassionate approach, we can better support individuals with Somatization Disorder and improve their overall well-being and quality of life.

In conclusion, Somatization Disorder is a complex condition characterized by the presence of multiple physical symptoms without any underlying medical explanation. It can cause significant distress and impairment in daily functioning. Through a multidisciplinary approach that includes psychotherapy, medication, supportive counseling, and education, individuals with Somatization Disorder can manage their symptoms and improve their overall well-being. It is crucial to address the challenges and stigma associated with this condition and promote understanding and support within society.

Conversion Disorder

Conversion disorder, also known as functional neurological symptom disorder, is a condition that involves the presence of neurological symptoms without any identifiable organic cause. These symptoms are often associated with significant distress or impairment in functioning. Conversion disorder is classified as a somatic symptom disorder in the Diagnostic and Statistical Manual of Mental Disorders (DSM-5).

Background

Conversion disorder has a long and complex history, with descriptions dating back to ancient times. The term "conversion" was first used by Sigmund Freud, who believed that the symptoms were a way of converting psychological distress into physical manifestations. Freud's conceptualization of conversion disorder centered around the unconscious conflict and the need to protect oneself from emotional pain.

Diagnosis and Symptoms

The diagnosis of conversion disorder is primarily clinical, based on the presence of certain criteria outlined in the DSM-5. These criteria include the presence of one or more symptoms of altered voluntary motor or sensory functioning, the absence of any medical condition that could account for the symptoms, and evidence of a psychological or behavioral factor affecting the symptoms or their severity.

Symptoms of conversion disorder can vary widely and may include, but are not limited to, paralysis or weakness in limbs, blindness or visual disturbances, difficulty swallowing or speaking, and loss of sensation or abnormal movement in certain body parts. The symptoms often do not conform to known anatomical or physiological pathways, leading to confusion and frustration among both patients and healthcare professionals.

Theoretical Explanations

The exact cause of conversion disorder is not fully understood. However, several theoretical explanations have been proposed to explain the development and maintenance of symptoms:

- **Psychodynamic theory**: Building on Freud's earlier work, psychodynamic theories suggest that conversion disorder is a defense mechanism, allowing individuals to cope with unconscious conflicts or traumatic experiences by converting them into physical symptoms. The symptoms serve as a symbolic expression of inner distress.

- **Sociocultural factors**: Some researchers argue that sociocultural factors, such as the influence of the media and cultural beliefs about illness, can play a role in the development of conversion disorder. For example, in certain cultures, physical symptoms may be more acceptable and less stigmatizing than psychological symptoms, leading individuals to convert their distress into bodily complaints.

- **Cognitive explanations**: Cognitive theories propose that individuals with conversion disorder have difficulties processing and expressing emotions. The conversion symptoms serve as a way to channel these emotional distresses into physical manifestations that are more easily recognizable and understood.

Treatment Approaches

The treatment of conversion disorder involves a multidisciplinary approach, which may include medical, psychological, and rehabilitative interventions. The primary goal of treatment is to alleviate symptoms and improve functioning.

- **Psychotherapy**: Psychotherapy, particularly psychodynamic therapy, is often used to explore the underlying psychological conflicts or traumatic experiences that may be contributing to the conversion symptoms. Cognitive-behavioral therapy (CBT) may also be beneficial in helping individuals change maladaptive thought patterns and behaviors associated with the symptoms.

- **Physical therapy:** Physical therapy and occupational therapy may play a crucial role in the treatment of conversion disorder. These approaches focus on improving physical functioning and helping individuals regain control and confidence in their movements. Gradual exposure and desensitization techniques may also be used to address fear or avoidance associated with specific bodily movements or sensations.

- **Education and support:** Providing education and support to individuals with conversion disorder and their families is essential. Understanding the nature of the condition, dispelling myths and misconceptions, and offering practical strategies for managing symptoms can help reduce distress and improve overall well-being.

Contemporary Challenges and Future Directions

Despite advancements in our understanding and treatment of conversion disorder, several challenges persist. Stigma surrounding mental health and the mind-body connection can impede timely diagnosis and appropriate care. Misdiagnosis and unnecessary medical procedures are also common, highlighting the need for improved education and training among healthcare professionals.

Future research in conversion disorder should focus on further elucidating the underlying mechanisms and potential biomarkers of the condition. The development of more effective interventions, such as targeted pharmacological treatments or neurostimulation techniques, may also be explored.

Ultimately, a comprehensive and integrated approach that combines psychological, social, and medical perspectives is crucial for the successful management of conversion disorder. By recognizing the complex interplay of biological, psychological, and social factors, we can provide more informed and compassionate care to individuals with this condition.

Illness Anxiety Disorder

Illness Anxiety Disorder (IAD), also known as hypochondriasis, is a mental health disorder characterized by excessive worry and fear about having a serious medical condition. Individuals with IAD often misinterpret normal bodily sensations as signs of a severe illness, leading to constant preoccupation with their health and seeking medical attention repeatedly.

Symptoms and Diagnosis

The key feature of Illness Anxiety Disorder is the persistent fear of having a serious medical condition, despite having little or no medical evidence to support the belief. Individuals with IAD may exhibit the following symptoms:

- Constant worry about having a specific illness

- Dread or preoccupation with bodily sensations and physical symptoms

- Frequent doctor visits, medical tests, and seeking reassurance

- Excessive internet searching about medical conditions

- Hypersensitivity to minor physical changes

- Obsession with illness-related information, such as reading medical journals or articles

- Anxiety and distress related to the fear of having a serious illness

To diagnose Illness Anxiety Disorder, mental health professionals rely on criteria outlined in the Diagnostic and Statistical Manual of Mental Disorders (DSM-5). The DSM-5 criteria include:

1. Preoccupation with having a serious medical condition for at least six months

2. Absence or minimal medical evidence to support the belief of having a medical condition

3. High level of anxiety and distress about health concerns

4. Excessive health-related behaviors, such as doctor visits or medical tests

5. Not better explained by another mental health disorder

It is important to note that IAD is different from somatic symptom disorder, where individuals experience real physical symptoms, but the symptoms are not fully explained by a medical condition.

Theory and Explanations

The exact cause of Illness Anxiety Disorder is unclear; however, several factors may contribute to its development:

- Cognitive Factors: Individuals with IAD often have distorted beliefs and catastrophic interpretations of bodily sensations. They may excessively focus on physical symptoms and interpret them as signs of a severe illness.

- Family History: There might be a genetic component to IAD, as individuals with a family history of anxiety disorders or health-related fears are more likely to develop the disorder.

- Childhood Experiences: Traumatic events related to illness, either personal experiences or witnessing an illness in a family member, can contribute to the development of IAD.

- Anxiety Sensitivity: Individuals with high levels of anxiety sensitivity may be more prone to developing IAD. Anxiety sensitivity refers to the fear of anxiety symptoms and the belief that those symptoms indicate something harmful.

Treatment Approaches

Treatment for Illness Anxiety Disorder typically involves a combination of psychotherapy, medication, and cognitive-behavioral approaches. The goal of treatment is to reduce anxiety, change maladaptive thoughts and behaviors, and improve overall functioning. Some common treatment approaches for IAD include:

- Cognitive-Behavioral Therapy (CBT): CBT helps individuals identify and challenge their irrational thoughts and beliefs about illness. It also helps them develop healthier coping strategies and reduce avoidance behaviors.

- Exposure and Response Prevention (ERP): ERP is a type of therapy that gradually exposes individuals to their feared situations or scenarios related to health concerns. It helps them learn to tolerate uncertainty and reduce the need for reassurance-seeking behaviors.

- Medication: In some cases, medication such as selective serotonin reuptake inhibitors (SSRIs) may be prescribed to help reduce anxiety and obsessive thoughts related to health concerns.

Real-World Example

Consider Sarah, a 35-year-old woman who constantly worries about having a heart attack. She experiences occasional chest pain, which she interprets as a sign of an impending heart attack. Despite multiple visits to the doctor and being reassured that her heart is healthy, Sarah constantly searches for information online about heart disease and fears that her symptoms are being overlooked. This preoccupation with her health causes significant distress and interferes with her daily life.

To address Sarah's Illness Anxiety Disorder, a therapist might use a combination of CBT and exposure therapy. The therapist would help Sarah recognize and challenge her catastrophic thoughts about her symptoms, gradually expose her to situations that trigger her anxiety, and teach her healthier coping strategies. Over time, Sarah may learn to manage her anxiety, reduce her preoccupation with health concerns, and regain control over her life.

Caveats and Considerations

While the treatments mentioned above have shown to be effective for many individuals with IAD, it is essential to tailor the treatment approach to meet each individual's specific needs. Additionally, it is crucial to rule out any underlying medical conditions that may contribute to the symptoms before making a diagnosis of IAD.

It is also important to address any comorbid mental health conditions that may be present alongside IAD, such as anxiety disorders or depression. Treating these conditions in conjunction with IAD can greatly improve overall well-being and reduce symptom severity.

Furthermore, involving the patient's support system, such as family or close friends, can help provide a supportive environment and assist in the recovery process.

Conclusion

Illness Anxiety Disorder is a complex mental health condition characterized by excessive worry about having a serious medical condition. Proper diagnosis, understanding of the underlying factors, and an individualized treatment approach can help individuals with IAD regain control over their lives and reduce their preoccupation with health concerns. With appropriate support, psychotherapy, and sometimes medication, individuals with IAD can learn to manage their anxiety and improve their overall well-being.

By addressing Illness Anxiety Disorder in a comprehensive and empathetic manner, we can work towards a sustainable mental health future where individuals are empowered to overcome their fears and live fulfilling lives.

The Role of Mind-Body Connection in Psychosomatic Disorders

Psychosomatic disorders are conditions in which psychological factors play a significant role in the development, progression, or symptomatology of physical illnesses. These disorders, also known as psychophysiological disorders or somatoform disorders, highlight the intricate relationship between the mind and body. Understanding the role of the mind-body connection is crucial in the diagnosis, treatment, and management of psychosomatic disorders.

Background

The mind-body connection refers to the bidirectional communication and interaction between our thoughts, emotions, beliefs, and physical health. Traditional medical models often separated mental and physical health, treating them as distinct entities. However, research in recent decades has highlighted the interconnectedness of psychological and physical well-being.

Psychosomatic disorders typically present with physical symptoms that cannot be explained by known medical conditions, leading healthcare professionals to consider the influence of psychological and emotional factors. The mind-body connection in psychosomatic disorders involves both physiological and psychological mechanisms.

Physiological Mechanisms

Psychosomatic disorders involve a complex interplay between the central nervous system (CNS), autonomic nervous system (ANS), endocrine system, and immune system. Stress, one of the primary contributors to psychosomatic disorders, triggers the release of stress hormones like cortisol, adrenaline, and norepinephrine, resulting in physiological changes.

For example, chronic stress can lead to increased sympathetic nervous system activity, causing elevated heart rate, blood pressure, and altered immune function. These physiological changes can contribute to the development of various psychosomatic symptoms, such as gastrointestinal disturbances, headaches, and cardiovascular problems.

Moreover, the brain-gut axis, a bidirectional communication system between the brain and the gut, plays a crucial role in psychosomatic disorders. Stress and emotional factors can disrupt this axis, leading to gastrointestinal symptoms like irritable bowel syndrome (IBS). The gut also produces neurotransmitters, such as serotonin, that influence mood and emotions, further emphasizing the interconnection between the mind and body.

Psychological Mechanisms

Psychological factors play a significant role in the development and exacerbation of psychosomatic disorders. Emotional distress, such as chronic anxiety, depression, or unresolved trauma, can manifest as physical symptoms. The mind-body connection operates through various psychological mechanisms:

- **Somatization:** Somatization is the psychological process in which emotional distress is expressed as physical symptoms. Individuals with psychosomatic disorders may have difficulty recognizing and appropriately expressing their emotions, leading to the conversion of emotional distress into physical complaints.

- **Psychological Defense Mechanisms:** Defense mechanisms, such as repression, denial, or displacement, can contribute to the development of psychosomatic symptoms. These mechanisms operate unconsciously to protect the individual from distressing emotions, leading to physical symptom manifestation.

- **Cognitive Factors:** Negative thought patterns, irrational beliefs, and catastrophic thinking can impact the experience of physical symptoms. For example, individuals with health anxiety may misinterpret benign bodily sensations as signs of serious illness, leading to heightened anxiety and exacerbation of physical symptoms.

- **Emotional Regulation:** Difficulties in emotional regulation, such as difficulties in identifying and managing emotions, can influence psychosomatic symptoms. Suppressing or overly expressing emotions can both contribute to physical symptomatology.

Treatment Approaches

Addressing the mind-body connection is a fundamental aspect of managing psychosomatic disorders. Treatment approaches for psychosomatic disorders aim to integrate psychological and physical interventions to promote healing and well-being. Some effective strategies include:

- **Cognitive-Behavioral Therapy (CBT):** CBT is a widely used therapeutic approach that focuses on identifying and modifying maladaptive thoughts, beliefs, and behaviors. CBT can help individuals with psychosomatic disorders recognize and challenge negative thoughts, develop healthier coping mechanisms, and strengthen the mind-body connection.

- **Mindfulness-Based Interventions:** Mindfulness practices, such as meditation and body scans, can help individuals with psychosomatic disorders develop present-moment awareness and non-judgmental acceptance of physical and emotional experiences. Mindfulness-based interventions have shown promising results in reducing physical symptoms and improving psychological well-being.

- **Stress Management Techniques:** Learning effective stress management techniques can empower individuals to better cope with stressors and minimize their impact on physical health. Techniques such as relaxation exercises, breathing exercises, and time management strategies can help restore balance to the mind-body connection.

- **Psychopharmacological Interventions:** In some cases, psychopharmacological interventions may be necessary to manage underlying mood or anxiety disorders that contribute to psychosomatic symptoms. Medications, such as selective serotonin reuptake inhibitors (SSRIs) or anxiolytics, may be prescribed in conjunction with psychotherapy.

- **Complementary and Alternative Therapies:** Complementary and alternative therapies, like acupuncture, yoga, or massage therapy, can complement traditional treatments by promoting relaxation, reducing stress, and improving overall well-being. These therapies may help restore balance to the mind-body connection.

Case Study: The Mind-Body Connection in Somatization Disorder

Let's consider the case of Mark, a 35-year-old man who frequently experiences multiple physical symptoms, such as headaches, digestive problems, and muscle pain. After a thorough medical evaluation, no underlying medical conditions are found to explain his symptoms. Mark's symptoms are severe and significantly impact his daily life. He also reports high levels of stress and anxiety due to work-related pressures and relationship difficulties.

In this case, Mark's physical symptoms may be a manifestation of somatization disorder, a psychosomatic disorder characterized by the presence of multiple unexplained physical symptoms. The mind-body connection in somatization disorder involves the interplay of physiological and psychological factors.

Physiologically, Mark's chronic stress activates his sympathetic nervous system, leading to increased muscle tension, headaches, and gastrointestinal disturbances. The release of stress hormones further exacerbates his physical symptoms. Additionally, alterations in the brain-gut axis may contribute to his digestive symptoms.

Psychologically, Mark's high levels of stress and anxiety may contribute to the development and perpetuation of his physical symptoms. His emotional distress may be somatized, resulting in a greater focus on physical sensations and heightened symptom perception. Cognitive factors, such as catastrophic thinking or health anxiety, may also amplify his perceptions of physical symptoms.

Treatment for Mark would involve a comprehensive approach that addresses both the physiological and psychological aspects of his condition. Cognitive-behavioral therapy can help Mark identify and challenge negative thought patterns and develop healthier coping strategies. Stress management techniques, relaxation exercises, and mindfulness-based interventions can assist in managing his stress levels and improving the mind-body connection.

By addressing the mind-body connection, Mark can gain a better understanding of the underlying factors contributing to his psychosomatic symptoms. With appropriate interventions, he can learn to manage his stress, improve psychological well-being, and ultimately reduce his physical symptoms.

Resources

- National Alliance on Mental Illness (NAMI) – www.nami.org
- American Psychosomatic Society – www.psychosomatic.org
- The Mind-Gut Connection by Emeran Mayer
- The Body Keeps the Score by Bessel van der Kolk

Key Takeaways

- The mind-body connection involves bidirectional communication and interaction between psychological factors and physical health.

- Physiological mechanisms involving the CNS, ANS, endocrine system, and immune system contribute to the development and progression of psychosomatic disorders.

- Psychological mechanisms, such as somatization, defense mechanisms, cognitive factors, and emotional regulation, play significant roles in psychosomatic disorders.

- Treatment approaches for psychosomatic disorders include cognitive-behavioral therapy, mindfulness-based interventions, stress management techniques, and complementary therapies.

- Understanding and addressing the mind-body connection is crucial in effectively managing psychosomatic disorders and promoting overall well-being.

In conclusion, recognizing and addressing the role of the mind-body connection in psychosomatic disorders is essential in providing comprehensive and effective care. By integrating psychological and physiological approaches, healthcare professionals can help individuals regain balance and improve their overall well-being. Through ongoing research and a holistic perspective, we can continue to enhance our understanding and treatment of psychosomatic disorders, ensuring a sustainable mental health future.

Sleep Disorders

Insomnia

Insomnia is a common sleep disorder characterized by difficulty falling asleep, staying asleep, or experiencing non-restorative sleep. It affects millions of people worldwide and can have a significant impact on overall health and well-being. In this section, we will explore the causes, consequences, and potential treatment options for insomnia.

Understanding Insomnia

Insomnia can be classified into two main types: acute and chronic. Acute insomnia is usually short-term and often occurs in response to a specific event or circumstance, such as stress, travel, or illness. Chronic insomnia, on the other hand, persists for at least three nights a week for three months or more and is typically not directly related to a specific trigger.

There are several factors that can contribute to the development of insomnia. These include:

- Psychological factors: Stress, anxiety, depression, and other mental health disorders can disrupt sleep and contribute to insomnia.

- Medical conditions: Chronic pain, respiratory disorders, gastrointestinal issues, and hormonal imbalances can all interfere with sleep and lead to insomnia.

- Sleep-related disorders: Insomnia can also be a symptom of other sleep disorders such as sleep apnea or restless legs syndrome.

- Lifestyle habits: Poor sleep hygiene, such as irregular sleep schedules, excessive caffeine or alcohol consumption, and exposure to electronic devices before bed, can contribute to insomnia.

Consequences of Insomnia

The consequences of chronic insomnia extend beyond feeling tired during the day. Persistent sleep disturbances can have a significant impact on various aspects of life, including:

- Impaired cognitive function: Insomnia can affect memory, attention, concentration, and problem-solving abilities, making it difficult to perform daily tasks effectively.

- Mood disturbances: Chronic sleep deprivation can contribute to the development or exacerbation of mental health conditions such as anxiety and depression.

- Decreased quality of life: Insomnia can lead to decreased productivity, fatigue, irritability, and a reduced overall sense of well-being.

- Increased risk of accidents and injuries: Sleep deprivation due to insomnia can impair judgment, coordination, and reaction times, increasing the risk of accidents at home, work, or while driving.

- Negative impact on physical health: Chronic insomnia has been associated with an increased risk of developing various health conditions, including cardiovascular disease, obesity, and diabetes.

Treatment Approaches for Insomnia

The treatment of insomnia typically involves a combination of lifestyle changes, behavioral interventions, and, in some cases, medication. Here are some approaches that can be effective in managing insomnia:

- Sleep hygiene: Establishing a consistent sleep routine, creating a comfortable sleep environment, and avoiding stimulating activities before bed can improve sleep quality.

- Cognitive-behavioral therapy for insomnia (CBT-I): CBT-I is a highly effective, evidence-based approach that helps individuals identify and change negative thoughts and behaviors that contribute to insomnia.

- Relaxation techniques: Practices such as deep breathing exercises, progressive muscle relaxation, and guided imagery can help calm the mind and promote better sleep.

- Stimulus control: This technique involves associating the bed and bedroom with sleep and relaxation, rather than wakefulness and anxiety.

- Sleep restriction: Restricting the time spent in bed to the actual amount of sleep obtained can help consolidate sleep and regulate the sleep schedule.

- Medications: In some cases, doctors may prescribe sleep medications for short-term use to help manage insomnia. However, these should be used judiciously and under medical supervision due to the potential for dependence and other side effects.

It is worth noting that the treatment of insomnia should be tailored to each individual, taking into account their unique circumstances, underlying causes, and preferences. A comprehensive approach that addresses the root causes and promotes healthy sleep habits is crucial for long-term management of insomnia.

Example Case Study

To illustrate the impact of insomnia on an individual's life, let's consider the case of Sarah, a 35-year-old working professional experiencing chronic insomnia. Sarah struggles to fall asleep most nights, often finds herself waking up multiple times during the night, and feels tired and unrefreshed in the morning. As a result, she struggles with daytime sleepiness, difficulty concentrating at work, and heightened irritability.

Sarah seeks help from a sleep specialist who conducts a thorough evaluation to identify the underlying factors contributing to her insomnia. The specialist works with Sarah to develop a personalized treatment plan, which includes implementing good sleep hygiene practices, practicing relaxation techniques before bed, and engaging in cognitive-behavioral therapy for insomnia.

Over time, as Sarah consistently follows the recommended treatment plan, she begins to experience improvements in her sleep quality and daytime functioning. She starts feeling more rested, regains her ability to concentrate, and notices a reduction in her irritability levels. With ongoing support, Sarah learns to manage her insomnia effectively and regain control over her sleep.

Key Takeaways

Insomnia is a prevalent sleep disorder that can significantly impact an individual's well-being and daily functioning. It is important to address the underlying causes and implement appropriate treatment strategies to manage insomnia effectively. A multimodal approach that combines lifestyle changes, behavioral interventions, and, if necessary, medication, can help individuals attain better sleep and improve their overall quality of life. It is crucial to consult with healthcare professionals to receive an accurate diagnosis and develop an individualized treatment plan that suits specific needs and preferences.

Narcolepsy

Narcolepsy is a neurological disorder that disrupts the normal sleep-wake cycle. It is characterized by excessive daytime sleepiness, sudden onset of sleep, and cataplexy, which is a sudden loss of muscle tone often triggered by strong emotions. This section will explore the causes, symptoms, diagnosis, and treatment options for narcolepsy.

Understanding Narcolepsy

Narcolepsy affects approximately 1 in every 2,000 people worldwide and typically manifests during adolescence or early adulthood. The exact cause of narcolepsy is not fully understood, but it is believed to be a result of genetic and environmental factors. It is important to note that narcolepsy is not caused by laziness or a lack of sleep hygiene.

Individuals with narcolepsy often experience excessive daytime sleepiness, even after getting a full night's sleep. They may have difficulty staying awake during normal daytime activities, such as working, studying, or socializing. This excessive sleepiness can be debilitating and interfere with daily functioning.

Cataplexy is another hallmark symptom of narcolepsy. It is characterized by a sudden loss of muscle tone, leading to temporary muscle weakness or paralysis. Cataplexy is often triggered by strong emotions, such as laughter, surprise, or anger. The severity of cataplexy episodes can vary, from a brief muscle weakness to a complete collapse.

Other symptoms of narcolepsy may include sleep paralysis, which is a temporary inability to move or speak while falling asleep or waking up, and hallucinations, which are vivid and often frightening experiences during sleep-wake transitions.

Diagnosing Narcolepsy

Diagnosing narcolepsy can be challenging, as its symptoms are often mistaken for other sleep disorders or attributed to stress and fatigue. However, a thorough evaluation by a sleep specialist is crucial for an accurate diagnosis.

The diagnostic process usually involves a comprehensive medical history, including a detailed description of symptoms and their impact on daily life. A sleep diary may also be recommended to track sleep patterns and daytime sleepiness.

In some cases, a multiple sleep latency test (MSLT) may be conducted. This test measures how quickly a person falls asleep during the day and assesses the presence of rapid eye movement (REM) sleep. People with narcolepsy tend to enter REM sleep more quickly than individuals without the condition.

Genetic testing may also be done to identify specific gene variations associated with narcolepsy. However, genetic testing is not widely available and is not necessary for diagnosis in most cases.

Treatment for Narcolepsy

While there is no cure for narcolepsy, treatment options are available to manage its symptoms and improve quality of life.

Stimulant medications, such as modafinil and methylphenidate, are commonly prescribed to help promote wakefulness and reduce excessive daytime sleepiness. These medications work by stimulating the central nervous system.

Selective serotonin reuptake inhibitors (SSRIs), such as fluoxetine and venlafaxine, may be used to manage cataplexy and other symptoms of narcolepsy. SSRIs can help regulate emotions and reduce the frequency and severity of cataplexy episodes.

Lifestyle modifications can also play a significant role in managing narcolepsy. Maintaining a consistent sleep schedule, practicing good sleep hygiene, and taking short naps during the day can help alleviate excessive sleepiness. Avoiding alcohol, caffeine, and heavy meals close to bedtime can also support better sleep quality.

In addition to medication and lifestyle changes, behavioral therapy and counseling may be beneficial for individuals with narcolepsy. Cognitive-behavioral therapy (CBT) can help address any emotional or psychological challenges associated with the condition and develop coping strategies for managing symptoms.

Real-World Example

To better understand the impact of narcolepsy on individuals and their daily lives, let's consider the case of Sarah. Sarah is a 25-year-old woman who was recently diagnosed with narcolepsy. Before her diagnosis, she struggled with excessive daytime sleepiness, often falling asleep at work and during social gatherings. She also experienced several cataplexy episodes, causing her to lose muscle strength and fall.

After her diagnosis, Sarah started taking prescribed medications to manage her symptoms. She learned relaxation techniques to help control her emotions and reduce the frequency of cataplexy episodes. Sarah also worked with a sleep specialist to develop a sleep schedule and incorporate short naps into her daily routine.

With the right treatment and support, Sarah was able to regain control of her life. She now manages her narcolepsy symptoms effectively, allowing her to continue pursuing her career and enjoying social activities with her friends and family.

Summary

Narcolepsy is a neurological disorder characterized by excessive daytime sleepiness, cataplexy, sleep paralysis, and hallucinations. It can significantly impact an individual's quality of life and daily functioning. While there is no cure for narcolepsy, treatment options, including medication, lifestyle modifications, and therapy, can help manage symptoms and improve overall well-being. A thorough evaluation by a sleep specialist is essential for an accurate diagnosis and personalized treatment plan.

Restless Legs Syndrome

Restless Legs Syndrome (RLS) is a neurological disorder characterized by an irresistible urge to move the legs, usually accompanied by uncomfortable sensations in the legs. These sensations are often described as crawling, tingling, itching, or burning, and can range from mild to severe. Individuals with RLS typically experience worsening of symptoms during periods of rest or inactivity, such as when sitting or lying down, and find relief by moving their legs or walking. RLS can significantly disrupt sleep and quality of life.

Signs and Symptoms

The primary symptoms of Restless Legs Syndrome include:

- Uncomfortable sensations in the legs, often described as crawling, tingling, itching, or burning

- Urge to move the legs, usually accompanied by an involuntary movement

- Worsening of symptoms during periods of rest or inactivity

- Temporary relief by moving the legs or walking

These symptoms tend to occur or worsen in the evening or at night, leading to sleep disturbances and insomnia. RLS can also cause significant distress, anxiety, and depression.

Causes and Risk Factors

The exact cause of Restless Legs Syndrome is still uncertain, but several factors are believed to contribute to its development. Research suggests a strong genetic component, with RLS often running in families. Other potential risk factors include:

- Iron deficiency: Low levels of iron in the brain may disrupt dopamine signaling, which is involved in the movement control and the regulation of bodily sensations.

- Dopamine dysfunction: Imbalances in dopamine, a neurotransmitter, may play a role in RLS.

- Chronic diseases and conditions: Certain conditions such as kidney failure, diabetes, and peripheral neuropathy have been associated with the development of RLS.

- Pregnancy: RLS symptoms can occur or worsen during pregnancy, particularly in the third trimester.

- Medications: Some medications, including certain antidepressants, antipsychotics, and antihistamines, can exacerbate RLS symptoms.

- Lifestyle factors: Excessive caffeine intake, smoking, and alcohol consumption may increase the risk of developing RLS.

Diagnosis

To diagnose Restless Legs Syndrome, healthcare professionals typically rely on the following criteria:

- An overwhelming urge to move the legs, usually accompanied by uncomfortable sensations

- Symptoms that worsen during periods of rest or inactivity

- Symptoms that improve with movement

- Symptoms that occur primarily or exclusively in the evening or at night

In addition, healthcare professionals may inquire about the frequency, duration, and intensity of symptoms, as well as their impact on sleep and daily activities. Blood tests may be conducted to assess iron levels and rule out other underlying conditions.

Treatment

Although there is no cure for Restless Legs Syndrome, several treatment options are available to manage symptoms and improve quality of life. The treatment approach may vary depending on the severity and frequency of symptoms, as well as the underlying causes.

1. **Lifestyle Modifications:** Making certain lifestyle changes can help alleviate RLS symptoms. These may include avoiding caffeine and alcohol, practicing good sleep hygiene, exercising regularly but not too close to bedtime, and applying heat or cold therapy to the legs.

2. **Medications:** In more severe cases, medications may be prescribed to reduce symptoms. Dopamine agonists, opioids, anticonvulsants, and sleep medications are commonly used to manage RLS symptoms. However, medication should be used judiciously and under the supervision of a healthcare professional due to potential side effects and risks.

3. **Iron Supplementation:** If blood tests reveal iron deficiency, iron supplements may be prescribed to improve symptoms. This is particularly effective for individuals with low iron levels.

4. **Complementary Therapies:** Some individuals find relief from RLS symptoms through complementary therapies such as massage, acupuncture, yoga, or relaxation techniques. These approaches can help reduce stress and promote relaxation, which may alleviate symptoms.

The Impact of Restless Legs Syndrome

Restless Legs Syndrome can have a significant impact on an individual's life, affecting their physical and mental well-being. The disruptive nature of the symptoms can lead to chronic sleep deprivation, fatigue, and daytime drowsiness, impairing cognitive function and overall productivity. The emotional toll of RLS, including frustration, anxiety, and depression, should not be overlooked.

Furthermore, the discomfort and distress associated with RLS can affect personal relationships, work performance, and social activities. Individuals with RLS may find it challenging to sit or stay still for extended periods, which may limit their ability to participate in certain activities or professions.

Current Research and Future Directions

Research into Restless Legs Syndrome is ongoing, focusing on understanding the underlying mechanisms and identifying new treatment strategies. Some areas of investigation include:

- Further exploring the role of genetics and familial inheritance in RLS.
- Investigating the relationship between iron metabolism and RLS.
- Investigating the impact of dopamine dysfunction on RLS symptoms.
- Developing non-pharmacological interventions, such as transcranial magnetic stimulation, for symptom management.

It is essential to continue raising awareness and educating healthcare professionals about Restless Legs Syndrome to improve early diagnosis and treatment. By further understanding the complex interplay between genetics, brain function, and lifestyle factors in RLS, we can develop more targeted and effective interventions to improve the lives of individuals affected by this condition.

Summary

Restless Legs Syndrome is a neurological disorder characterized by an irresistible urge to move the legs, often accompanied by uncomfortable sensations. While the exact cause is not fully understood, factors such as genetics, iron deficiency, and dopamine dysfunction are thought to contribute to its development. The diagnosis is based on specific criteria related to the urge to move the legs and the worsening of symptoms at rest. Treatment options include lifestyle modifications, medications, iron supplementation, and complementary therapies. RLS can significantly impact an individual's quality of life, affecting sleep, cognitive function, and emotional well-being. Ongoing research aims to deepen our understanding of RLS and develop more effective treatments for symptom relief.

Sleep Hygiene and Treatment Approaches for Sleep Disorders

Sleep is a fundamental physiological process that is essential for our overall well-being and functioning. Adequate and quality sleep is vital for maintaining optimal physical and mental health. However, many individuals struggle with sleep-related issues and disorders that can significantly impact their daily lives. In this section, we will explore the concept of sleep hygiene and various treatment approaches for sleep disorders.

Sleep Hygiene

Sleep hygiene refers to a series of practices and habits that promote healthy sleep patterns and improve sleep quality. By adopting good sleep hygiene practices, individuals can create an optimal sleep environment and establish a consistent bedtime routine, which can help regulate their sleep-wake cycle. Here are some key elements of sleep hygiene:

- **Maintain a consistent sleep schedule:** Go to bed at the same time every night and wake up at the same time every morning, even on weekends. This helps regulate the body's internal clock and promotes better sleep quality.

- **Create a sleep-friendly environment:** Make your bedroom a calm, comfortable, and dark environment that is conducive to sleep. Remove electronic devices that emit blue light, such as smartphones and tablets, as they can disrupt the production of melatonin, a hormone that regulates sleep.

- **Establish a bedtime routine:** Engage in relaxing activities before bed to signal to your body that it is time to sleep. This can include reading a book, taking a warm bath, practicing deep breathing exercises, or listening to calming music. Avoid stimulating activities, such as working or exercising, close to bedtime.

- **Limit exposure to stimuli:** Reduce your consumption of caffeine, nicotine, and alcohol, especially in the evening. These substances can interfere with sleep patterns and reduce sleep quality. Additionally, avoid large meals, spicy foods, and excessive fluid intake before bedtime to minimize discomfort and nocturnal awakenings.

- **Create a comfortable sleep environment:** Invest in a supportive mattress and pillows, and use breathable and comfortable bedding materials. Adjust the room temperature to a cool and pleasant level, as extreme temperatures can disrupt sleep.

- **Manage stress and anxiety:** Practice stress reduction techniques, such as mindfulness meditation or journaling, to help calm the mind before bed. Consider developing a worry journal to write down any concerns or anxieties before sleeping, which can help ease your mind.

By incorporating these sleep hygiene practices into your daily routine, you can improve your sleep quality and overall well-being. However, for individuals who experience persistent sleep disturbances or have diagnosed sleep disorders, additional treatment approaches may be necessary.

Treatment Approaches for Sleep Disorders

Sleep disorders can manifest in various forms, including insomnia, sleep apnea, narcolepsy, and restless legs syndrome, among others. These disorders can significantly impact an individual's quality of life and overall health. Treatment approaches for sleep disorders aim to address the underlying causes and alleviate symptoms. Here are some common treatment options:

- **Cognitive-Behavioral Therapy for Insomnia (CBT-I):** CBT-I is a structured therapeutic approach that focuses on changing thoughts and behaviors that contribute to insomnia. It involves techniques such as sleep restriction, stimulus control, relaxation training, and cognitive restructuring. CBT-I has been shown to be highly effective in improving sleep quality and reducing insomnia symptoms.

- **Continuous Positive Airway Pressure (CPAP):** CPAP therapy is the gold standard treatment for obstructive sleep apnea. It involves wearing a mask over the nose or nose and mouth while sleeping, which delivers a continuous flow of air to keep the airway open. CPAP therapy helps alleviate symptoms such as snoring and daytime sleepiness, improving the quality of sleep and overall well-being.

- **Medication:** In cases where lifestyle modifications and non-pharmacological treatments are insufficient, medication may be prescribed to manage sleep disorders. For example, hypnotic medications can be prescribed for short-term management of insomnia, while stimulant medications may be used to treat excessive daytime sleepiness associated with narcolepsy.

- **Alternative Therapies:** Some individuals may find relief from their sleep disorders through alternative therapies such as acupuncture, aromatherapy, or herbal supplements. While the evidence for the effectiveness of these treatments is limited, they may be worth exploring under the guidance of a healthcare professional.

- **Sleep Study and Diagnosis:** In cases where the underlying cause of the sleep disorder is unknown, a sleep study may be recommended. A sleep study, also known as polysomnography, involves monitoring various physiological parameters during sleep, such as brain waves, eye movements, and oxygen levels. This evaluation can help identify the specific sleep disorder and guide appropriate treatment.

It is essential to consult with a healthcare professional or a sleep specialist for an accurate diagnosis and individualized treatment plan. They can assess the nature and severity of the sleep disorder and recommend the most appropriate treatment options for your specific needs.

Promoting Healthy Sleep Habits

In addition to sleep hygiene practices and treatment approaches, there are several general strategies that can promote healthy sleep habits and improve sleep quality:

- **Regular exercise:** Engaging in regular physical activity can promote better sleep. However, it is important to avoid vigorous exercise close to bedtime, as it can increase alertness and make it difficult to fall asleep. Aim for at least 30 minutes of moderate-intensity exercise most days of the week.

- **Limit daytime napping:** If you have trouble sleeping at night, try to limit daytime napping or avoid it altogether. If you must nap, keep it short (around 20-30 minutes) and avoid napping too close to bedtime.

- **Manage light exposure:** Exposure to natural light during the day can help regulate your sleep-wake cycle. Try to spend time outdoors or near windows during the daytime. In the evening, minimize exposure to bright lights, particularly blue light emitted by electronic devices. Consider using blue light-blocking glasses or installing screen filters to reduce exposure.

- **Avoid clock-watching:** Constantly checking the clock during the night can increase anxiety and make it harder to fall back asleep. If you have trouble sleeping, try turning your clock away from your line of sight or placing it in a location where you cannot easily check the time.

- **Journaling:** Keeping a sleep diary can help identify patterns or triggers that may be affecting your sleep. Each night, record the time you go to bed, the time you wake up, and any factors that may have influenced your sleep, such as caffeine intake, stress levels, or emotional state.

- **Relaxation techniques:** Practice relaxation techniques, such as deep breathing exercises, progressive muscle relaxation, or guided imagery, before bed. These techniques can help calm your mind and body, promoting a state of relaxation conducive to sleep.

By adopting these healthy sleep habits and addressing any underlying sleep disorders or issues, you can enhance the quality of your sleep and promote overall well-being.

Conclusion

Sleep hygiene practices and treatment approaches for sleep disorders play a significant role in promoting healthy sleep patterns and improving sleep quality. By adopting good sleep hygiene practices, seeking appropriate treatment when necessary, and implementing strategies to promote healthy sleep habits, individuals can optimize their sleep and enhance their overall physical and mental health.

Remember, adequate and quality sleep is vital for our overall functioning and well-being. If you are experiencing persistent sleep problems or suspect you may have a sleep disorder, it is essential to consult with a healthcare professional or a sleep specialist to receive a proper diagnosis and personalized treatment plan. Sleep well and prioritize your sleep for a healthier and happier life!

Other Psychological Challenges

Dissociative Disorders

In this section, we will explore the concept of dissociative disorders, which are a group of mental health conditions characterized by disturbances in a person's identity, memory, and consciousness. Dissociative disorders can have a profound impact on an individual's daily functioning and overall well-being. We will discuss the different types of dissociative disorders, their causes, symptoms, diagnosis, and treatment options.

Types of Dissociative Disorders

There are several types of dissociative disorders, each with its own unique set of symptoms and characteristics. The main types include:

1. **Dissociative Identity Disorder (DID):** Formerly known as multiple personality disorder, this condition is characterized by the presence of two or more distinct identities or personality states within an individual. These identities may have their own behaviors, memories, and emotions. Individuals with DID often experience gaps in memory for important personal information, as well as significant distress and impairment in daily functioning.

2. **Dissociative Amnesia:** This disorder is characterized by the inability to recall important personal information, usually of a traumatic or stressful nature. The memory loss is typically selective and may be specific to certain

periods of time, events, or people. Dissociative amnesia is not due to normal forgetfulness and is often related to psychological factors.

3. **Depersonalization-Derealization Disorder:** Individuals with this disorder often have recurrent episodes of feeling detached from their own body (depersonalization) and/or a sense of unreality or detachment from their surroundings (derealization). These experiences may feel as if they are living in a dream or observing themselves from outside their body. Depersonalization-derealization disorder can significantly disrupt a person's sense of self and their ability to engage in everyday activities.

Causes and Risk Factors

The exact causes of dissociative disorders are not fully understood. However, researchers believe that a combination of genetic, biological, and environmental factors may contribute to their development. Some potential causes and risk factors include:

- **Severe childhood trauma:** Many individuals with dissociative disorders have a history of childhood abuse, neglect, or other forms of trauma. The dissociation may serve as a coping mechanism to escape from the overwhelming psychological pain associated with these traumatic experiences.

- **Biological factors:** Certain brain regions and neurotransmitters have been implicated in the development of dissociative disorders. Differences in brain structure and function, as well as alterations in serotonin and norepinephrine levels, may contribute to the symptoms experienced by individuals with dissociative disorders.

- **Stress and psychological distress:** High levels of chronic stress, such as those experienced in war zones or natural disasters, can increase the risk of developing dissociative disorders. Additionally, individuals with other mental health conditions, such as post-traumatic stress disorder (PTSD) or borderline personality disorder, may be more susceptible to developing dissociative disorders.

Symptoms and Diagnosis

The symptoms of dissociative disorders can vary depending on the specific type. However, there are some common signs and symptoms that may indicate the presence of a dissociative disorder, including:

- **Memory gaps or blackouts:** Individuals may have difficulty remembering important personal information, significant events, or periods of time.

- **Identity confusion or identity alteration:** In dissociative identity disorder, individuals may exhibit marked changes in their identity, including behaviors, mannerisms, and preferences.

- **Depersonalization and derealization:** Patients with depersonalization-derealization disorder may describe feeling detached from their own body or experiencing the world as if it were unfamiliar or artificial.

- **Emotional and psychological distress:** Dissociative disorders often cause significant distress and impairment in daily functioning. Individuals may experience anxiety, depression, mood swings, or other emotional challenges.

To diagnose dissociative disorders, mental health professionals use various assessment tools, including clinical interviews, psychological evaluations, and standardized tests. Diagnosis can be challenging due to the overlap of symptoms with other mental health conditions. A comprehensive assessment is essential to rule out other potential causes of the symptoms.

Treatment Approaches

The treatment of dissociative disorders typically involves a multimodal approach, tailored to the individual's specific symptoms and needs. Treatment may include:

- **Psychotherapy:** Psychotherapy, particularly trauma-focused approaches, is the primary treatment for dissociative disorders. Techniques such as cognitive-behavioral therapy (CBT), psychodynamic therapy, and eye movement desensitization and reprocessing (EMDR) may be used to help individuals process traumatic memories, manage symptoms, improve coping skills, and integrate dissociated identities.

- **Medication:** In some cases, medications such as antidepressants, anxiolytics, or antipsychotics may be prescribed to manage specific symptoms, such as depression, anxiety, or psychosis.

- **Stabilization and safety planning:** Ensuring the safety and stability of the individual is crucial, particularly if there are any concerns regarding self-harm or suicidal ideation. This may involve developing safety plans, providing crisis intervention, and coordinating care with other healthcare providers.

- **Supportive therapies:** Adjunctive therapies, such as art therapy, music therapy, or animal-assisted therapy, may be used to provide additional support and enhance the overall therapeutic process.

It is important to note that the treatment of dissociative disorders can be complex and may require long-term therapy. A collaborative and multidisciplinary approach involving psychiatrists, psychologists, social workers, and other healthcare professionals is often necessary to provide comprehensive care.

Case Example

Consider the case of Sarah, a 28-year-old woman who presents with dissociative amnesia. Sarah reports experiencing significant memory loss for the past three months and is unable to recall important events, such as her sister's wedding. She feels detached from her own identity and describes living in a fog, as if she is watching her life from afar. Sarah is also experiencing anxiety and depression.

Sarah's therapist conducts a thorough assessment, which includes a clinical interview, psychological evaluation, and consultation with other professionals involved in her care. The assessment reveals a history of childhood trauma, including physical and emotional abuse. The therapist develops a treatment plan focused on trauma-focused therapy, utilizing CBT techniques and incorporating mindfulness-based practices to help Sarah process her traumatic experiences and regain a sense of self.

Over time, Sarah's treatment progresses, and she begins to make significant improvements. She starts to recover memories and develop effective coping strategies to manage her anxiety and depression. With ongoing therapy and support, Sarah gradually learns to reintegrate her dissociated experiences and build a stronger connection with her identity, ultimately improving her overall well-being and functionality.

Unconventional Example: Virtual Reality Therapy

In recent years, emerging technologies, such as virtual reality (VR), have shown promise as a therapeutic tool for individuals with dissociative disorders. VR therapy can create immersive environments that simulate real-life situations, allowing individuals to safely confront and process traumatic memories or trigger situations. By exposing individuals to controlled virtual environments, therapists can facilitate desensitization and reprocessing of traumatic memories, reducing distress and promoting healing.

For example, a therapist may use VR to recreate a scene similar to the traumatic event experienced by a person with dissociative amnesia. The individual can then revisit the virtual environment, gradually processing the traumatic memories and emotions associated with the event. Through repeated exposure and therapeutic support, VR therapy can help individuals with dissociative disorders break free from the grip of traumatic memories and promote healing and resilience.

Conclusion

Dissociative disorders are complex mental health conditions that require a comprehensive and multidimensional approach to assessment and treatment. Through a combination of psychotherapy, medication, and supportive therapies, individuals with dissociative disorders can find relief from their symptoms, regain a sense of self, and rebuild their lives. As the field of mental health continues to evolve, incorporating innovative approaches such as virtual reality therapy may further enhance the treatment outcomes for individuals with dissociative disorders.

Obsessive-Compulsive Disorder (OCD)

Obsessive-Compulsive Disorder (OCD) is a debilitating mental health condition characterized by the presence of obsessions and/or compulsions that significantly interfere with a person's daily life. In this section, we will explore the various aspects of OCD, including its symptoms, causes, diagnosis, and treatment approaches.

Understanding OCD

OCD is often misunderstood and portrayed as a personality quirk or a desire for cleanliness. However, it is a much more complex and distressing condition that goes beyond mere perfectionism.

Symptoms of OCD: People with OCD experience intrusive thoughts, images, or urges known as obsessions, which elicit significant distress. These obsessions are usually accompanied by repetitive behaviors or mental acts called compulsions that individuals feel compelled to perform to reduce anxiety or prevent perceived harm.

Common obsessions: Obsessions in OCD can vary widely but often revolve around themes of contamination, symmetry, orderliness, aggressive or sexual thoughts, and religious or moral concerns.

Common compulsions: Compulsions are repetitive behaviors that individuals with OCD feel driven to perform to alleviate anxiety. They can include actions like excessive handwashing, checking behaviors, ordering or arranging objects, repeating specific phrases or prayers, or seeking reassurance from others.

Impact on daily life: OCD symptoms can be time-consuming and can interfere with a person's ability to maintain relationships, engage in productive work or academic activities, and enjoy a fulfilling life.

Causes of OCD

The exact cause of OCD is not yet fully understood. However, research suggests that a combination of genetic, biological, and environmental factors contribute to its development.

Biological factors: There is evidence to suggest that imbalances in certain brain chemicals, primarily serotonin, play a role in the development of OCD. Additionally, abnormalities in certain brain regions involved in decision-making, such as the orbitofrontal cortex and basal ganglia, have also been observed in individuals with OCD.

Genetic factors: OCD tends to run in families, indicating a genetic predisposition. Several genes have been identified as potentially contributing to the development of OCD, although more research is needed to fully understand their role.

Environmental factors: Stressful life events, trauma, and childhood adversity may increase the risk of developing OCD in susceptible individuals. In some cases, OCD symptoms can be triggered or exacerbated by specific life events or situations.

Diagnosis and Assessment

Diagnosing OCD involves a comprehensive assessment by a mental health professional. The diagnosis is based on the presence of obsessions and/or compulsions that consume a significant amount of time, cause distress, and interfere with daily functioning.

Clinical interview: A mental health professional will conduct a detailed clinical interview to gather information about the nature and severity of symptoms, their impact on daily life, and any associated distress.

Assessment tools: Psychological assessments, such as self-report measures and structured interviews, may be used to supplement the clinical interview and provide further insights into the specific symptoms and impairment related to OCD.

Differential diagnosis: It is crucial to distinguish OCD from other mental health conditions that may share some similarities in symptoms, such as anxiety disorders, hoarding disorder, or body dysmorphic disorder.

Treatment Approaches

OCD is a treatable condition, and early intervention significantly improves outcomes. The most effective treatments for OCD combine medication, specifically selective serotonin reuptake inhibitors (SSRIs), with psychotherapy.

Cognitive-Behavioral Therapy (CBT): CBT, particularly a specialized form called Exposure and Response Prevention (ERP), is considered the gold standard treatment for OCD. ERP involves gradually exposing individuals to situations that trigger their obsessions while preventing the accompanying compulsive behaviors. This exposure helps individuals learn to tolerate anxiety without resorting to rituals.

Medication: SSRIs, which are commonly used to treat depression and anxiety, have also been found to be effective in reducing OCD symptoms. These medications help to increase serotonin levels in the brain, which can help alleviate obsessions and compulsions.

Other therapies: In some cases, additional therapies such as Acceptance and Commitment Therapy (ACT) or Dialectical Behavior Therapy (DBT) may be beneficial, especially if there are co-occurring conditions like depression or difficulties with emotional regulation.

Challenges and Future Directions

While significant progress has been made in understanding and treating OCD, there are still several challenges and areas for improvement in the field.

Access to treatment: Many individuals with OCD face challenges in accessing timely and appropriate treatment due to factors such as stigma, financial barriers, or limited availability of qualified mental health professionals.

Co-occurring conditions: OCD frequently co-occurs with other mental health conditions, such as depression, anxiety disorders, or substance use disorders. Treating these comorbid conditions concurrently can be crucial for achieving optimal outcomes in OCD treatment.

Personalized approaches: Further research is needed to identify subtypes of OCD, predict treatment response, and develop more personalized treatment approaches tailored to individual needs.

Prevention strategies: Efforts to prevent the development of OCD or to intervene early in high-risk individuals hold promise. Identifying risk factors, promoting resilience, and implementing preventive interventions are areas of ongoing research.

In conclusion, OCD is a complex and distressing mental health condition characterized by obsessions and compulsions. Through a combination of medication, therapy, and ongoing support, individuals with OCD can achieve significant symptom reduction and improved quality of life. Ongoing research and advocacy efforts are crucial to address the challenges associated with OCD and to promote a sustainable mental health future.

Schizophrenia

Schizophrenia is a chronic and severe mental disorder characterized by disruptions in thought processes, perceptions, emotions, and behavior. It affects approximately 1

Symptoms of Schizophrenia

The symptoms of schizophrenia can be categorized into three main groups: positive symptoms, negative symptoms, and cognitive symptoms.

- **Positive symptoms:** These symptoms represent an excess or distortion of normal behavior. They include hallucinations, delusions, disorganized thinking and speech, and abnormal motor behavior. Hallucinations are sensory experiences that are not based in reality, such as hearing voices that others cannot hear. Delusions are false beliefs that are firmly held despite evidence to the contrary. Disorganized thinking and speech may manifest as difficulty organizing thoughts, jumping between unrelated topics, or providing answers that do not make sense. Abnormal motor behavior can range from agitated body movements to catatonia, a state of immobility and unresponsiveness.

- **Negative symptoms:** These symptoms reflect a decrease or absence of normal behavior. They include reduced emotional expression, social withdrawal, lack of motivation or pleasure, diminished speech, and difficulty in initiating and sustaining activities. Negative symptoms can significantly impair a person's ability to engage in relationships, work, and self-care.

- **Cognitive symptoms:** These symptoms involve deficits in cognitive functioning, such as problems with attention, memory, and executive functioning. Individuals with schizophrenia may have difficulty focusing, remembering information, and making decisions. These cognitive impairments can have a profound impact on daily functioning and overall quality of life.

Causes of Schizophrenia

The exact cause of schizophrenia is still unknown, but it is believed to be a result of a combination of genetic, environmental, and neurobiological factors.

- **Genetic factors:** Schizophrenia tends to run in families, suggesting a genetic predisposition. However, no single gene has been identified as the sole cause of the disorder. It is likely that multiple genes interact with each other and with environmental factors to increase the risk of developing schizophrenia.

- **Environmental factors:** Prenatal exposure to viral infections, maternal malnutrition, and complications during childbirth have been linked to an increased risk of developing schizophrenia. Additionally, exposure to certain psychoactive substances, such as cannabis or stimulants, during adolescence or early adulthood can increase the risk of developing the disorder.

- **Neurobiological factors:** Imbalances in brain chemicals (neurotransmitters) such as dopamine and glutamate have been implicated in the development of schizophrenia. Structural and functional abnormalities in specific brain regions, such as the prefrontal cortex and hippocampus, have also been observed in individuals with schizophrenia.

Diagnosis and Treatment

Diagnosing schizophrenia involves a comprehensive evaluation of the individual's symptoms, medical history, and family history. A psychiatrist or other mental health professional will conduct interviews and assessments to determine if the diagnostic criteria for schizophrenia are met.

Treatment for schizophrenia typically involves a combination of medication, psychosocial interventions, and support services.

- **Medication:** Antipsychotic medications are the primary treatment for schizophrenia. They help to reduce the intensity of psychotic symptoms, such as hallucinations and delusions. Newer atypical antipsychotic medications have fewer side effects compared to older typical antipsychotics, but they still carry risks and may cause side effects. It is important for individuals to work closely with a healthcare provider to find the most effective medication at the lowest possible dose.

- **Psychosocial interventions:** Various psychosocial interventions can complement medication and help individuals with schizophrenia manage their symptoms and improve their overall functioning. Cognitive-behavioral therapy (CBT) can help individuals challenge and change their delusional beliefs or cope with hallucinations. Family therapy can improve communication and support within the family unit. Social skills training can help individuals develop and enhance their social interaction and communication skills. Supported employment and education programs can provide opportunities for individuals to engage in meaningful work or studies.

- **Support services:** Support services are crucial in providing ongoing assistance to individuals with schizophrenia. These services may include case management, housing assistance, vocational rehabilitation, and community support programs.

Challenges and Future Directions

While treatment options for schizophrenia have improved over the years, several challenges persist in providing optimal care for individuals with this disorder.

- **Stigma:** Stigma surrounding mental illness, including schizophrenia, can lead to discrimination and social exclusion. This stigma can discourage individuals from seeking help and hinder their ability to access appropriate care and support.

- **Treatment adherence:** Medication adherence can be a significant challenge for individuals with schizophrenia. Some may experience side effects or have difficulty understanding the benefits of medication, leading to discontinuation or inconsistent use. Improving medication adherence through education, support, and shared decision-making is an ongoing focus of research and clinical practice.

- **Preventing relapses:** Schizophrenia is a chronic condition, and managing the risk of relapse is essential. Developing strategies to identify early signs of relapse, engaging individuals in treatment during prodromal phases, and promoting continuous care and support are areas of ongoing research.

- **Personalized medicine:** Advances in genetics and neuroscience hold promise for the development of personalized treatment approaches for schizophrenia. Identifying biomarkers and using genetic information to tailor interventions could enhance treatment outcomes and minimize side effects.

- **Recovery-oriented approaches:** Shifting the focus from solely managing symptoms to supporting recovery and overall wellbeing is gaining recognition in the field of schizophrenia treatment. Recovery-oriented approaches emphasize empowerment, community integration, and the development of individual strengths and goals. These approaches aim to improve quality of life and enable individuals to lead fulfilling lives.

In conclusion, schizophrenia is a complex mental disorder that requires a comprehensive understanding of its symptoms, causes, and treatment options. Ongoing research and advancements in the field of schizophrenia offer hope for improving outcomes and providing holistic care to individuals with this condition. By addressing the challenges and embracing new directions in schizophrenia treatment, we can work towards a future that promotes the well-being and recovery of those affected by this disorder.

Bipolar Disorder

Bipolar disorder, also known as manic-depressive illness, is a psychiatric condition characterized by extreme mood swings, including episodes of mania and depression. These mood swings can vary in intensity and duration, affecting a person's thoughts, emotions, behaviors, and overall functioning. Understanding bipolar disorder requires knowledge of its symptoms, etiology, diagnosis, treatment, and management.

Symptoms of Bipolar Disorder

The symptoms of bipolar disorder can be divided into two main phases: the manic phase and the depressive phase.

During the manic phase, individuals may experience:

- Abnormally elevated mood or irritability

- Increased energy levels and restlessness

- Decreased need for sleep without feeling tired

- Racing thoughts and rapid speech
- Impulsive and risky behavior, such as excessive spending, reckless driving, or substance abuse
- Grandiose beliefs or inflated self-esteem

In contrast, during the depressive phase, individuals may experience:

- Persistent feelings of sadness, hopelessness, or emptiness
- Loss of interest in previously enjoyed activities
- Fatigue or decreased energy levels
- Sleep disturbances, either insomnia or excessive sleep
- Changes in appetite and weight
- Difficulty concentrating or making decisions
- Thoughts of death or suicide

It's important to note that the frequency, duration, and severity of these mood episodes can vary widely among individuals with bipolar disorder. Some may experience more frequent and severe episodes, while others may have longer periods of stability between episodes.

Etiology of Bipolar Disorder

The exact cause of bipolar disorder is not fully understood, but research suggests that it is a complex interaction of genetic, biological, and environmental factors.

Genetic factors play a significant role in the development of bipolar disorder. Studies have shown that individuals with a family history of bipolar disorder are at a higher risk of developing the condition themselves. Specific genetic variations related to neurotransmitter systems and the regulation of mood have also been identified.

Biological factors, such as imbalances in brain chemicals (neurotransmitters) and abnormal brain structure or function, are believed to contribute to bipolar disorder. Neurotransmitters like dopamine, serotonin, and norepinephrine play a crucial role in regulating mood, and any disruption in their normal functioning can lead to mood instability.

Environmental factors, including traumatic life events, significant stress, and substance abuse, can trigger or exacerbate bipolar episodes in individuals with a genetic predisposition. Additionally, disruptions in sleep patterns and seasonal changes have been linked to the onset of mood episodes in some individuals.

Diagnosis of Bipolar Disorder

Diagnosing bipolar disorder involves a comprehensive assessment of symptoms, medical history, and family history. It typically requires the presence of both manic and depressive episodes to establish a diagnosis.

A healthcare professional, such as a psychiatrist or psychologist, will conduct a thorough psychiatric evaluation, which includes:

- Interviewing the individual and their family members to gather detailed information about symptoms and their impact on daily life

- Evaluating the duration, frequency, and intensity of mood episodes

- Assessing for the presence of other medical or psychiatric conditions that may mimic or coexist with bipolar disorder

Diagnostic criteria outlined in the Diagnostic and Statistical Manual of Mental Disorders (DSM-5) are commonly used as guidelines for diagnosing bipolar disorder. The DSM-5 defines several subtypes of bipolar disorder, including bipolar I disorder, bipolar II disorder, cyclothymic disorder, and other specified and unspecified bipolar and related disorders.

Treatment and Management of Bipolar Disorder

Bipolar disorder is a chronic condition that requires long-term treatment and management. The goals of treatment include stabilizing mood, managing symptoms, preventing relapse, and improving overall functioning and quality of life.

Treatment of bipolar disorder often involves a combination of:

- Medication: Mood stabilizers, such as lithium, anticonvulsants, and atypical antipsychotics, are commonly prescribed to manage mood swings. Antidepressants may be used cautiously during depressive episodes, but they are typically avoided during manic episodes to prevent triggering a switch to mania.

- Psychotherapy: Talk therapies, such as cognitive-behavioral therapy (CBT), interpersonal therapy, and family-focused therapy, can help individuals understand and cope with their illness, manage stress, and improve communication and relationship skills.

- Psychoeducation: Educating individuals and their families about bipolar disorder, its symptoms, and treatment options is essential for promoting self-management and adherence to treatment plans.

- Lifestyle modifications: Adopting a regular sleep schedule, engaging in regular exercise, managing stress, avoiding substance abuse, and maintaining a healthy diet can all contribute to mood stability and overall wellbeing.

The management of bipolar disorder also involves monitoring for potential complications or comorbidities, such as substance abuse, anxiety disorders, or physical health problems. Regular follow-up appointments with healthcare providers are crucial for assessing treatment response, adjusting medications, and addressing any emerging concerns.

Promising Research and Unconventional Approaches

In recent years, several novel approaches to the treatment and management of bipolar disorder have emerged:

- Chronotherapy: This approach involves manipulating sleep-wake cycles and light exposure to stabilize mood and reduce depressive symptoms in individuals with bipolar disorder.

- Nutritional interventions: Some research suggests that certain dietary modifications, such as increasing omega-3 fatty acids and consuming a balanced, nutrient-rich diet, may have a positive impact on mood stability.

- Transcranial magnetic stimulation (TMS): TMS is a non-invasive procedure that uses magnetic fields to stimulate specific areas of the brain. It has shown promise in reducing depressive symptoms in individuals with bipolar disorder.

- Mindfulness-based interventions: Practices like mindfulness meditation and yoga have been studied for their potential benefits in reducing stress, improving emotion regulation, and promoting overall wellbeing in individuals with bipolar disorder.

While these approaches show promise, further research is needed to establish their efficacy and safety in the context of bipolar disorder.

Conclusion

Bipolar disorder is a complex psychiatric condition characterized by significant mood swings and impacts on a person's daily life. Understanding the symptoms, etiology, diagnosis, and treatment of bipolar disorder is crucial for providing effective care and support to individuals living with this condition. Ongoing research and exploration of unconventional approaches offer hope for enhanced treatment outcomes and improved quality of life for individuals with bipolar disorder. By advancing our knowledge and implementing evidence-based practices, we can work towards a sustainable mental health future that addresses the holistic needs of individuals with bipolar disorder and promotes their overall wellbeing.

Postpartum Depression

Postpartum depression is a common mental health disorder that affects women after childbirth. It is characterized by feelings of sadness, hopelessness, and exhaustion, which can interfere with a woman's ability to care for herself and her newborn. Postpartum depression is different from the "baby blues," which are mild mood swings that many women experience after giving birth. While the baby blues usually resolve within a couple of weeks, postpartum depression can last for months or even longer if left untreated.

Understanding Postpartum Depression

Postpartum depression is a complex condition with a variety of contributing factors. The hormonal changes that occur after childbirth, including a drop in estrogen and progesterone levels, can contribute to the development of postpartum depression. Additionally, psychological and social factors, such as a history of depression or anxiety, lack of social support, and high levels of stress, can increase the risk of experiencing postpartum depression.

It is important to recognize that postpartum depression is not a sign of weakness or a character flaw. It is a medical condition that can affect any woman, regardless of her socioeconomic status or personal circumstances. Understanding this can help reduce the stigma associated with postpartum depression and encourage women to seek help without feeling ashamed or guilty.

Identifying Symptoms and Diagnosing Postpartum Depression

Recognizing the symptoms of postpartum depression is essential for early intervention and treatment. Some common symptoms include:

- Persistent feelings of sadness, hopelessness, or emptiness
- Extreme fatigue or loss of energy
- Difficulty sleeping or sleeping too much
- Changes in appetite and weight (eating too little or too much)
- Loss of interest or pleasure in activities once enjoyed
- Feelings of worthlessness or guilt
- Difficulty concentrating or making decisions
- Thoughts of death or suicide

It is important to note that postpartum depression can also manifest with physical symptoms such as headaches, stomachaches, or muscle pain. These physical symptoms are often overlooked or attributed to the challenges of new motherhood, which can lead to a delay in diagnosing and treating postpartum depression.

Diagnosing postpartum depression involves a comprehensive assessment of symptoms and may include screening tools such as the Edinburgh Postnatal Depression Scale (EPDS). This questionnaire helps healthcare providers evaluate a woman's mental health and identify the presence and severity of postpartum depression. It is a valuable tool for initiating conversations about postpartum mental health and guiding appropriate treatment plans.

Treatment and Support for Postpartum Depression

Fortunately, postpartum depression is a highly treatable condition, and with the right support, women can fully recover. Treatment options for postpartum depression may include a combination of the following:

- Therapy: Individual therapy, such as cognitive-behavioral therapy (CBT), can help women identify and address negative thought patterns and develop coping strategies. Couples or family therapy can also be beneficial for improving communication and support within the family unit.
- Medication: Antidepressant medications, such as selective serotonin reuptake inhibitors (SSRIs), may be prescribed to alleviate the symptoms of postpartum depression. It is important for women to discuss their options

with a healthcare provider to determine the best course of action based on their individual needs.

- Support groups: Participating in peer-led support groups can provide a sense of belonging and validation, reducing feelings of isolation and stigma. Sharing experiences with other women who have gone through or are going through postpartum depression can be comforting and empowering.

- Lifestyle changes: Adopting a healthy lifestyle can have a positive impact on mental health. Engaging in regular physical activity, maintaining a balanced diet, and ensuring adequate sleep can improve overall well-being and support the recovery process.

- Social support: Strong social support is crucial for women experiencing postpartum depression. Partner involvement, family support, and connections with other new mothers can provide emotional support and practical assistance in caring for the newborn.

It is important to note that treatment plans may vary depending on the severity of symptoms and the individual's preferences. Women should work closely with their healthcare providers to develop a personalized treatment plan that aligns with their needs and goals.

The Role of Healthcare Professionals

Healthcare professionals, including obstetricians, pediatricians, and mental health providers, play a vital role in the identification, assessment, and treatment of postpartum depression. They have a responsibility to screen women for postpartum depression during pregnancy and after childbirth and make appropriate referrals for further evaluation and treatment.

In addition to clinical care, healthcare professionals can also provide education and support to women and their families. They can help dispel misunderstandings about postpartum depression, offer guidance on coping strategies, and provide information on community resources and support groups.

The Importance of Self-Care for Mothers

Mothers experiencing postpartum depression often find it challenging to prioritize self-care while navigating the demands of caring for a newborn. However, self-care is crucial for their well-being and recovery. Here are some self-care strategies that can help women manage postpartum depression:

- Rest and sleep: Getting enough rest and sleep can improve mood and overall functioning. Taking short naps when the baby sleeps and asking for help with nighttime feedings can provide much-needed rest.

- Nutrition: Eating a balanced diet can support physical and mental well-being. Opting for nutritious meals and snacks rich in fruits, vegetables, whole grains, and lean proteins can positively impact mood and energy levels.

- Exercise: Engaging in gentle exercises, such as walking or yoga, can boost mood and energy levels. Even short bursts of physical activity throughout the day can have a positive impact on mental health.

- Time for oneself: Carving out time for activities that bring joy and relaxation is essential for mental well-being. Whether it's reading a book, taking a bath, or pursuing a hobby, making self-care a priority can help alleviate symptoms of postpartum depression.

- Seeking support: Reaching out for support from loved ones, friends, or support groups can provide a sense of validation and understanding. It is important for women to communicate their needs and feelings openly and let others provide help and support.

By prioritizing self-care, women can better manage the challenges of postpartum depression and cultivate a healthier and more fulfilling postpartum experience.

Conclusion

Postpartum depression is a serious yet treatable mental health disorder that requires attention and support. By understanding the symptoms, seeking appropriate treatment, and practicing self-care, women can overcome postpartum depression and thrive during the transformative journey of motherhood. It is essential for healthcare professionals, families, and communities to provide support and resources to ensure the well-being of new mothers and their families. Together, we can create a supportive and nurturing environment for women experiencing postpartum depression.

Historical Perspectives on Mental Illness

The Asylum Era

The Asylum Era marks a significant period in the history of mental health care, characterized by the establishment of mental asylums or psychiatric hospitals. This era, which lasted from the late 18th century to the early 20th century, had a profound impact on the perception and treatment of mental illness.

Origins of the Asylum Movement

The origins of the Asylum Era can be traced back to the social and cultural context of the time. The industrial revolution, urbanization, and changes in societal attitudes towards mental illness all contributed to the emergence of asylums as a solution to the challenges posed by the increasing numbers of mentally ill individuals.

One of the pioneers of the asylum movement was Philippe Pinel, a French physician who believed in humane treatment for the mentally ill. In 1793, Pinel was appointed as the head physician at La Bicêtre, a notorious asylum in Paris. His approach shifted the focus from strict confinement and physical punishment to a more compassionate and therapeutic approach. Pinel advocated for the removal of chains, better living conditions, and the provision of moral treatment for the patients.

Characteristics of the Asylum Era

During the Asylum Era, mental asylums became institutionalized, with large-scale facilities being built to house and treat individuals with mental illness. These asylums aimed to provide care, protection, and treatment for the mentally ill, but their actual conditions varied greatly.

The asylums were often overcrowded, with limited resources and a lack of qualified staff. Many patients were subject to neglect and abuse, and the segregation of individuals based on the severity of their illness became common practice. The emphasis was on containment rather than active treatment or rehabilitation.

Moral Treatment Movement

Despite the shortcomings of the asylums, the Asylum Era also saw the emergence of the Moral Treatment Movement. This movement advocated for a more humane and compassionate approach to mental health care. The moral treatment philosophy emphasized the importance of benevolent and respectful interactions with patients, providing them with dignity and a sense of purpose.

Advocates of the moral treatment movement believed that mental illness was not a moral failing but rather a medical condition that could be treated. They promoted activities such as work, education, and recreation as means of therapy and social integration. Several asylums began to implement these principles, which marked a significant shift in the approach to mental health care.

Critiques of the Asylum Era

While the establishment of asylums represented a significant step forward in recognizing the need for specialized mental health care, it was not without its criticisms. The conditions within asylums often failed to live up to the lofty ideals of the moral treatment movement. Overcrowding, unsanitary conditions, and the lack of trained personnel undermined the aspirations of providing effective care and rehabilitation for the mentally ill.

Furthermore, the asylum system perpetuated the stigma and social exclusion associated with mental illness. Patients were often isolated from society, and their confinement reinforced the perception that mental illness was a mark of shame or moral failure.

Legacies of the Asylum Era

The Asylum Era left a lasting impact on the field of mental health care. It laid the foundation for the development of psychiatric hospitals and the professionalization of mental health care providers. The moral treatment movement, despite its shortcomings, paved the way for more patient-centered approaches to treatment and rehabilitation.

However, the Asylum Era also serves as a cautionary tale. It highlights the dangers of institutionalization and the need to balance the provision of care with the preservation of individual rights and autonomy. The deficiencies of the asylums underscore the importance of ongoing efforts to improve mental health care and combat stigma in contemporary society.

Contemporary Reflections

As mental health care continues to evolve, it is crucial to critically reflect on the lessons from the Asylum Era. While the shift towards community-based care and the deinstitutionalization movement has led to positive changes, challenges such as resource limitations, access to care, and stigma still persist. Understanding the

HISTORICAL PERSPECTIVES ON MENTAL ILLNESS

historical context of the Asylum Era can inform modern efforts to build a more equitable and effective mental health care system for all individuals.

Key Takeaways:

- The Asylum Era was characterized by the establishment of mental asylums or psychiatric hospitals for the care and treatment of mentally ill individuals.

- The moral treatment movement emerged during this era, advocating for a more compassionate and humane approach to mental health care.

- Asylums faced challenges such as overcrowding, lack of resources, and abuse, which led to critiques of the system.

- The legacy of the Asylum Era includes the professionalization of mental health care providers and a shift towards patient-centered approaches.

- Reflection on the Asylum Era informs contemporary efforts to improve mental health care, combat stigma, and ensure the provision of equitable and effective care.

Discussion Questions:

1. What were the major factors that contributed to the emergence of the Asylum Era?

2. How did the moral treatment movement challenge the prevailing attitudes towards mental illness during the Asylum Era?

3. In what ways did the Asylum Era fall short of its goals in providing effective care and treatment for the mentally ill?

4. What lessons can be learned from the Asylum Era in terms of improving mental health care in contemporary society?

Further Readings:

- Foucault, M. (1961). *Madness and Civilization: A History of Insanity in the Age of Reason*. Vintage.

- Grob, G. N. (1994). *The Mad Among Us: A History of the Care of America's Mentally Ill*. Simon and Schuster.

- Micale, M. S. (2008). *Mental Illness in America: A History*. Princeton University Press.

- Shorter, E. (1997). *A History of Psychiatry: From the Era of the Asylum to the Age of Prozac*. John Wiley & Sons.

Exercises

1. Research and discuss the contributions of other key figures in the Asylum Era, besides Philippe Pinel, in advancing the humane treatment of the mentally ill.

2. Visit a local museum or historical archive to explore artifacts or documents related to the Asylum Era. Reflect on the impact and significance of these historical relics.

3. Interview a mental health care professional about their perspectives on the historical context of the Asylum Era and its influence on current practices.

Notes

The Asylum Era is a significant period in the history of mental health care. It highlights the evolution of societal attitudes towards mental illness, the emergence of asylums, and the subsequent challenges and critiques of the asylum system. Reflecting on this era can inform our understanding of contemporary mental health care and inspire improvements in the field.

Moral Treatment Movement

The Moral Treatment Movement was a significant development in the history of mental health care that emerged in the late 18th century and continued into the 19th century. This movement emphasized a more humane and compassionate approach to the treatment of individuals with mental illness, focusing on moral and social reformation rather than punitive measures.

Background

Before the advent of the Moral Treatment Movement, individuals with mental illness were often subjected to harsh and inhumane treatment. They were commonly confined in asylums or prisons, where they suffered neglect, abuse, and isolation. The prevailing belief was that mental illness was a sign of moral weakness or demonic possession, and therefore, the treatment involved punishment and confinement rather than therapeutic interventions.

The Enlightenment era, with its emphasis on reason, science, and human rights, laid the groundwork for a change in the perception and treatment of mental illness. Advocates of this movement believed that individuals with mental illness were not fundamentally different from those without mental illness, and that their condition could be treated with kindness, respect, and understanding.

Principles of the Moral Treatment Movement

The Moral Treatment Movement was based on several key principles:

1. Individualized Care: This approach recognized the uniqueness of each person's experience with mental illness. It emphasized the importance of tailoring treatment to meet the specific needs of each individual, rather than employing a one-size-fits-all approach. Personalized care involved considering the individual's background, personality, and circumstances to provide the most appropriate treatment.

2. Therapeutic Environment: The movement emphasized the creation of a therapeutic environment that promoted healing and recovery. Asylums were transformed into more homelike settings, with well-maintained grounds, adequate living conditions, and opportunities for social interaction. The aim was to provide a nurturing and supportive environment conducive to the restoration of mental health.

3. Occupation and Activity: The Moral Treatment Movement recognized the value of engaging individuals with mental illness in meaningful activities. Workshops, craft programs, and other occupational activities were introduced to provide a sense of purpose, structure, and personal accomplishment. Engaging in productive work was believed to enhance self-esteem, promote socialization, and provide a distraction from symptoms.

4. Social Interaction: The movement advocated for the integration of individuals with mental illness into society through social interaction. This involved organizing social events, promoting group activities, and encouraging community involvement. The aim was to reduce the stigma and isolation associated with mental illness, fostering a sense of belonging and inclusion.

Approaches and Practices

Various therapeutic approaches and practices were implemented during the Moral Treatment Movement. These included:

1. Moral Therapy: Moral therapy was the cornerstone of the movement. It emphasized the importance of establishing a trusting therapeutic relationship between caregivers and individuals with mental illness. The primary goal of moral therapy was to guide and encourage patients to adopt socially appropriate behaviors and attitudes through moral suasion, moral discipline, and moral reasoning.

2. Occupational Therapy: Occupational therapy played a crucial role in the treatment of mental illness during this period. It involved engaging patients in purposeful and meaningful activities, such as gardening, farming, arts and crafts, and manual labor. Occupational therapy aimed to improve cognitive functioning, enhance self-esteem, and promote a sense of accomplishment.

3. Recreational Activities: Recreation and leisure activities were considered essential for the well-being of individuals with mental illness. These activities provided opportunities for relaxation, enjoyment, and social interaction. Sports, games, music, and dance were often included as part of the treatment regimen.

4. Family Involvement: The Moral Treatment Movement recognized the importance of family support and involvement in the treatment process. Families were encouraged to visit and support their loved ones in the asylums, and efforts were made to educate them about mental illness and its treatment. The involvement of families helped to reduce stigma and foster a sense of community support.

Impact and Legacy

The Moral Treatment Movement had a profound impact on the treatment of mental illness. It challenged the prevailing notion that individuals with mental illness were incurable and dangerous, and instead emphasized the potential for recovery and reintegration into society. The movement laid the foundation for modern mental health care by establishing the importance of compassionate, person-centered care.

The principles and practices of the Moral Treatment Movement continue to influence contemporary mental health care. Today, the focus on individualized care, therapeutic environments, meaningful activities, and social interaction remains central to the delivery of mental health services. The movement also paved the way for the development of occupational therapy and the recognition of the importance of holistic approaches to mental health.

However, it is important to acknowledge that not all aspects of the Moral Treatment Movement were without flaws. Some institutions fell short of providing adequate resources and support, leading to overcrowding and neglect.

Additionally, the movement did not address the underlying social and structural factors that contribute to mental health disparities.

Nevertheless, the Moral Treatment Movement represents a significant milestone in the history of mental health care, promoting humane treatment, compassion, and the belief in the potential for recovery and resilience in individuals with mental illness. Its legacy continues to guide and inspire modern approaches to mental health care, striving for holistic, person-centered practices that prioritize the well-being and dignity of each individual.

Community Mental Health Centers

Community mental health centers play a vital role in providing accessible and comprehensive mental health care to individuals in their local communities. These centers serve as a hub for delivering a wide range of services, including assessment, diagnosis, treatment, and support for individuals of all ages who are experiencing mental health challenges. In this section, we will explore the history, functions, and benefits of community mental health centers, as well as some of the challenges they face.

History of Community Mental Health Centers

The concept of community mental health centers emerged as a response to the deinstitutionalization movement that gained momentum in the mid-20th century. Before the 1950s, mental health care largely relied on large, centralized psychiatric institutions known as asylums. However, these institutions were often overcrowded, and the treatment provided was often inadequate and inhumane.

The deinstitutionalization movement aimed to shift the focus of mental health care from institutionalization to community-based care. It recognized the importance of integrating individuals with mental illnesses into their communities and providing them with support to lead fulfilling lives. Community mental health centers were established as a key component of this movement, serving as local resources for individuals in need of mental health services.

Functions of Community Mental Health Centers

Community mental health centers offer a wide range of services to meet the diverse needs of individuals in their communities. Some of the key functions of these centers include:

1. Assessment and Diagnosis: Community mental health centers provide comprehensive assessments to evaluate individuals' mental health needs. This

involves conducting interviews, administering psychological tests, and gathering information from various sources to inform the diagnostic process.

2. Treatment and Therapy: These centers offer evidence-based interventions for various mental health disorders. Treatment modalities can include individual therapy, group therapy, family therapy, and medication management. The goal is to help individuals manage symptoms, develop coping skills, and improve their overall well-being.

3. Crisis Intervention: Community mental health centers are equipped to provide immediate support and intervention during mental health crises. They offer crisis hotlines, emergency counseling, and access to psychiatric services to ensure individuals receive the urgent care they need.

4. Prevention and Early Intervention: These centers play a crucial role in preventive efforts by promoting mental health awareness, providing education and outreach programs, and identifying individuals at risk of developing mental health problems. Early intervention services aim to address symptoms at their onset and prevent the progression of mental health disorders.

5. Case Management and Support Services: Community mental health centers often provide case management services to individuals with complex mental health needs. Case managers help coordinate and advocate for services, ensure access to community resources, and provide ongoing support to promote recovery and community integration.

Benefits of Community Mental Health Centers

Community mental health centers offer several benefits that contribute to the overall well-being of individuals and the community at large. Some of these benefits include:

1. Accessibility: By being located within the community, these centers are easily accessible to individuals seeking mental health services. This proximity reduces barriers to care, such as transportation issues and stigma associated with visiting distant psychiatric institutions.

2. Holistic and Person-Centered Care: Community mental health centers adopt a holistic approach to mental health care, considering the unique needs and preferences of each individual. They emphasize person-centered care, promoting the active involvement of individuals in treatment planning and decision-making.

3. Integrated Care: These centers often collaborate with other healthcare providers, including primary care physicians, social workers, and specialty care providers. This integrated approach ensures that individuals receive comprehensive care that addresses both their mental and physical health needs.

4. Continuity of Care: Community mental health centers offer ongoing support and follow-up care to individuals, promoting continuity of care. This continuity helps prevent relapses, ensures individuals receive necessary interventions and support, and facilitates their recovery journey.

5. Community Integration: By providing services within the community, these centers support the integration of individuals with mental illnesses into their social networks and community activities. This integration reduces isolation, improves social support, and enhances overall quality of life.

Challenges Facing Community Mental Health Centers

While community mental health centers play a crucial role in enhancing mental health care delivery, they face several challenges that can impact their effectiveness. Some of the key challenges include:

1. Funding and Resources: Community mental health centers often struggle with limited funding and resources to meet the growing demand for services. Insufficient funding can lead to staff shortages, inadequate infrastructure, and limited access to specialized interventions.

2. Stigma and Discrimination: Stigma surrounding mental health remains a significant barrier to accessing care in many communities. Community mental health centers must work to reduce stigma, raise awareness, and educate the public about the importance of mental health.

3. Fragmented Systems: In some cases, coordination and collaboration between different sectors, such as mental health, primary care, and social services, can be challenging. Integration of services across systems is crucial to ensure seamless and comprehensive care for individuals with mental health needs.

4. Limited Specialty Services: While community mental health centers offer a wide range of services, they may have limitations in providing specialized care for complex or rare mental health conditions. Referrals to specialty providers and ensuring timely access to these services can be a challenge.

5. Workforce Shortages: Community mental health centers often struggle to recruit and retain qualified mental health professionals. Shortages in psychiatrists, psychologists, and other mental health professionals can limit the capacity of these centers to meet the needs of their communities.

Addressing these challenges requires sustained efforts from governments, policymakers, communities, and mental health professionals. Adequate funding, improved training and workforce development, collaboration between different sectors, and destigmatization campaigns are essential for the success and sustainability of community mental health centers.

Case Study: The Assertive Community Treatment (ACT) Model

One prominent example of an innovative community mental health care model is the Assertive Community Treatment (ACT) model. ACT is an evidence-based, interdisciplinary approach that provides comprehensive and intensive community-based care for individuals with severe and persistent mental illnesses, such as schizophrenia and bipolar disorder.

The ACT model revolves around a multidisciplinary team that includes psychiatrists, nurses, case managers, social workers, and vocational specialists. These teams work collaboratively to provide a range of services, including medication management, crisis intervention, psychosocial rehabilitation, housing support, and employment assistance.

The key principles of the ACT model include:

1. Accessibility and availability of services 2. Multidisciplinary and integrated care approach 3. Individualized and person-centered care 4. Comprehensive and long-term support 5. Assertive outreach to individuals in their communities 6. Emphasis on community integration and recovery-oriented care

Studies have shown that the ACT model improves outcomes for individuals with severe mental illness, including reduced hospitalizations, increased housing stability, improved quality of life, and enhanced community integration. This model highlights the importance of community mental health centers in delivering effective and holistic care for individuals with complex mental health needs.

Conclusion

Community mental health centers play a critical role in providing accessible, comprehensive, and person-centered care to individuals in their local communities. These centers offer a range of services, including assessment, treatment, crisis intervention, prevention, and support, with the goal of promoting recovery and community integration. Despite the challenges they face, community mental health centers have the potential to significantly impact the well-being of individuals and contribute to building sustainable mental health futures. By addressing funding and resource limitations, reducing stigma, promoting integration and collaboration, and investing in a skilled and diverse workforce, we can ensure that community mental health centers continue to thrive and meet the evolving mental health needs of our communities.

Contemporary Approaches to Mental Illness

In recent years, there has been a significant shift in how we understand and approach mental illness. Contemporary approaches to mental illness are guided by the recognition that it is a complex and multifaceted phenomenon that requires a holistic and person-centered approach. These approaches aim to empower individuals, promote recovery, and enhance their overall wellbeing. In this section, we will explore some of the key contemporary approaches to mental illness and their implications for mental health care.

Recovery-Oriented Approach

One of the central principles of contemporary approaches to mental illness is the recovery-oriented approach. This approach emphasizes the potential for individuals with mental illness to recover and lead meaningful and fulfilling lives. It recognizes that recovery is a unique and personal journey for each individual and places emphasis on their strengths, resilience, and self-determination.

A recovery-oriented approach involves a collaborative partnership between the individual and their healthcare providers, ensuring that their goals and preferences are taken into account. It promotes a holistic view of mental health, addressing not only the symptoms of mental illness but also the individual's social, emotional, and physical wellbeing. This approach also focuses on reducing the stigma and discrimination experienced by individuals with mental illness, promoting inclusivity, and encouraging community integration.

Person-Centered Care

Person-centered care is another important contemporary approach to mental illness. It recognizes that mental health care should be individualized and tailored to the unique needs and preferences of each person. This approach emphasizes the importance of establishing a therapeutic alliance between the individual and their healthcare provider, built on trust, respect, and empathy.

Person-centered care involves actively engaging individuals in decision-making about their care, treatment, and recovery. It recognizes their expertise in their own experiences and values their input in developing personalized care plans. This approach also takes into account the social and cultural context of the individual, considering their background, beliefs, and values in the delivery of care.

Integrated Care

Integrated care is a contemporary approach that recognizes the interconnectedness of mental health with physical health and other psychosocial aspects. It involves the integration of mental health services with primary care, ensuring a coordinated and seamless approach to healthcare delivery. This approach aims to address the physical, mental, and social determinants of health that influence mental illness.

By integrating mental health services with primary care, individuals with mental illness can receive comprehensive and holistic care that addresses their mental health needs alongside their physical health needs. Integrated care promotes early identification and intervention for mental illness, reducing the burden on individuals and improving overall health outcomes.

Strengths-Based Approach

The strengths-based approach is another contemporary approach that focuses on identifying and building upon an individual's strengths, abilities, and resources. Rather than solely focusing on symptoms and deficits, this approach shifts the focus towards nurturing and maximizing the individual's existing strengths.

By identifying and leveraging an individual's strengths, the strengths-based approach aims to enhance their resilience, self-efficacy, and overall wellbeing. This approach encourages individuals to actively participate in their own recovery by setting goals, developing skills, and cultivating positive coping strategies. It recognizes that every individual has unique strengths and potentials, even in the face of mental illness.

Culturally Competent Care

Culturally competent care is an essential aspect of contemporary approaches to mental illness, recognizing the importance of cultural diversity and cultural factors in mental health. This approach acknowledges that culture influences an individual's perception of mental illness, help-seeking behaviors, and treatment preferences.

Culturally competent care involves healthcare providers being knowledgeable about and sensitive to the cultural background, beliefs, and values of the individuals they serve. It requires actively engaging individuals in a culturally responsive and respectful manner, incorporating cultural practices and traditions into the delivery of care. This approach aims to reduce disparities in mental health care and improve access and outcomes for diverse populations.

Technology-Based Interventions

With the rapid advancement of technology, contemporary approaches to mental illness increasingly incorporate technology-based interventions. These interventions utilize digital tools, such as mobile apps, online platforms, virtual reality, and wearable devices, to support mental health care and promote wellbeing.

Technology-based interventions provide individuals with accessible and convenient resources for self-management, psychoeducation, and symptom tracking. They also enable remote delivery of mental health services, improving access particularly for those in underserved areas. However, it is important to ensure that these interventions are evidence-based, ethically designed, and culturally sensitive to maximize their effectiveness.

In conclusion, contemporary approaches to mental illness recognize the complexity of mental health and the importance of comprehensive and person-centered care. These approaches promote recovery, empower individuals, and enhance their overall wellbeing. By embracing the principles of recovery-oriented care, person-centered care, integrated care, strengths-based care, culturally competent care, and technology-based interventions, mental health care can be transformed to meet the evolving needs of individuals with mental illness and promote sustainable mental health for all.

Chapter 3: Promoting Holistic Health

Chapter 3: Promoting Holistic Health

Chapter 3: Promoting Holistic Health

In this chapter, we will explore the concept of holistic health and its application in mental health care. Holistic health refers to an integrated approach that considers the physical, mental, emotional, and spiritual dimensions of an individual's well-being. It recognizes the interconnectedness of these aspects and aims to address them comprehensively to promote optimal mental health. By incorporating various modalities and practices, holistic health approaches seek to enhance overall wellness and resilience.

The Biopsychosocial Model

A key framework in understanding holistic health is the biopsychosocial model. This model acknowledges the influence of biological, psychological, and social factors on mental health. It emphasizes that mental health is not solely determined by genetic or biological factors, but also by psychological and social determinants.

According to this model, mental health disorders arise from a combination of biological vulnerabilities, psychological factors (such as thoughts, emotions, and behaviors), and social factors (including relationships, culture, and environment). By adopting a biopsychosocial perspective, mental health professionals can develop a broader understanding of a person's mental health needs and tailor interventions accordingly.

Integrative Medicine in Mental Health Care

Integrative medicine combines conventional medical approaches with complementary and alternative therapies to promote holistic health. In the context of mental health care, integrative medicine integrates evidence-based psychological interventions with complementary therapies such as yoga, acupuncture, and mindfulness meditation.

Yoga, for example, has been found to reduce symptoms of anxiety and depression by combining physical postures (asanas), breath control (pranayama), and meditation. Acupuncture, another complementary therapy, involves the insertion of thin needles into specific points of the body to restore balance and stimulate healing. Studies have shown that acupuncture can be effective in reducing symptoms of depression and anxiety.

Mindfulness meditation, a practice derived from Buddhist traditions, has gained significant attention in recent years for its positive effects on mental health. It involves paying attention to the present moment non-judgmentally, which can help individuals reduce stress, depression, and anxiety. Mindfulness-based interventions have been incorporated into various mental health treatment approaches, such as Mindfulness-Based Cognitive Therapy (MBCT) and Mindfulness-Based Stress Reduction (MBSR).

Integrative medicine recognizes the importance of addressing the whole person and empowering individuals to actively participate in their own healing process. By combining evidence-based practices with complementary therapies, integrative medicine offers a comprehensive and personalized approach to mental health care.

Complementary and Alternative Therapies

Complementary and alternative therapies encompass a range of non-conventional approaches to mental health care. These therapies are often used alongside conventional treatments and can provide additional support for individuals experiencing mental health challenges.

Some common complementary and alternative therapies include:

1. Herbal and nutritional supplements: Certain herbs and supplements, such as St. John's wort and omega-3 fatty acids, have been studied for their potential benefits in treating depression, anxiety, and other mental health conditions. It is important to note that these supplements should be used under the guidance of healthcare professionals, as they may interact with medications or have side effects.

2. Aromatherapy: Aromatherapy involves the use of essential oils derived from plants to promote relaxation and emotional well-being. Essential oils can be used in

various ways, such as through inhalation or in massage oils.

3. Massage therapy: Massage therapy can help reduce muscle tension, promote relaxation, and alleviate symptoms of stress and anxiety. It can be particularly beneficial for individuals experiencing physical and emotional distress.

4. Art therapy: Art therapy involves the use of creative processes, such as painting, drawing, and sculpting, to explore and express emotions. This therapeutic approach can help individuals gain insight into their mental health challenges and facilitate healing and self-discovery.

5. Music therapy: Music therapy utilizes the power of music to address emotional, cognitive, and social needs. It can be particularly effective in reducing stress, promoting relaxation, and enhancing self-expression.

It is important to note that while these therapies may provide valuable support, they should not be considered as standalone treatments for severe or acute mental health conditions. They should be integrated into a comprehensive treatment plan under the guidance of trained professionals.

Mind-Body Connection in Holistic Health

Holistic health approaches often emphasize the connection between the mind and body in promoting overall well-being. The mind-body connection refers to the dynamic interaction between thoughts, emotions, behavior, and physical health.

Stress, for example, can have profound effects on both mental and physical health. Chronic stress can contribute to the development or exacerbation of mental health disorders, such as anxiety and depression. It can also lead to physical health problems, including high blood pressure, cardiovascular disease, and compromised immune function.

Mind-body practices, such as meditation, yoga, and tai chi, aim to harness the mind-body connection to promote healing and well-being. These practices can help individuals cultivate awareness of their thoughts, emotions, and bodily sensations, and develop greater control over their responses to stressors. By reducing stress and promoting relaxation, mind-body practices play a significant role in holistic health approaches to mental health care.

Summary

Promoting holistic health is essential in mental health care to address the multidimensional nature of well-being. The biopsychosocial model provides a comprehensive framework for understanding the interplay between biological, psychological, and social factors. Integrative medicine and complementary and alternative therapies offer additional tools to support mental health through a personalized and holistic approach. By recognizing the mind-body connection and incorporating practices that promote relaxation and self-awareness, individuals can enhance their overall well-being and resilience.

Holistic Approaches to Mental Health

The Biopsychosocial Model

The biopsychosocial model is a comprehensive framework that takes into account the biological, psychological, and social factors that influence an individual's health and well-being. It recognizes that health and illness are influenced by a complex interaction of various factors, including biological processes, psychological factors, and social determinants. This model provides a holistic approach to understanding and addressing mental health issues, emphasizing the interconnectedness of these different domains.

Biological Factors

Biological factors refer to the physiological processes and genetic factors that contribute to an individual's mental health. These include the functioning of the brain, neurotransmitter imbalances, hormonal changes, and genetic predispositions. For example, conditions such as depression may be linked to imbalances in neurotransmitters like serotonin, while schizophrenia may be associated with abnormal brain structure or functioning.

Understanding the biological factors involved in mental health is crucial for diagnosis and treatment. Advances in neuroscience and genetics have provided valuable insights into the biological basis of mental disorders, leading to the development of targeted interventions such as medication and brain stimulation techniques. For example, selective serotonin reuptake inhibitors (SSRIs) are commonly prescribed to treat depressive disorders by restoring serotonin balance in the brain.

Psychological Factors

Psychological factors refer to individual cognitive and emotional processes that contribute to mental health. These include thoughts, beliefs, emotions, personality traits, and coping strategies. Psychological factors interact with biological processes and social factors to shape an individual's mental well-being. For example, cognitive distortions and negative thinking patterns are often associated with depression and anxiety disorders.

Psychological interventions aim to promote mental health by addressing these cognitive and emotional processes. Therapeutic approaches such as cognitive-behavioral therapy (CBT) and psychodynamic therapy help individuals identify and modify maladaptive thoughts and behaviors, thereby promoting positive mental health outcomes. Additionally, developing emotional intelligence and coping skills can enhance resilience and well-being.

Social Factors

Social factors refer to the social, cultural, and environmental influences on mental health. These encompass various aspects, including family dynamics, social support networks, socioeconomic status, education, employment, and access to healthcare. Social determinants can have a significant impact on mental health outcomes, affecting the risk of developing mental disorders and the ability to seek help and treatment.

For instance, individuals from low socioeconomic backgrounds may face higher stress levels, limited access to resources, and reduced opportunities for mental health promotion. Social isolation and lack of support networks can also contribute to poor mental health outcomes. Recognizing the influence of social factors is crucial for addressing disparities and creating equitable mental health services for all individuals.

Integration of the Biopsychosocial Model

The biopsychosocial model recognizes that mental health and well-being are multifaceted and complex phenomena. It emphasizes the interaction between biological, psychological, and social factors, emphasizing that a comprehensive understanding of mental health requires considering all these dimensions. By integration, practitioners can develop individualized treatment plans that address the unique needs and circumstances of each person.

This model provides a framework for collaboration among healthcare providers from various disciplines, including psychiatrists, psychologists, social workers, and other professionals. It promotes a holistic approach to mental health care, recognizing that no single factor operates in isolation. For example, medication may be necessary to address certain biological factors, but pairing it with therapy that addresses psychological and social factors can enhance treatment outcomes.

The biopsychosocial model also highlights the importance of prevention and early intervention. By addressing biological, psychological, and social factors proactively, we can promote mental health and prevent the development of more severe mental disorders. This emphasizes the need for comprehensive mental health policies that address all dimensions of the model and provide accessible and equitable mental health services for all individuals.

Example: Depression and the Biopsychosocial Model

To illustrate the application of the biopsychosocial model, let's consider the example of depression. According to this model, depression may have biological factors such as imbalances in neurotransmitters like serotonin, psychological factors such as negative thinking patterns, and social factors such as lack of social support or adverse life events.

In terms of treatment, the biopsychosocial model suggests a multidimensional approach. Medications, such as selective serotonin reuptake inhibitors (SSRIs), may be prescribed to address the biological component of depression. However, it would also be important to incorporate psychological interventions such as cognitive-behavioral therapy (CBT) to address maladaptive thought patterns and social support interventions to build a supportive network.

Additionally, the biopsychosocial model emphasizes the importance of prevention and early intervention. By recognizing the various factors that contribute to depression, strategies can be implemented to prevent its onset or intervene at an early stage. This may involve promoting healthy lifestyles, educating individuals about recognizing early symptoms, and addressing social determinants such as reducing stigma and improving access to mental health services.

In conclusion, the biopsychosocial model provides a comprehensive framework for understanding and addressing mental health issues. It considers the interplay between biological, psychological, and social factors, emphasizing the need for a holistic approach to mental health care. By using this model, healthcare practitioners and policymakers can develop strategies that promote the well-being and resilience of individuals and communities.

Integrative Medicine in Mental Health Care

Integrative medicine is an approach that combines conventional medical treatments with complementary and alternative therapies to promote overall health and well-being. In the context of mental health care, integrative medicine focuses on incorporating evidence-based holistic interventions alongside traditional psychiatric treatments. This section explores the principles, benefits, and applications of integrative medicine in mental health care.

Principles of Integrative Medicine

Integrative medicine recognizes the interconnectedness of the mind, body, and spirit and seeks to address all aspects of a person's well-being. The following principles guide the practice of integrative medicine in mental health care:

1. **Holistic Perspective:** Integrative medicine views mental health as more than just the absence of disease. It emphasizes the balance and integration of physical, emotional, mental, social, and spiritual aspects of an individual's life.

2. **Patient-Centered Approach:** Integrative medicine prioritizes collaboration between the patient and healthcare team. It values the patient's preferences and includes them in the decision-making process.

3. **Evidence-Informed Therapies:** Integrative medicine incorporates therapies that have scientific evidence supporting their efficacy and safety. It also values personalized treatments tailored to the individual's unique needs.

4. **Emphasis on Prevention:** Integrative medicine promotes proactive strategies to prevent mental health issues and improve overall well-being. It recognizes the importance of lifestyle modifications, stress reduction techniques, and early intervention.

5. **Integration of Multiple Disciplines:** Integrative medicine draws from various healthcare disciplines, including conventional medicine, psychology, nutrition, mind-body practices, and complementary therapies. It encourages a collaborative and multidisciplinary approach to patient care.

6. **Promotion of Self-Healing:** Integrative medicine recognizes the inherent healing capacity within individuals. It aims to support and enhance the body's natural ability to heal by addressing underlying imbalances and supporting optimal functioning.

Benefits of Integrative Medicine in Mental Health Care

Integrative medicine offers several benefits for individuals seeking mental health care. Some key advantages include:

- **Comprehensive Treatment:** Integrative medicine combines conventional treatments such as medications and psychotherapy with complementary and alternative therapies. This approach addresses a broader range of mental health challenges and provides more comprehensive care.

- **Personalized Approach:** Integrative medicine recognizes that mental health is unique to each individual, and there is no one-size-fits-all solution. By incorporating personalized treatments, it enables tailored interventions that resonate with the patient's specific needs and preferences.

- **Reduced Side Effects:** Integrative medicine often includes non-pharmacological interventions, which can minimize the reliance on medications and reduce the risk of associated side effects. This approach can be particularly beneficial for individuals who prefer a more natural and holistic approach to mental health care.

- **Enhanced Well-being:** Integrative medicine focuses on promoting overall well-being, not just symptom management. By addressing various aspects of a person's life, such as diet, exercise, stress reduction, and social support, it aims to improve mental health and enhance quality of life.

- **Empowerment and Engagement:** Integrative medicine encourages active participation and self-care. Patients are often involved in decision-making and empowered to take charge of their mental health. This approach fosters a sense of ownership and enables individuals to become active agents in their healing process.

Applications of Integrative Medicine in Mental Health Care

Integrative medicine offers a wide range of therapeutic approaches that can be employed in mental health care. Some common applications include:

1. **Nutrition:** Proper nutrition plays a crucial role in mental health. Integrative medicine incorporates dietary interventions, such as a balanced diet rich in nutrients, to support brain function and emotional well-being.

2. **Mind-Body Practices:** Techniques like mindfulness meditation, yoga, and tai chi promote relaxation, reduce stress, and enhance self-awareness. Integrative medicine often includes these practices to manage symptoms of anxiety, depression, and other mental health disorders.

HOLISTIC APPROACHES TO MENTAL HEALTH

3. **Supplements and natural remedies:** Certain supplements and herbal remedies have shown promise in managing mental health conditions. Integrative medicine utilizes evidence-based natural therapies, such as omega-3 fatty acids, St. John's Wort, and lavender, to complement conventional treatments.

4. **Acupuncture:** Based on traditional Chinese medicine, acupuncture involves the insertion of thin needles into specific points on the body. Integrative medicine may incorporate acupuncture to alleviate symptoms of anxiety, depression, and post-traumatic stress disorder (PTSD).

5. **Art and Music Therapy:** Creative arts therapies, such as art therapy and music therapy, provide expressive outlets for emotional healing and self-expression. Integrative medicine utilizes these modalities to complement traditional talk therapies in the treatment of mental health disorders.

6. **Exercise and Physical Activity:** Regular exercise has been shown to have positive effects on mental health. Integrative medicine may recommend exercise as an adjunctive therapy to reduce symptoms of depression, anxiety, and stress.

Considerations and Challenges

While integrative medicine offers valuable contributions to mental health care, several considerations and challenges should be recognized:

- **Evidence-Based Practice:** It is essential to ensure that the complementary and alternative therapies included in integrative medicine are well-researched and evidence-based. Robust scientific evidence is necessary to support their use and make informed decisions about their suitability for individual patients.

- **Safety and Regulation:** Integrative medicine encompasses a wide range of interventions, including dietary supplements, herbs, and other natural remedies. It is crucial to ensure their safety, quality, and appropriate regulation to protect patients from potential harm or interactions with other treatments.

- **Collaborative Communication:** Effective communication and collaboration between conventional healthcare providers and practitioners of complementary therapies are essential. This coordination ensures comprehensive and cohesive care for patients and minimizes the risk of potential interactions or conflicts.

- **Patient Education and Informed Consent:** Patients should be well-informed about the risks, benefits, and limitations of integrative medicine approaches. Informed consent and ongoing education empower patients to make informed decisions and actively engage in their treatment plans.

By embracing the principles of integrative medicine and incorporating evidence-based complementary and alternative therapies, mental health care can become more comprehensive, personalized, and holistic. It is essential for practitioners, researchers, and policymakers to continue exploring the potential of integrative medicine in promoting mental health and well-being.

Example Problem:

Imagine a patient with anxiety disorder who is interested in exploring integrative medicine approaches. Discuss one evidence-based complementary therapy that may be beneficial for managing anxiety symptoms and explain how it can be incorporated into their treatment plan.

Solution:

One evidence-based complementary therapy for managing anxiety symptoms is mindfulness meditation. Mindfulness involves intentionally paying attention to the present moment, without judgment. Numerous studies have shown that mindfulness meditation can reduce anxiety and improve overall well-being.

Incorporating mindfulness into the patient's treatment plan can be done through various means:

1. **Guided Meditation:** The patient can attend mindfulness-based stress reduction (MBSR) classes or use smartphone applications that provide guided mindfulness meditation sessions. These resources offer step-by-step instructions and allow individuals to practice mindfulness in a structured and supportive environment.

2. **Daily Practice:** The patient can allocate a specific time each day to engage in mindfulness meditation. Even just a few minutes of mindful breathing or body scan exercises can help reduce anxiety symptoms over time. Encouraging regular practice is crucial for experiencing the benefits of mindfulness.

3. **Integration into Daily Activities:** Mindfulness can be incorporated into various daily activities, such as eating, walking, or taking a shower. The patient can

practice being fully present and non-judgmental during these moments, focusing on the sensory experiences and their breath.

4. **Group Support:** The patient may benefit from joining mindfulness meditation groups or support groups where they can share experiences and insights with like-minded individuals. Group settings can foster a sense of connection and provide additional support during the mindfulness journey.

Before recommending mindfulness meditation, it is important to assess the patient's readiness and willingness to engage in this practice. Some individuals may find it challenging to sit still or struggle with racing thoughts during meditation. In such cases, it can be helpful to start with shorter sessions or explore other complementary therapies that might better suit their needs and preferences.

Overall, mindfulness meditation is one example of an evidence-based complementary therapy that can be integrated into a comprehensive treatment plan for anxiety disorders. Its inclusion in mental health care highlights the principle of integrative medicine, which recognizes the importance of addressing the mind-body connection for promoting holistic well-being.

Complementary and Alternative Therapies

Complementary and alternative therapies, also known as CAM therapies, are non-conventional approaches to healthcare that aim to promote health and well-being. These therapies are often used alongside traditional medical treatments to enhance their effectiveness or to address specific aspects of a person's health that may not be adequately addressed by conventional medicine alone.

Background

The use of complementary and alternative therapies dates back to ancient times, and many traditional healing practices have been incorporated into modern CAM approaches. These therapies acknowledge the interconnectedness of the mind, body, and spirit and emphasize the importance of treating the whole person rather than just the symptoms of a specific illness or condition.

In recent years, there has been a growing interest in CAM therapies as individuals seek more holistic and natural approaches to their health and well-being. These therapies can encompass a wide range of practices, including herbal medicine, acupuncture, chiropractic care, massage therapy, yoga, meditation, and many others.

Principles of Complementary and Alternative Therapies

Complementary and alternative therapies are guided by several principles that differentiate them from conventional medicine:

1. Holistic Approach: CAM therapies focus on treating the whole person, taking into account their physical, mental, emotional, and spiritual aspects. They recognize that health is a complex interplay of various factors and aim to restore balance and harmony within the individual.

2. Individualized Treatment: CAM therapies emphasize personalized care, tailoring treatments to each person's unique needs. Practitioners spend more time with patients, obtaining a comprehensive understanding of their health history, lifestyle, and goals in order to develop a targeted and effective treatment plan.

3. Natural and Non-Invasive: CAM therapies often utilize natural substances or techniques to support the body's inherent healing abilities. They aim to stimulate self-healing processes, minimize side effects, and promote the body's own capacity for well-being.

4. Integration with Conventional Medicine: CAM therapies are typically used alongside traditional medical treatments, with the goal of enhancing overall outcomes. They can complement the benefits of conventional treatments, provide additional support, and help manage side effects or improve quality of life.

Common Complementary and Alternative Therapies

There is a wide array of complementary and alternative therapies available, each with its own unique principles and benefits. Here, we discuss some of the most commonly used therapies:

Herbal Medicine Herbal medicine, also known as botanical medicine, utilizes plant extracts, herbs, and other natural substances to promote health and treat illnesses. Traditional knowledge about the medicinal properties of plants forms the basis of herbal medicine. These natural substances can be taken orally, applied topically, or used in various preparations, such as teas, tinctures, or capsules. Some examples of commonly used herbs include echinacea, ginkgo biloba, and St. John's wort.

Acupuncture Acupuncture is an ancient Chinese therapy that involves the insertion of thin needles into specific points on the body. These acupuncture points are believed to be connected through energy channels or meridians, and stimulation of these points is thought to restore the flow of energy and promote healing. Acupuncture is commonly used for pain management, stress reduction, and overall well-being.

Chiropractic Care Chiropractic care focuses on the diagnosis and treatment of musculoskeletal disorders, primarily those affecting the spine. Chiropractors use manual techniques, such as spinal manipulation and adjustment, to alleviate pain, improve joint function, and enhance the body's ability to heal itself. Chiropractic care is often sought for conditions such as back pain, neck pain, and headaches.

Massage Therapy Massage therapy involves the manipulation of soft tissues in the body, such as muscles, tendons, and ligaments, to promote relaxation, relieve tension, and improve overall well-being. Various techniques, including Swedish massage, deep tissue massage, and aromatherapy massage, are used depending on the individual's needs and preferences. Massage therapy can help reduce stress, alleviate pain, and improve circulation.

Yoga and Meditation Yoga is a mind-body practice that combines physical postures, breathing exercises, and meditation to enhance physical strength, flexibility, and mental well-being. It promotes mindfulness, relaxation, and self-awareness, and has been shown to have numerous health benefits, including stress reduction, improved sleep, and increased overall vitality. Meditation, on the other hand, involves focusing one's attention and eliminating the stream of thoughts to achieve a state of mental clarity and relaxation.

Safety and Efficacy Considerations

While many complementary and alternative therapies are safe and effective when used appropriately, it is important to approach them with caution and consult qualified practitioners. Here are some important considerations:

- Education and Certification: Ensure that practitioners of CAM therapies have proper education, certification, and experience in their field. This helps ensure that they adhere to standard practices and ethical guidelines.

- Communication with Conventional Healthcare Providers: It is crucial to inform your healthcare provider about any CAM therapies you are considering or currently undergoing. This enables them to provide comprehensive and coordinated care, considering potential interactions, contraindications, or any other relevant considerations.

- Individual Variability: Each person may respond differently to complementary and alternative therapies. What works for one individual may not work for another. It is important to be open-minded and patient while exploring different approaches to find what best suits your needs and preferences.

- Evidence-Informed Decision Making: Seek evidence-based information about the safety and effectiveness of specific CAM therapies. Look for credible sources, such as reputable scientific journals, systematic reviews, or recommendations from trusted healthcare organizations.

It is worth noting that while some complementary and alternative therapies have a growing body of scientific evidence supporting their efficacy, others may have limited research or conflicting findings. More research is needed to better understand the mechanisms of action, optimal uses, and potential risks associated with these therapies.

Conclusion

Complementary and alternative therapies offer a diverse range of approaches to promote health and well-being. When used alongside conventional medicine, these therapies can enhance the overall effectiveness of healthcare practices and provide individuals with additional tools to support their physical, mental, and emotional well-being. However, it is important to approach these therapies with an informed and cautious mindset, considering safety, efficacy, and individual variability. By integrating complementary and alternative therapies into a comprehensive healthcare plan, individuals can work towards achieving a more holistic and sustainable approach to their mental health and overall well-being.

Mind-Body Connection in Holistic Health

The mind and body are interconnected, and this relationship forms the basis of holistic health practices. In the context of mental health, the mind-body connection emphasizes the influence of psychological factors on physical well-being and vice versa. This section explores the concept of the mind-body connection, its role in holistic health, and its implications for mental health care.

Understanding the Mind-Body Connection

The mind-body connection refers to the dynamic interaction between the mind (including thoughts, emotions, and beliefs) and the body (including physiological processes and physical health). This connection is bidirectional, meaning that changes in the mind can impact the body, and changes in the body can impact the mind.

According to the biopsychosocial model, which considers biological, psychological, and social factors in health and illness, the mind and body are intertwined. This model recognizes that mental health issues can manifest physically and that physical health problems can affect mental well-being. For example, chronic stress and anxiety can lead to physical symptoms like headaches, muscle tension, and digestive issues.

The Role of Psychoneuroimmunology

Psychoneuroimmunology is a field of study that explores the relationships between psychological processes, the central nervous system, and the immune system. It examines how psychological factors, such as stress and emotions, can impact immune function and overall health.

Research in psychoneuroimmunology has shown that stress hormones, such as cortisol, can suppress immune function and increase susceptibility to illness. Conversely, positive emotions and practices like mindfulness and meditation have been found to boost immune system activity and enhance overall well-being.

Implications for Holistic Health Care

Recognizing the mind-body connection has important implications for holistic health care. Holistic approaches aim to address the whole person, including their physical, mental, emotional, and spiritual well-being. By considering the mind-body connection, practitioners can develop comprehensive treatment plans that target both physical and psychological aspects of health.

In mental health care, interventions that leverage the mind-body connection can be effective in managing various conditions. For example, mindfulness-based stress reduction techniques have been shown to reduce symptoms of anxiety and depression by promoting self-awareness, improving emotion regulation, and reducing physiological arousal.

Additionally, integrating mind-body practices like yoga and Tai Chi into treatment plans can enhance overall well-being. These practices combine physical movement, breath control, and meditation, promoting relaxation, stress reduction, and mind-body integration.

Promoting the Mind-Body Connection

To promote the mind-body connection in holistic health, individuals can engage in self-care practices that nurture both their mental and physical well-being. Some strategies to consider include:

- Regular physical activity: Engaging in physical exercise not only benefits the body but also supports mental health by reducing stress, boosting mood, and improving sleep.

- Mindfulness and meditation: Taking time for mindfulness exercises or meditation can help individuals become more attuned to their thoughts, emotions, and bodily sensations, fostering a stronger mind-body connection.

- Nutrition and hydration: Consuming a balanced diet and staying hydrated are essential for optimal physical and mental health. Proper nourishment supports brain function and overall well-being.

- Adequate sleep: Getting enough quality sleep is crucial for mental and physical restoration. Poor sleep can negatively impact mood, cognitive function, and immune system functioning.

- Social support: Cultivating positive social connections and seeking support from others can contribute to mental and physical health. Social support provides a sense of belonging and emotional well-being.

Case Study: Mind-Body Connection in Chronic Pain Management

Chronic pain is a multifaceted condition that can significantly impact a person's physical and mental well-being. In a holistic approach to chronic pain management, addressing the mind-body connection is crucial.

For example, a patient with chronic lower back pain may benefit from a comprehensive treatment plan that includes physical therapy to address the underlying physical issues, along with psychological interventions like cognitive-behavioral therapy to manage pain-related thoughts and emotions.

Mind-body practices such as yoga or meditation can also be integrated to promote relaxation, reduce muscle tension, and enhance overall well-being.

By recognizing the mind-body connection in chronic pain management, healthcare providers can improve treatment outcomes and empower patients to take an active role in their own healing process.

Conclusion

Understanding and harnessing the mind-body connection is essential in promoting holistic health. By recognizing the bidirectional relationship between the mind and body, practitioners and individuals can develop effective strategies to support mental and physical well-being. Incorporating mind-body practices into holistic health care can enhance overall resilience and contribute to sustainable mental health. Embracing the mind-body connection is a key step towards a comprehensive and effective approach to mental health and well-being in contemporary society.

Nutrition and Mental Health

Sure! Here's an example of how you can write the content of the section "3.3.1 The Gut-Brain Connection":

The Gut-Brain Connection

The gut-brain connection refers to the bidirectional communication system between the gastrointestinal tract (the gut) and the brain. It involves complex interactions between the central nervous system (CNS), enteric nervous system (ENS), and the gut microbiota. This connection plays a crucial role in maintaining mental health and overall well-being.

Background

The gut-brain connection has been recognized for centuries, with ancient Greek philosophers contemplating the link between emotions and digestion. However, it is only in recent years that scientific research has shed light on the intricate mechanisms underlying this relationship.

The gut and the brain are connected through the vagus nerve, a cranial nerve that carries signals from the gut to the brain and vice versa. Additionally, the ENS, often referred to as the "second brain," is a complex network of neurons located within the walls of the gastrointestinal tract. The ENS can operate independently, but it also communicates with the brain through the vagus nerve.

Principles of the Gut-Brain Connection

Several key principles govern the gut-brain connection:

1. Neurotransmitters: The gut produces and releases various neurotransmitters, including serotonin, dopamine, and gamma-aminobutyric acid (GABA). These neurotransmitters play essential roles in regulating mood, emotions, and cognition.

2. Microbiota: The gut is inhabited by trillions of microorganisms collectively known as the gut microbiota. This diverse ecosystem of bacteria, viruses, and fungi can influence brain development, behavior, and mental health. The microbiota produces metabolites and neurotransmitters that can directly affect the central nervous system.

3. Immune System: The gut is closely linked to the immune system, and immune activation in the gut can impact the brain. Chronic inflammation in the gut has been associated with an increased risk of mental health disorders, such as depression and anxiety.

The Impact of Gut Health on Mental Health

Emerging research suggests that disruptions in the gut-brain connection can contribute to the development of mental health disorders. For example:

- Depression and Anxiety: Alterations in gut microbiota composition have been observed in individuals with depression and anxiety disorders. Furthermore, studies have shown that probiotics and prebiotics, which positively modulate gut microbiota, can improve symptoms of these disorders.

- Stress Response: The gut-brain connection plays a crucial role in modulating the body's stress response. Chronic stress can disrupt the balance of gut microbiota and increase the production of stress hormones, leading to an increased susceptibility to stress-related disorders.

- Neurodegenerative Diseases: Growing evidence suggests that the gut-brain axis is involved in the development and progression of neurodegenerative diseases, such as Alzheimer's and Parkinson's disease. Dysregulation of gut microbiota and inflammation in the gut have been implicated in the pathogenesis of these conditions.

Interventions to Improve Gut Health and Mental Well-being

Taking care of gut health is crucial for promoting mental well-being. Here are some strategies to improve gut health:

- Healthy Diet: Consuming a diet rich in fiber, fruits, vegetables, and fermented foods supports a diverse and healthy gut microbiota. Avoiding excessive sugar, processed foods, and artificial additives is also important.

- Probiotics and Prebiotics: Probiotics are live microorganisms that can confer health benefits when consumed, while prebiotics are dietary fibers that promote the growth of beneficial gut bacteria. Including probiotic-rich foods (e.g., yogurt, kefir) and prebiotic-rich foods (e.g., onions, garlic) in the diet can support a healthy gut microbiota.

- Mind-Body Practices: Stress management techniques, such as meditation, mindfulness, and relaxation exercises, can help regulate the stress response and improve gut health. These practices promote a state of calmness, which positively influences gut function and microbiota.

- Physical Activity: Regular exercise has been associated with a more diverse gut microbiota and improved mental health outcomes. Engaging in aerobic and resistance exercises can positively influence gut health and overall well-being.

Conclusion

Understanding and nurturing the gut-brain connection is vital for promoting mental health and overall well-being. By adopting a holistic approach that encompasses diet, lifestyle, and psychological interventions, individuals can optimize their gut health and support their mental well-being. Ongoing research in this field holds promise for the development of innovative treatments and interventions targeting the gut-brain connection.

Nutritional Psychiatry

Nutritional psychiatry is an emerging field that explores the relationship between diet and mental health. It focuses on the impact of nutrition on brain function and the development, prevention, and treatment of mental disorders. This section will delve into the principles of nutritional psychiatry, dietary recommendations for mental health, and the role of nutrition in the management of mental health disorders.

Principles of Nutritional Psychiatry

The field of nutritional psychiatry is based on several key principles:

1. **The Gut-Brain Axis:** The gut and brain are interconnected through a bidirectional communication system known as the gut-brain axis. This axis involves the complex interactions between the central nervous system, the enteric nervous system, and the gut microbiota. The gut microbiota play a crucial role in regulating brain function, behavior, and mental health.

2. **Inflammation and Oxidative Stress:** Inflammation and oxidative stress are implicated in the development and progression of mental health disorders. Diet can modulate these processes, either exacerbating or mitigating their impact on mental health. A diet rich in anti-inflammatory and antioxidant nutrients can help reduce inflammation and oxidative stress, promoting better mental health.

3. **Neurotransmitter Production:** Neurotransmitters, such as serotonin and dopamine, play a critical role in mood regulation and mental well-being. Certain nutrients, such as tryptophan and tyrosine, are precursors for neurotransmitter production. Adequate intake of these nutrients is essential for optimal brain function.

4. **Micronutrient Status:** Micronutrients, including vitamins, minerals, and omega-3 fatty acids, are essential for brain health and function. Deficiencies in these micronutrients have been linked to an increased risk of mental health disorders. A well-balanced diet that includes a variety of nutrient-dense foods can help maintain optimal micronutrient status.

Dietary Recommendations for Mental Health

Research suggests that certain dietary patterns are associated with improved mental health outcomes. While individual nutritional needs may vary, the following recommendations can serve as a general guide:

1. **Mediterranean Diet:** The Mediterranean diet, characterized by high consumption of fruits, vegetables, legumes, whole grains, fish, and healthy fats (such as olive oil and nuts), has been consistently linked to a reduced risk of depression and other mental health disorders. This dietary pattern provides important nutrients and antioxidants that support brain health.

2. **Anti-inflammatory Diet:** Chronic low-grade inflammation has been associated with mental health disorders. Following an anti-inflammatory diet, which includes foods rich in omega-3 fatty acids (such as fatty fish), colorful fruits and vegetables, whole grains, and healthy fats, can help reduce inflammation and support mental well-being.

3. **Probiotics and Prebiotics:** Probiotics are beneficial bacteria that promote a healthy gut microbiota. Consuming foods rich in probiotics, such as yogurt and fermented vegetables, or taking probiotic supplements may help support mental health. Prebiotics, on the other hand, are indigestible fibers that serve as food for probiotics. Including prebiotic-rich foods, like bananas, onions, and garlic, can help nurture a healthy gut microbiota.

4. **Avoid or Limit Processed Foods:** Processed foods, which are often high in added sugars, unhealthy fats, and artificial additives, have been associated with an increased risk of mental health disorders. Limiting the consumption of processed foods and focusing on whole, unprocessed foods is beneficial for mental health.

5. **Hydration:** Dehydration can negatively impact cognitive function and mood. Staying adequately hydrated by drinking water and consuming hydrating foods, such as fruits and vegetables with high water content, is essential for optimal brain function.

The Role of Nutrition in Mental Health Disorders

Nutritional interventions can play a significant role in the management of mental health disorders. While they should never replace conventional treatments, they can be complementary and beneficial in promoting better mental well-being. Here are some examples:

1. **Depression:** Research suggests that certain nutrients, such as omega-3 fatty acids, B vitamins, vitamin D, and folate, may have a positive impact on depressive symptoms. Incorporating sources of these nutrients into the diet, such as fatty fish, leafy green vegetables, legumes, and fortified foods, may help support individuals with depression.

2. **Anxiety:** Some studies have shown that magnesium, zinc, and certain herbal supplements, such as passionflower and chamomile, may help reduce anxiety symptoms. Additionally, avoiding caffeine and incorporating relaxation-promoting foods, like herbal teas, can contribute to a calmer state of mind.

3. **ADHD:** While there is no specific "ADHD diet," some evidence suggests that increasing the intake of omega-3 fatty acids, iron, zinc, and magnesium may help manage ADHD symptoms. Including foods like fatty fish, lean meats, whole grains, and dark chocolate can provide these essential nutrients.

4. **Schizophrenia:** Some research has explored the potential benefits of certain nutrients, such as omega-3 fatty acids and antioxidants, in managing symptoms of schizophrenia. A well-rounded diet that includes fatty fish, nuts, seeds, fruits, and vegetables can support overall mental health in individuals with schizophrenia.

5. **Eating Disorders:** Nutritional rehabilitation is a critical component of eating disorder treatment. Registered dietitians play a crucial role in developing individualized meal plans, focusing on balanced nutrition, and addressing any nutrient deficiencies. Supporting a positive and healthy relationship with food is essential in the recovery process.

Overall, focusing on a nutritious, well-balanced diet is essential for optimal mental health. Nutritional psychiatry offers a holistic approach that complements traditional mental health interventions, emphasizing the importance of nutrition in promoting mental well-being. By incorporating these principles and dietary recommendations, individuals can support their mental health and overall quality of life.

Dietary Recommendations for Mental Health

In recent years, there has been increasing interest in the connection between nutrition and mental health. It is now widely recognized that the foods we consume can have a significant impact on our mental well-being. In this section, we will explore the role of diet in promoting mental health and discuss dietary recommendations that can support optimal mental well-being.

The Gut-Brain Connection

Before diving into specific dietary recommendations, it is crucial to understand the gut-brain connection. The gut and the brain are intricately connected, and they communicate through a bidirectional pathway known as the gut-brain axis. This axis involves the nervous system, immune system, and endocrine system, and it plays a crucial role in regulating our emotions, mood, and cognitive function.

The gut microbiota, which consists of trillions of microorganisms residing in our digestive system, plays a crucial role in this communication. These microorganisms help break down food, produce essential nutrients, and modulate key neurotransmitters involved in mood regulation, such as serotonin and dopamine.

A healthy gut microbiota has been linked to improved mental health, while an imbalance in the gut microbial composition, known as dysbiosis, has been associated with mental health disorders such as depression and anxiety. Therefore, optimizing gut health through diet can have a significant impact on mental well-being.

Nutritional Psychiatry

The emerging field of nutritional psychiatry focuses on the relationship between diet and mental health. Research has found that certain nutrients can influence brain function and play a role in the development and management of mental health conditions.

Here are some dietary recommendations that can support mental health:

- **Eat a balanced diet:** A balanced diet that includes a variety of whole foods is essential for overall well-being, including mental health. Aim to consume a wide range of fruits, vegetables, whole grains, lean proteins, and healthy fats.

- **Increase omega-3 fatty acids:** Omega-3 fatty acids, found in fatty fish (such as salmon and sardines), walnuts, flaxseeds, and chia seeds, have been shown to have antidepressant and anti-inflammatory effects. Including these foods in your diet can help support brain health and reduce symptoms of depression and anxiety.

- **Consume adequate antioxidants:** Antioxidants protect against oxidative stress, which can contribute to mental health disorders. Include foods rich in antioxidants, such as berries, dark chocolate, spinach, and nuts, in your diet.

- **Ensure sufficient B vitamins:** B vitamins play a vital role in brain health and the production of neurotransmitters. Include foods rich in B vitamins, such as whole grains, legumes, leafy greens, and eggs, in your diet.

- **Moderate caffeine and alcohol intake:** While caffeine can provide a temporary energy boost, excessive consumption can disrupt sleep and contribute to anxiety. Similarly, excessive alcohol intake can worsen mood symptoms. It is important to consume these substances in moderation.

- **Stay hydrated:** Dehydration can affect cognitive function and mood. Make sure to drink enough water throughout the day to maintain proper hydration.

- **Consider probiotics:** Probiotics are beneficial bacteria that can help restore and maintain a healthy gut microbiota. Including probiotic-rich foods, such as yogurt, kefir, sauerkraut, and kimchi, in your diet can support gut health and potentially improve mental well-being.

It is important to note that while nutrition can play a significant role in mental health, it is not a standalone treatment for mental health disorders. It should be considered as part of a comprehensive treatment plan, including therapy, medication (if necessary), and lifestyle changes.

Practical Tips and Caveats

Incorporating dietary recommendations for mental health into your daily life can be challenging. Here are some practical tips to help you implement these recommendations:

- **Plan ahead:** Plan your meals and snacks in advance to ensure you have access to nutritious options throughout the day.

- **Cook at home:** Cooking meals at home gives you more control over the ingredients and allows you to make healthier choices.

- **Be mindful of portion sizes:** While certain foods are beneficial for mental health, it is essential to consume them in appropriate portion sizes to maintain a balanced diet.

- Seek professional guidance: If you have specific dietary restrictions or conditions, such as allergies or chronic illnesses, consider consulting a registered dietitian or healthcare provider for personalized recommendations.

It is also important to note that individual responses to dietary interventions may vary, and it may take time to notice significant changes in mental well-being. It is essential to listen to your body and make adjustments that work best for you.

Conclusion

Nutrition plays a crucial role in mental health, and adopting a balanced diet that supports the gut-brain connection can have positive effects on overall well-being. The dietary recommendations discussed in this section provide a starting point for creating a nutritionally sound diet that supports mental health. Remember, small changes in your diet can lead to significant improvements in your mental well-being.

Nutritional Interventions for Mental Health Disorders

Nutrition plays a crucial role in maintaining overall health and well-being. It not only affects physical health but also has a significant impact on mental health. Research has shown that certain nutritional interventions can be beneficial in the prevention and management of mental health disorders. In this section, we will explore the role of nutrition in mental health and highlight some key interventions that can help in the treatment of various mental health disorders.

The Gut-Brain Connection

The gut-brain connection refers to the bidirectional communication between the gastrointestinal system and the brain. The gut, often referred to as the "second brain," contains a complex network of neurons that communicate with the central nervous system. This communication occurs via various pathways, including the vagus nerve, hormones, and neurotransmitters.

Emerging evidence suggests that the gut microbiota, the diverse community of microorganisms residing in the gastrointestinal tract, plays a crucial role in this connection. The gut microbiota produces neurotransmitters, such as serotonin and dopamine, that are essential for maintaining stable mood and cognitive function. It also influences the production of inflammatory molecules and regulates the body's stress response.

Research has shown that alterations in the gut microbiota composition, known as dysbiosis, are associated with an increased risk of mental health disorders, including depression, anxiety, and autism spectrum disorder. Therefore, targeting the gut microbiota through dietary interventions is a promising approach for improving mental health outcomes.

Nutritional Psychiatry

Nutritional psychiatry is an emerging field that focuses on the relationship between diet and mental health. It explores the impact of food and nutrients on brain structure, function, and mental well-being. Several dietary patterns have been identified as beneficial for mental health, including the Mediterranean diet, the DASH (Dietary Approaches to Stop Hypertension) diet, and the traditional Japanese diet.

Key components of these dietary patterns include:

- **Whole foods:** Emphasizing the consumption of minimally processed foods, such as fruits, vegetables, whole grains, legumes, nuts, and seeds. These foods are rich in essential nutrients, antioxidants, and fiber, which support brain health and reduce inflammation.

- **Omega-3 fatty acids:** Found in fatty fish, walnuts, flaxseeds, and chia seeds, omega-3 fatty acids have been shown to have antidepressant and anti-inflammatory effects. They are essential for brain development and function.

- **Probiotics and fermented foods:** Probiotics, such as those found in yogurt and fermented foods like kimchi and sauerkraut, can help restore gut microbiota balance and positively influence mental health. They may alleviate symptoms of depression and anxiety by modulating neurotransmitter production and reducing inflammation.

- **Antioxidants:** Found in colorful fruits and vegetables, antioxidants protect against oxidative stress and inflammation. They are thought to have a neuroprotective effect and may reduce the risk of mental health disorders.

Dietary Recommendations for Mental Health

While there is no one-size-fits-all dietary recommendation for mental health, incorporating the following principles into your diet can have a positive impact on mental well-being:

- **Balance and moderation:** Maintain a balanced diet that includes a variety of nutrient-dense foods. Avoid extreme diets or restrictive eating patterns, as they may lead to nutrient deficiencies or imbalances.

- **Reduce processed foods and added sugars:** Processed foods, including sugary snacks, sugary drinks, and refined grains, have been associated with an increased risk of mental health disorders. Limiting their consumption can help support mental well-being.

- **Stay hydrated:** Dehydration can negatively affect mood and cognitive function. Ensure an adequate intake of water and limit the consumption of sugary beverages and alcohol.

- **Personalize your diet:** Consider individual preferences, cultural backgrounds, and specific dietary needs when making food choices. Consulting with a registered dietitian can help develop a personalized nutrition plan.

Nutritional Interventions for Specific Mental Health Disorders

While a healthy diet is beneficial for overall mental health, specific nutritional interventions can also target certain mental health disorders. Here, we will discuss a few examples:

- **Depression and anxiety:** Supplementation with omega-3 fatty acids, particularly eicosapentaenoic acid (EPA) and docosahexaenoic acid (DHA), has shown promise in reducing depressive symptoms. Other nutrients, such as B vitamins, magnesium, and zinc, may also play a role in managing depression and anxiety.

- **Schizophrenia:** Individuals with schizophrenia often have higher levels of oxidative stress and inflammation. Antioxidant-rich foods, such as fruits and vegetables, may help reduce these markers and improve symptoms related to schizophrenia.

- **Bipolar disorder:** Ensuring a consistent intake of omega-3 fatty acids and maintaining stable blood sugar levels through regular, balanced meals may help manage mood swings and stabilize symptoms associated with bipolar disorder.

- **ADHD:** Limited evidence suggests that omega-3 fatty acid supplementation may improve attention and reduce hyperactivity in individuals with ADHD. Additionally, a well-balanced diet that includes sufficient protein, complex carbohydrates, and micronutrients may support optimal cognitive function.

Caution and Consultation

While nutritional interventions can be beneficial, it is important to approach them with caution. Individual responses to dietary changes may vary, and it is recommended to consult with a healthcare professional, such as a registered dietitian or a mental health provider, before making significant changes to your diet or starting any supplementation.

Additionally, nutritional interventions should not be used as a substitute for evidence-based treatments for mental health disorders. They should be seen as complementary approaches that can support overall well-being and mental health.

Conclusion

Nutritional interventions can be valuable in promoting mental health and managing mental health disorders. The gut-brain connection, along with the emerging field of nutritional psychiatry, highlights the importance of a well-balanced diet in maintaining mental well-being. By incorporating nutrient-dense foods, omega-3 fatty acids, probiotics, and antioxidants, individuals can support their mental health and enhance overall resilience. However, it is crucial to approach nutritional interventions with caution and consult with healthcare professionals to develop personalized and evidence-based strategies.

Exercise and Mental Health

The Benefits of Physical Activity on Mental Health

Physical activity has long been recognized for its positive effects on physical health, but its importance in promoting mental health is equally significant. Engaging in regular exercise has been shown to have numerous benefits for mental well-being, including reducing symptoms of depression and anxiety, improving mood and self-esteem, and enhancing overall cognitive function.

The Link Between Physical Activity and Mental Health

Physical activity has a direct impact on the brain and its functioning. When we engage in exercise, our bodies release endorphins, which are often referred to as "feel-good" hormones. These endorphins interact with receptors in the brain, reducing our perception of pain and triggering positive feelings. This release of endorphins during exercise contributes to an increased sense of well-being and improved mood.

Furthermore, physical activity stimulates the production of neurotransmitters such as serotonin and dopamine, which are involved in regulating mood and emotions. Serotonin, in particular, plays a crucial role in reducing symptoms of depression and anxiety. Regular exercise has been shown to increase serotonin levels, leading to a more positive mental state.

Reducing Symptoms of Depression and Anxiety

One of the most significant mental health benefits of physical activity is its ability to reduce symptoms of depression and anxiety. Numerous studies have consistently demonstrated that engaging in regular exercise can be as effective as medication or therapy in alleviating symptoms of depression.

Exercise not only increases the production of endorphins and neurotransmitters but also promotes changes in the brain's neural pathways. It helps to modulate stress responses, regulate emotions, and enhance the brain's ability to cope with anxiety and stress. Additionally, physical activity provides a sense of accomplishment and mastery, which can improve self-esteem and confidence.

Example: Research conducted at Harvard Medical School showed that individuals who engaged in a regular exercise routine experienced a significant decrease in symptoms of depression and anxiety after just 12 weeks compared to those who did not exercise.

Improving Mood and Self-esteem

Regular physical activity has been shown to improve mood and enhance overall well-being. Exercise helps to increase self-esteem and body image perception, which are crucial aspects of mental health. Engaging in physical activity not only improves physical fitness but also contributes to a positive self-perception and body satisfaction.

Furthermore, exercise provides an opportunity for social interaction and engagement with others, which can enhance social support and relationships.

Participating in group activities or team sports creates a sense of belonging and can help individuals overcome feelings of isolation or loneliness.

Enhancing Cognitive Function

In addition to its effects on mood and mental well-being, physical activity has also been shown to enhance cognitive function. Regular exercise improves memory, attention, and problem-solving skills, ultimately boosting overall cognitive performance.

Exercise increases blood flow to the brain, delivering oxygen and nutrients that are essential for optimal brain function. It also promotes the growth of new neurons and strengthens neural connections, particularly in areas of the brain associated with memory and learning.

Example: A study conducted at the University of Illinois found that students who engaged in regular physical activity performed better on cognitive tasks and had improved memory compared to their sedentary peers.

Incorporating Physical Activity into Daily Life

Integrating physical activity into daily life doesn't necessarily require a rigorous exercise routine. Simple activities such as walking, cycling, or gardening can provide mental health benefits. It's important to find an activity that you enjoy and that suits your lifestyle to ensure long-term adherence.

Tip: Consider incorporating physical activity into your daily routine by taking the stairs instead of the elevator, going for a short walk during lunch breaks, or participating in active hobbies such as dancing or swimming.

Conclusion

Physical activity is not only vital for physical health but also plays a crucial role in promoting mental well-being. The benefits of regular exercise on mental health are extensive, ranging from reducing symptoms of depression and anxiety to improving mood, self-esteem, and cognitive function.

By incorporating physical activity into our daily lives, we can enhance our mental well-being and overall quality of life. Whether it's engaging in structured exercise programs or incorporating more movement into our routines, the positive impact on mental health is well worth the effort. So, let's get moving and prioritize our mental health through physical activity.

Remember, always consult with a healthcare professional before starting any exercise regimen, especially if you have any pre-existing health conditions.

Exercise as an Adjunctive Treatment for Mental Illness

Exercise has long been recognized for its positive impact on physical health. However, recent research has shown that exercise can also have significant benefits for mental health. In fact, exercise is now recognized as an adjunctive treatment for various mental illnesses, including depression, anxiety disorders, bipolar disorder, and schizophrenia. In this section, we will explore the effects of exercise on mental health and how it can be integrated into mental health care.

The Impact of Exercise on Mental Health

Regular physical activity has been shown to have numerous benefits for mental health. Exercise can improve mood, reduce symptoms of depression and anxiety, boost self-esteem, enhance cognitive function, and improve sleep quality. These effects are thought to be due to the release of endorphins, neurotransmitters that promote feelings of happiness and well-being.

Moreover, exercise has been found to have neuroprotective effects on the brain. It can increase the production of brain-derived neurotrophic factor (BDNF), a protein that helps support and promote the growth of new neurons. BDNF plays a crucial role in neuroplasticity, the brain's ability to adapt and change in response to new experiences and challenges. By enhancing neuroplasticity, exercise can help protect against cognitive decline and improve overall brain health.

Exercise as an Adjunctive Treatment

Exercise is not meant to replace traditional treatments for mental illnesses, but rather to complement them. It can be used as an adjunctive treatment to enhance the effectiveness of other interventions such as medication and therapy.

For individuals with depression, research has consistently shown that exercise can be as effective as antidepressant medication in reducing symptoms. Exercise increases the production of serotonin, a neurotransmitter involved in regulating mood, which can help alleviate depressive symptoms. Additionally, engaging in physical activity provides individuals with a sense of accomplishment and mastery, which can boost self-esteem and improve overall well-being.

In the case of anxiety disorders, exercise has been found to reduce symptoms by promoting relaxation and reducing the physiological effects of anxiety. Physical activity can help individuals manage stress, which is often a trigger for anxiety symptoms. Moreover, exercise can serve as a distraction from anxious thoughts and provide individuals with a sense of control over their body and mind.

For individuals with bipolar disorder, exercise can help stabilize mood and reduce the severity and frequency of mood swings. Regular exercise can regulate sleep patterns, increase energy levels, and improve overall functioning. It is important, however, for individuals with bipolar disorder to work closely with their healthcare provider to monitor their exercise routine and ensure that it is balanced and not triggering manic or hypomanic episodes.

In the case of schizophrenia, exercise has been shown to improve cognitive function, reduce negative symptoms, and enhance social functioning. Physical activity can help individuals with schizophrenia regain a sense of control over their body, improve their self-confidence, and promote social interaction. Importantly, exercise programs for individuals with schizophrenia should be tailored to their individual needs and abilities.

Integrating Exercise into Mental Health Care

To effectively integrate exercise into mental health care, a multidisciplinary approach is essential. Mental health professionals, such as psychiatrists, psychologists, and social workers, should collaborate with exercise specialists, such as physical therapists or certified trainers, to develop personalized exercise programs for individuals with mental illnesses.

It is important to assess the individual's physical health and fitness level before prescribing an exercise routine. This can be done through a comprehensive evaluation that includes a medical history, physical examination, and, if necessary, fitness tests. Based on the assessment, an exercise program can be designed to meet the individual's specific needs and goals.

The exercise program should be tailored to the individual's preferences and abilities to ensure adherence and sustainability. It should include a combination of aerobic exercise, such as walking, jogging, or cycling, and strength training exercises to improve muscular strength and endurance. Additionally, incorporating enjoyable activities, such as dancing or team sports, can help enhance motivation and long-term adherence.

To support individuals in incorporating exercise into their daily routine, it can be helpful to provide education and resources on physical activity and mental health. This can include information on the benefits of exercise, tips for overcoming barriers to exercise, and strategies for maintaining motivation. Additionally, providing access to fitness facilities, group exercise classes, or community-based exercise programs can facilitate engagement and social support.

Case Study: Exercise as an Adjunctive Treatment for Depression

Sarah, a 35-year-old woman, has been struggling with depression for the past year. Despite receiving therapy and medication, she continues to experience low mood, lack of motivation, and fatigue. Sarah's therapist suggests incorporating exercise into her treatment plan as an adjunctive treatment.

Sarah starts by engaging in regular brisk walking for 30 minutes a day, five days a week. She gradually increases the intensity and duration of her exercise, incorporating jogging and strength training exercises. Sarah finds that exercise boosts her mood, increases her energy levels, and provides a sense of accomplishment.

In addition to the physical benefits, exercise also helps Sarah manage stress and improve her sleep quality. She notices that her depressive symptoms decrease, and she feels more engaged in her therapy sessions. Sarah continues to work closely with her therapist and healthcare provider to monitor her progress and adjust her treatment plan as needed.

Conclusion

Exercise is a powerful adjunctive treatment for mental illnesses, offering numerous benefits for individuals' mental well-being. It can improve mood, reduce symptoms of depression and anxiety, enhance cognitive function, and promote overall brain health. By integrating exercise into mental health care, individuals can take an active role in their treatment and experience enhanced overall outcomes. The collaboration between mental health professionals and exercise specialists is key to developing personalized exercise programs that address individuals' unique needs and goals. With a multidisciplinary approach, exercise can play a crucial role in promoting mental health and well-being.

Integrating Exercise into Mental Health Care

Exercise has long been recognized for its physical health benefits, but its positive impact on mental health is becoming increasingly evident. Integrating exercise into mental health care has shown promising results in improving overall well-being and functioning. In this section, we will explore the benefits of exercise for mental health, discuss different ways to incorporate exercise into a mental health care plan, and provide practical strategies for promoting regular physical activity.

The Benefits of Exercise for Mental Health

Engaging in regular exercise has been found to have numerous benefits for mental health. Physical activity can help reduce symptoms of depression, anxiety, and stress. It has also been shown to improve mood, enhance cognitive function, boost self-esteem, and promote better sleep.

Exercise has a positive impact on the brain and neurotransmitter activity, leading to the release of endorphins, also known as "feel-good" hormones. These endorphins act as natural mood lifters and can help alleviate symptoms of depression and anxiety. Additionally, exercise increases blood flow to the brain, promoting the growth of new neurons and improving cognitive function.

Incorporating exercise into a mental health care plan can also contribute to the overall sense of empowerment and self-efficacy in individuals. When individuals engage in regular exercise and witness the positive effects it has on their mental well-being, they gain a sense of control over their mental health and feel more confident in managing their symptoms.

Strategies for Integrating Exercise into Mental Health Care

There are various strategies that mental health care providers can employ to promote the integration of exercise into treatment plans. Here are some practical approaches:

1. **Collaborative goal-setting:** Mental health care providers can work collaboratively with their clients to set realistic exercise goals tailored to their individual needs and preferences. This could involve discussing the types of activities they enjoy, their current fitness level, and any specific mental health symptoms they wish to target.

2. **Psychoeducation:** Providing psychoeducation on the benefits of exercise for mental health can help clients understand the rationale behind incorporating physical activity into their treatment plan. Explaining how exercise affects the brain, neurotransmitter activity, and overall well-being can increase motivation and engagement in exercise.

3. **Personalized exercise plans:** Developing personalized exercise plans for clients can help ensure that the prescribed activities are achievable and enjoyable for them. Taking into account their interests, physical abilities, and daily schedules can increase adherence and long-term sustainability.

4. **Group exercises:** Encouraging participation in group exercises can have additional social and motivational benefits. Group exercises, such as yoga classes or outdoor group walks, provide social support, foster a sense of community, and help individuals stay committed to their exercise routine.

5. **Mindful movement practices:** Integrating mindfulness into exercise routines can further enhance the mental health benefits. Mindful movement practices like yoga or tai chi combine physical activity with meditation and breathwork, promoting relaxation, stress reduction, and improved self-awareness.

6. **Incorporating exercise into daily routine:** Encouraging clients to find opportunities to incorporate physical activity into their daily routine is crucial for long-term adherence. Simple modifications like taking the stairs instead of the elevator, walking or biking to work, or engaging in active hobbies can make exercise more accessible and sustainable.

Overcoming Barriers to Exercise

While exercise can be highly beneficial for mental health, there are common barriers that individuals may face when trying to incorporate physical activity into their routine. It is essential to address these barriers to ensure the success and sustainability of integrating exercise into mental health care.

Time constraints: Many individuals may perceive a lack of time as a major barrier to exercise. Mental health care providers can work with clients to identify time-saving strategies, such as short bursts of physical activity throughout the day, incorporating exercise into daily tasks, or finding time-efficient workout routines.

Motivation and self-efficacy: Some individuals may struggle with low motivation or a lack of confidence in their ability to exercise. Providers can help clients overcome these barriers by setting achievable goals, providing positive reinforcement, and offering support and guidance along the way.

Physical limitations: Physical limitations or chronic health conditions can pose challenges to engaging in certain types of exercise. Mental health care providers can collaborate with clients to find exercises that are safe and appropriate for their specific needs and abilities. Referrals to physical therapists or exercise specialists may be necessary in some cases.

Environmental factors: Environmental factors such as limited access to safe and affordable exercise facilities or outdoor spaces can hinder engagement in physical activity. Providers can help clients explore alternative exercise options, such as home-based workouts, online fitness programs, or community resources available in their area.

Case Study: Integrating Exercise into a Mental Health Care Plan

To illustrate the practical application of integrating exercise into mental health care, let's consider the case of Sarah, a 30-year-old woman experiencing symptoms of anxiety and depression. Sarah seeks help from a mental health care provider and expresses an interest in incorporating exercise into her treatment plan.

The mental health care provider conducts an assessment to understand Sarah's current level of physical activity, exercise preferences, and any barriers she may encounter. Based on this information, they collaboratively set a realistic goal of engaging in 30 minutes of moderate-intensity aerobic exercise, such as brisk walking or cycling, three times a week.

The provider educates Sarah on how exercise can help alleviate symptoms of anxiety and depression by increasing the production of endorphins, promoting neuroplasticity, and reducing stress levels. They also discuss the potential benefits of exercising outdoors, such as exposure to nature, Vitamin D synthesis, and increased social interaction.

To enhance adherence and motivation, the provider suggests that Sarah join a local walking group that meets twice a week. This not only helps Sarah incorporate exercise into her routine but also provides a supportive social setting.

To address time constraints, the provider encourages Sarah to break down her exercise sessions into shorter bouts if needed. They explore options for incorporating physical activity into her daily routine, such as using active transportation for commuting or taking breaks for short walks during work hours.

Throughout the treatment process, the mental health care provider regularly monitors Sarah's progress, provides ongoing support and encouragement, and adjusts the exercise plan as necessary. They also collaborate with other healthcare professionals, such as a physical therapist or a nutritionist, to address any additional needs or concerns.

By integrating exercise into Sarah's mental health care plan, the provider helps her develop a holistic approach to managing her symptoms of anxiety and depression. Over time, Sarah experiences improvements in her mood, self-esteem, and overall well-being, leading to a more sustainable and resilient mental health outcome.

Conclusion

Integrating exercise into mental health care is a valuable and effective approach to promote holistic well-being. The benefits of exercise for mental health are well-documented, and incorporating physical activity into treatment plans can enhance the overall effectiveness of mental health interventions.

By employing strategies such as collaborative goal-setting, psychoeducation, personalized exercise plans, group exercises, and mindful movement practices, mental health care providers can assist individuals in reaping the mental health benefits of exercise. Overcoming barriers to exercise, such as time constraints, motivation, physical limitations, and environmental factors, is vital for successful integration.

Through a case study, we explored how exercise can be integrated into a mental health care plan, highlighting the importance of individualized approaches, ongoing monitoring, and multidisciplinary collaboration. By considering exercise as an essential component of mental health care, we can work towards a sustainable future that prioritizes the well-being of individuals as a whole.

Exercise Therapy for Mental Health Disorders

Exercise has long been recognized as a fundamental component of physical health. But its importance extends beyond just the physical aspects. Research has shown that exercise can have significant benefits for mental health as well. In this section, we will explore the role of exercise therapy in the treatment of mental health disorders.

The Mind-Body Connection

Before delving into the specifics of exercise therapy, it is important to understand the underlying concept of the mind-body connection. This concept recognizes the close interrelationship between our mental and physical well-being. Our mental state can influence our physical health, and vice versa.

Exercise therapy is grounded in the understanding that engaging in physical activity can have a positive impact on our mental well-being. When we exercise, our bodies release endorphins, which are often referred to as "feel-good" hormones. These endorphins can improve our mood, reduce feelings of stress and anxiety, and increase our overall sense of well-being.

Exercise as a Treatment for Mental Health Disorders

Exercise therapy involves the use of structured physical activity programs as an intervention for mental health disorders. It can be used as a standalone treatment or in combination with other forms of therapy, such as medication or counseling. Let's explore how exercise therapy can be beneficial for different mental health disorders:

1. **Depression and Anxiety:** Several studies have shown that regular exercise can be an effective treatment for depression and anxiety. Exercise stimulates the release of endorphins, which can improve mood and reduce feelings of sadness and anxiety. Furthermore, engaging in physical activity provides a distraction from negative thoughts and promotes a sense of accomplishment. Exercise therapy can involve a variety of activities, such as aerobic exercises, yoga, or strength training, tailored to the individual's preferences and capabilities.

2. **Stress and Trauma-related Disorders:** Exercise has been shown to reduce stress levels and help individuals cope with traumatic experiences. Physical activity can serve as an outlet for releasing tension and promoting a sense of control. Additionally, engaging in exercise can improve sleep quality, which is often disrupted in individuals with stress and trauma-related disorders. Exercise therapy for these disorders may include activities that promote relaxation and mindfulness, such as yoga or tai chi.

3. **Substance Use Disorders:** Exercise can play a valuable role in the treatment of substance use disorders. Regular physical activity can help individuals manage cravings and withdrawal symptoms, reduce stress and anxiety associated with recovery, and provide a healthy alternative to addictive behaviors. Exercise therapy programs for substance use disorders often involve a combination of cardiovascular exercise, strength training, and group physical activities that promote social support and accountability.

Designing an Exercise Therapy Program

When designing an exercise therapy program for individuals with mental health disorders, it is essential to consider individual needs, preferences, and capabilities. Here are some important factors to consider:

1. **Individual Assessment:** Before starting an exercise therapy program, a thorough assessment of the individual's physical and mental health is

necessary. This assessment can help determine any potential contraindications or limitations and guide the selection of appropriate exercises.

2. **Exercise Prescription:** Based on the individual's assessment, an exercise prescription can be developed. This prescription should include details such as the type of exercises recommended, frequency, intensity, and duration. It is important to strike a balance between challenging the individual and ensuring their safety and enjoyment.

3. **Progression and Adaptation:** Exercise therapy programs should be progressive and adaptable to the individual's changing needs and abilities. Gradually increasing the intensity or introducing new exercises can help individuals continue to benefit from the therapy.

4. **Incorporating Enjoyment:** To enhance adherence and motivation, it is crucial to include exercises that the individual enjoys. This may involve incorporating activities they find pleasurable, such as dancing, swimming, or hiking.

5. **Supervision and Support:** Depending on the individual's needs and capabilities, supervision and support from qualified professionals, such as exercise physiologists or mental health practitioners, may be necessary. This can ensure proper form, provide guidance, and address any concerns that may arise during the therapy.

Case Study: Exercise Therapy for Depression

To illustrate the potential benefits of exercise therapy for mental health disorders, let's consider a case study on exercise therapy for depression:

Sarah, a 35-year-old woman, has been diagnosed with major depressive disorder. She experiences persistent feelings of sadness, low energy levels, and a loss of interest in previously enjoyable activities. Sarah's therapist suggests incorporating exercise therapy into her treatment plan.

Sarah begins with a gentle walking routine for 30 minutes, three times a week. This allows her to gradually ease into physical activity while still experiencing the benefits of increased endorphin release. As Sarah's fitness level improves, she decides to try yoga classes as well.

After several weeks of consistent exercise therapy, Sarah notices improvements in her mood and overall well-being. She feels more energized, finds pleasure in daily activities, and experiences a reduction in depressive symptoms. Moreover, Sarah appreciates the mindfulness aspect of yoga, which helps her manage her negative thoughts and emotions.

The combination of aerobic exercise and mindfulness practices through yoga has provided Sarah with a holistic approach to her depression treatment. Exercise therapy has become an integral part of her ongoing mental health management.

Challenges and Considerations

While exercise therapy can be highly beneficial for individuals with mental health disorders, there are several challenges and considerations to keep in mind:

- **Individual Barriers:** Some individuals may face barriers to engaging in exercise therapy due to physical health limitations, lack of motivation, or time constraints. It is important to address these barriers and provide support and resources to overcome them.

- **Integration with Conventional Treatments:** Exercise therapy should be integrated into a comprehensive treatment plan that includes other evidence-based therapies, such as medication or psychotherapy. It is essential to coordinate care and ensure collaboration among healthcare professionals involved in the individual's treatment.

- **Safety Precautions:** For individuals with certain medical conditions or physical limitations, certain exercises may not be suitable or may require modifications. It is crucial to prioritize safety and consult with healthcare professionals when necessary.

- **Sustainability and Long-term Adherence:** Encouraging individuals to maintain regular exercise beyond the therapy period is crucial for long-term mental health benefits. Providing resources, support groups, and promoting enjoyable and varied physical activities can help individuals sustain their exercise routines.

Conclusion

Exercise therapy holds immense potential in the treatment of mental health disorders. By incorporating physical activity into treatment plans, individuals can experience improved mood, reduced symptoms, and enhanced overall well-being. It is crucial to tailor exercise therapy programs to individual needs, provide necessary support and supervision, and integrate it with other evidence-based treatments. With a comprehensive approach that includes exercise therapy, we can work towards a sustainable mental health future.

Key Takeaways:

- Exercise therapy involves the use of structured physical activity programs as an intervention for mental health disorders.
- Regular exercise can improve mood, reduce stress and anxiety, and promote overall well-being.
- Exercise therapy can be beneficial for various mental health disorders, including depression, anxiety, stress and trauma-related disorders, and substance use disorders.
- Designing exercise therapy programs requires individual assessment, exercise prescription, progression, adaptation, and incorporation of enjoyable activities.
- Exercise therapy should be integrated into comprehensive treatment plans and consider individual barriers, safety precautions, and long-term adherence.

Discussion Questions:

1. How can exercise therapy be incorporated into existing mental health treatment settings?
2. What strategies can be used to promote long-term adherence to exercise therapy programs?
3. How can exercise therapy be adapted to different populations, such as children, older adults, or individuals with physical limitations?
4. What are some potential challenges or barriers to implementing exercise therapy in community mental health settings?

Resources:

- American Psychological Association. (2018). Exercise: A treatment for depression and anxiety.
- National Institute of Mental Health. (2019). Exercise for mental health.
- The American Journal of Sports Medicine. (2020). Exercise and mental health.

Mind-Body Practices for Mental Wellbeing

Meditation and Mindfulness

Mindfulness and meditation practices have gained significant attention in recent years as effective tools for promoting mental health and overall well-being. In this section, we will explore the concepts of meditation and mindfulness, their benefits for mental health, and how they can be incorporated into holistic health practices.

Understanding Meditation

Meditation is a practice that involves training the mind to focus and redirect thoughts. It is an ancient practice that has roots in various religious and spiritual traditions, including Buddhism, Hinduism, and Taoism. However, in recent years, meditation has gained popularity outside of its traditional context and has been widely recognized for its mental health benefits.

There are different types of meditation techniques, including:

1. **Focused Attention Meditation:** This form of meditation involves focusing the attention on a single object, such as the breath, a sound, or a specific image. The goal is to develop concentration and mindfulness by maintaining focus and redirecting wandering thoughts.

2. **Loving-Kindness Meditation:** Also known as Metta meditation, this practice involves cultivating feelings of love, compassion, and kindness towards oneself and others. It aims to enhance positive emotions and develop a sense of connectedness with others.

3. **Body Scan Meditation:** This technique involves systematically focusing attention on different parts of the body, starting from the toes and moving up to the head. It helps in developing body awareness and promoting relaxation.

4. **Transcendental Meditation:** This type of meditation involves the repetition of a mantra, a specific word or phrase. It aims to quiet the mind and access a state of deep relaxation and heightened awareness.

Benefits of Meditation for Mental Health

Meditation has been shown to have numerous benefits for mental health. Some of the key benefits include:

1. **Stress Reduction:** Meditation helps in reducing perceived stress levels by activating the body's relaxation response and promoting a state of calm and relaxation.

2. **Improved Emotional Well-being**: Regular meditation practice can enhance emotional well-being by reducing symptoms of anxiety and depression. It cultivates awareness of emotions and helps individuals develop skills to respond to their emotions in a healthy manner.

3. **Enhanced Concentration and Focus**: Meditation improves attention and concentration by training the mind to stay focused and avoid distractions. It also enhances cognitive flexibility and problem-solving skills.

4. **Better Self-awareness**: Through meditation, individuals develop a heightened sense of self-awareness and self-compassion. It helps in recognizing and accepting thoughts, feelings, and bodily sensations without judgment.

5. **Improved Sleep**: Regular meditation practice has been associated with improved sleep quality and reduced insomnia symptoms. It helps in calming the mind and preparing it for restful sleep.

Incorporating Mindfulness into Daily Life

Mindfulness is often described as the practice of paying attention to the present moment without judgment. It involves cultivating a state of non-reactive awareness to the thoughts, emotions, and sensations that arise in the present moment. Mindfulness can be practiced formally through meditation, but it can also be incorporated into daily life activities.

Some ways to incorporate mindfulness into daily life include:

1. **Mindful Eating**: Paying close attention to the taste, texture, and sensations of eating, and savoring each bite mindfully.

2. **Mindful Walking**: Bringing awareness to the sensations of walking, such as the movement of the legs, the feeling of the ground beneath the feet, and the rhythm of breathing.

3. **Mindful Breathing**: Taking a few moments throughout the day to focus on the breath, observing its natural rhythm and sensations.

4. **Mindful Listening**: Engaging in active listening by fully focusing on the speaker without interrupting or formulating a response.

5. **Mindful Body Scan**: Taking a few minutes to scan the body from head to toe, noticing any areas of tension or discomfort with gentle awareness.

Practical Tips for Meditation and Mindfulness

Getting started with meditation and mindfulness can be intimidating for beginners. Here are some practical tips to help you incorporate these practices into your daily life:

1. **Start Small:** Begin with just a few minutes of meditation or mindfulness practice each day and gradually increase the duration as you become more comfortable.
2. **Create a Sacred Space:** Settle into a quiet and comfortable space free from distractions, where you can fully immerse yourself in the meditation or mindfulness practice.
3. **Be Patient and Non-judgmental:** It's natural for the mind to wander during meditation. Instead of being critical, gently redirect your attention back to the present moment without judgment.
4. **Experiment with Different Techniques:** Explore various meditation techniques to find the ones that resonate with you the most. Remember, there's no one-size-fits-all approach.
5. **Join a Meditation Group:** Consider joining a local meditation group or attending mindfulness workshops to learn from experienced practitioners and cultivate a sense of community.

Case Study: Mindfulness-Based Stress Reduction

One popular mindfulness program is Mindfulness-Based Stress Reduction (MBSR), developed by Dr. Jon Kabat-Zinn. MBSR is an eight-week program that combines mindfulness meditation, body awareness, and yoga. It has been widely studied and shown to be effective in reducing stress and improving overall well-being.

Participants in MBSR learn formal practices, including body scan meditation, sitting meditation, and gentle yoga. They also learn how to bring mindfulness into their daily lives through informal practices like mindful eating, walking, and communication. The program is typically facilitated by trained instructors and includes group sessions and home practice.

Research has shown that MBSR can benefit individuals with various mental health conditions, including anxiety, depression, chronic pain, and sleep disorders. It promotes resilience and equips individuals with skills to cope with stress and adversity.

Conclusion

Meditation and mindfulness offer valuable tools for promoting mental health and overall well-being. These practices cultivate present-moment awareness, enhance self-compassion, and reduce stress levels. By incorporating meditation and mindfulness into daily life, individuals can experience a greater sense of peace, clarity, and resilience. Whether practiced independently or as part of a structured program like MBSR, meditation and mindfulness have the potential to transform mental health for the better.

Yoga and Mental Health

In recent years, there has been a growing recognition of the effectiveness of yoga as a complementary therapy for mental health. Yoga is a mind-body practice that originated in ancient India and involves a combination of physical postures, breathing exercises, meditation, and relaxation. It aims to promote overall well-being and balance between the body and mind.

Yoga provides a holistic approach to mental health by addressing both the physical and psychological aspects of well-being. Through the practice of yoga, individuals can experience improved mental clarity, reduced stress and anxiety, enhanced self-awareness, and increased feelings of calm and relaxation.

Research studies have shown that yoga can have numerous positive effects on mental health. One of the key mechanisms through which yoga benefits mental health is by activating the body's relaxation response. This response counteracts the physiological effects of stress, such as elevated heart rate and blood pressure, and helps promote a sense of calm and well-being.

Yoga also helps regulate the autonomic nervous system, which plays a crucial role in stress response. By practicing yoga regularly, individuals can train their nervous systems to respond more adaptively to stress, leading to a reduction in symptoms of anxiety and depression.

Moreover, yoga promotes mindfulness, which is the practice of being fully present in the current moment without judgment. Mindfulness has been shown to be an effective technique for managing stress, improving mood, and enhancing overall well-being. Through yoga, individuals can cultivate mindfulness skills that can be applied to daily life, leading to increased resilience and improved mental health outcomes.

In addition to its physiological and psychological benefits, yoga can also address specific mental health conditions. For example, studies have shown that yoga can reduce symptoms of depression, particularly when combined with other treatment approaches such as medication or psychotherapy.

Yoga can also be effective in managing anxiety disorders, such as generalized anxiety disorder and panic disorder. The combination of physical postures, breathing exercises, and meditation in yoga helps individuals develop coping skills to manage anxiety symptoms and promote relaxation.

Furthermore, yoga has been shown to be beneficial for individuals with post-traumatic stress disorder (PTSD). The embodiment and grounding practices in yoga can help individuals build a sense of safety and stability in their bodies, reducing the hyperarousal and hypervigilance commonly associated with PTSD.

Integrating yoga into mental health care can be done in various settings, including individual therapy sessions, group therapy, or yoga classes specifically designed for mental health purposes. It is important to ensure that yoga instructors have an understanding of mental health and can adapt the practice to meet the unique needs of individuals with mental health conditions.

It's worth mentioning that yoga is not a replacement for traditional mental health treatments but rather a complementary therapy that can enhance overall well-being. It can be utilized in conjunction with other evidence-based treatments, such as medication and psychotherapy, to provide a comprehensive and holistic approach to mental health care.

In conclusion, yoga is a powerful tool for promoting mental health and well-being. Through its combination of physical postures, breathing exercises, and meditation, yoga can help individuals manage stress, improve mood, and cultivate resilience. By integrating yoga into mental health care, individuals can experience the multitude of benefits that yoga has to offer in enhancing their overall mental health and quality of life.

Tai Chi and Qigong

Tai Chi and Qigong are ancient Chinese practices that promote physical, mental, and spiritual well-being. Both practices involve a combination of gentle, flowing movements, deep breathing, and focused intention. While Tai Chi is primarily a martial art, Qigong focuses more on cultivating and balancing the body's vital energy, known as "Qi" or "Chi." In this section, we will explore the principles, benefits, and techniques of Tai Chi and Qigong.

Principles of Tai Chi and Qigong

Both Tai Chi and Qigong are rooted in the principles of traditional Chinese medicine and Taoist philosophy. The key principles include:

- **Qi flow:** The belief that energy flows throughout the body, and that blockages or imbalances in this energy can lead to illness. Tai Chi and Qigong aim to promote the smooth flow of Qi, restoring balance and enhancing vitality.

- **Yin-Yang balance:** Tai Chi and Qigong emphasize the importance of balancing Yin and Yang energies within the body. Yin represents the passive, receptive, and nurturing aspects, while Yang represents the active, dynamic, and expressive aspects. The practice helps achieve harmony between these opposing yet complementary forces.

- **Mind-body connection:** Both practices emphasize the integration of mind and body. By cultivating awareness and focusing the mind, practitioners can enhance their physical movements and connect with the present moment.

- **Softness and relaxation:** Tai Chi and Qigong teach practitioners to be soft and relaxed in their movements. Tension and rigidity are believed to impede the flow of Qi, while softness and relaxation allow for smooth energy circulation.

- **Alignment and posture:** Proper alignment and posture are essential in Tai Chi and Qigong. By aligning the body's structure, practitioners can facilitate the flow of energy and minimize strain on the joints.

Benefits of Tai Chi and Qigong

The regular practice of Tai Chi and Qigong offers numerous benefits for physical, mental, and emotional well-being. Some of the key benefits include:

- **Improved balance and coordination:** The slow and controlled movements of Tai Chi and Qigong help strengthen the muscles and improve balance and coordination. This is particularly beneficial for older adults in reducing the risk of falls.

- **Stress reduction:** The mindfulness and deep breathing techniques used in Tai Chi and Qigong promote relaxation and reduce stress. Regular practice can help lower cortisol levels and improve overall mental well-being.

- **Enhanced flexibility and strength:** The gentle stretching and weight-shifting movements in Tai Chi and Qigong help improve flexibility and strengthen muscles. This can lead to improved joint mobility and functional fitness.

- **Improved cardiovascular health:** Although Tai Chi and Qigong are low-impact exercises, they can still provide cardiovascular benefits. The slow, rhythmic movements help improve blood circulation, lower blood pressure, and reduce the risk of cardiovascular diseases.

- **Mind-body connection:** Practicing Tai Chi and Qigong helps cultivate a strong mind-body connection. This increased awareness can aid in managing emotions, reducing anxiety, and improving overall mental clarity.

Techniques and Practices

Tai Chi and Qigong can be practiced by people of all ages and fitness levels. Here are some common techniques and practices:

- **Tai Chi forms:** Tai Chi consists of a series of choreographed forms, which are specific movements and postures performed in a continuous, flowing sequence. Each form is designed to develop specific physical and energetic qualities.

- **Qigong exercises:** Qigong practices include a wide range of exercises designed to cultivate and balance Qi. These exercises may involve gentle movements, standing postures, breathing techniques, and meditation.

- **Meditation and breath control:** Both Tai Chi and Qigong incorporate meditation and breath control techniques. Focusing on the breath helps calm the mind, improve concentration, and regulate the flow of Qi.

- **Partner exercises:** Some Tai Chi and Qigong practices involve partner exercises, where individuals engage in gentle and synchronized movements together. This fosters connection, body awareness, and energetic exchange.

- **Daily practice:** Consistency is key in Tai Chi and Qigong. Practicing for at least 20-30 minutes a day can yield significant benefits. Finding a quiet and comfortable space, wearing loose and comfortable clothing, and selecting appropriate footwear are important considerations for practice.

Unconventional Approach: Tai Chi and Qigong with Everyday Objects

One unconventional approach to incorporating Tai Chi and Qigong into daily life is by using everyday objects as props. For example, you can perform standing Qigong exercises while waiting in line, using the wall or a chair for support. You can also practice Tai Chi forms while holding a broom, mimicking the movements and flow. This approach allows for integration of Tai Chi and Qigong principles into daily activities, making the practice more accessible and enjoyable.

Conclusion

Tai Chi and Qigong offer a holistic approach to promoting mental, physical, and spiritual well-being. By incorporating gentle movements, deep breathing, and focused intention, these practices help restore balance, reduce stress, and enhance overall vitality. Whether practicing traditional forms or exploring unconventional approaches, Tai Chi and Qigong provide valuable tools for cultivating resilience, mindfulness, and harmonious living.

Visualization and Imagery Techniques

In the field of mental health, visualization and imagery techniques are powerful tools that can be used to promote relaxation, reduce stress, and enhance overall wellbeing. Visualization involves creating mental images or scenarios that evoke a sense of calm and tranquility, while imagery techniques involve using images or objects to focus the mind and redirect thoughts. This section explores the principles behind visualization and imagery techniques, their benefits, and how they can be incorporated into daily practice.

Principles of Visualization

Visualization techniques are based on the principle that the mind and body are interconnected, and that mental images can have a profound impact on physical and emotional wellbeing. By focusing on positive and peaceful images, individuals can create a sense of relaxation and harmonize their mind and body.

To effectively engage in visualization, it is important to create a quiet and comfortable environment free from distractions. Close your eyes, take deep breaths, and allow your mind to wander to a serene and peaceful place. It could be a beautiful beach, a lush forest, or any other location that brings you a sense of calm. As you immerse yourself in the image, try to engage all your senses - what do you see, hear, taste, smell, and feel in this serene place? The more detailed and vivid your mental image, the more powerful the visualization will be.

Benefits of Visualization

Visualization techniques have been found to have numerous benefits for mental health and overall wellbeing. Some of the key benefits include:

1. Stress Reduction: Engaging in visualization can help calm the mind and reduce anxiety and stress. By focusing on positive images and sensations, individuals can shift their attention away from stressors and promote relaxation.

2. Improved Focus and Concentration: Visualization techniques can enhance concentration and focus by training the mind to stay present and engaged. By regularly practicing visualization, individuals can develop greater mental clarity and improve their ability to concentrate on the task at hand.

3. Emotional Regulation: Visualization can be used to regulate emotions and promote a positive outlook. By imagining positive scenarios or experiences, individuals can create a sense of joy, happiness, and gratitude, which can have a profound impact on overall mood and emotional wellbeing.

4. Enhanced Performance: Visualization has been widely used by athletes and performers to enhance performance. By mentally rehearsing and visualizing success, individuals can improve their confidence, motivation, and overall performance in various domains.

5. Relaxation and Sleep: Visualization techniques can be particularly useful for promoting relaxation and improving sleep quality. Engaging in a guided visualization before bedtime can help quiet the mind, reduce racing thoughts, and prepare the body for restful sleep.

Incorporating Visualization into Daily Practice

Incorporating visualization into your daily routine can be a simple yet powerful way to promote mental health and overall wellbeing. Here are some techniques to try:

1. Guided Visualization: There are numerous guided visualization exercises available online or in the form of apps. These guided exercises provide step-by-step instructions to help you create vivid mental images and engage your senses. Find a guided visualization that resonates with you and make it a regular part of your routine.

2. Create a Peaceful Visualization Space: Dedicate a quiet corner of your home as your visualization space. Decorate it with calming images, objects, or scents that help you relax and create a serene atmosphere. Use this space for your visualization practice, ensuring that it is free from distractions and interruptions.

3. Visualization Journals: Maintain a visualization journal to record your experiences and reflect on the emotions and sensations evoked during the practice. Writing down your visualizations can help deepen the experience and serve as a reference for future sessions.

4. Visualization as a Problem-Solving Tool: Visualization can also be used to explore solutions to problems or challenges. In this approach, visualize yourself successfully navigating a difficult situation or achieving a desired outcome. By mentally rehearsing success, you can enhance your problem-solving skills and boost self-confidence.

Case Study: Managing Test Anxiety through Visualization

Let's consider an example of how visualization can be used to manage test anxiety. Emily is a college student who experiences extreme anxiety before exams, which significantly impacts her performance. She decides to incorporate visualization techniques to help calm her nerves and improve her test-taking experience.

Before each exam, Emily finds a quiet space and practices deep breathing to relax her mind and body. She then begins her visualization practice by imagining herself in a peaceful and serene location. She visualizes herself confidently approaching the exam hall, feeling calm and focused. She sees herself answering each question with clarity and ease, feeling a sense of accomplishment with every correct answer. She imagines herself finishing the exam feeling satisfied and relieved.

By regularly practicing this visualization technique before each exam, Emily is able to reduce her test anxiety and approach exams with a greater sense of confidence. The positive images and sensations she engages in during visualization help her shift her focus away from anxiety-provoking thoughts and create a more relaxed mindset.

Resources for Visualization and Imagery Techniques

1. Apps: There are several smartphone apps available that offer guided visualization exercises, such as Headspace, Calm, and Insight Timer. These apps provide a variety of visualization options, making it easy to find guided exercises that suit your preferences and needs.

2. Books: There are numerous books available that provide guidance on visualization and imagery techniques. Some recommended books include "Creative Visualization" by Shakti Gawain and "The Healing Power of Visualization" by Gerald Epstein.

3. Online Resources: Many websites and online platforms offer free visualization exercises and resources. Some popular websites include Psychology Today, Mindful, and Health Journeys.

4. Professional Support: If you are facing significant mental health challenges or would like personalized guidance in incorporating visualization into your practice, consider seeking support from a mental health professional. They can provide tailored techniques and strategies to address your specific needs.

Exercise: Creating Your Personal Visualization Practice

Take a few moments to reflect on your current mental health and wellbeing. Identify an area of your life that could benefit from visualization and imagery techniques. It could be managing stress, improving sleep, boosting self-confidence, or any other aspect you wish to address.

Now, using the principles discussed in this section, create your personalized visualization practice. Consider the following questions:

1. What goal or outcome would you like to achieve through visualization?
2. What images, locations, or scenarios evoke a sense of calm and peace for you?
3. How can you engage all your senses in your visualization practice?
4. How often and when will you incorporate visualization into your daily routine?

Write down your personalized visualization practice and commit to incorporating it into your life. Make it a regular part of your self-care routine and notice the impact it has on your mental health and overall wellbeing.

Remember, the effectiveness of visualization and imagery techniques will vary from person to person. Be patient and kind to yourself as you explore and refine your practice.

Art and Music Therapy

The Therapeutic Power of Art

In the realm of mental health care, the use of art as a therapeutic tool has gained recognition and popularity in recent years. Art therapy, as it is commonly known, taps into the innate creative abilities of individuals to promote healing, self-expression, and personal growth. This section will explore the therapeutic power of art, its applications, and its effectiveness in enhancing mental well-being.

Understanding Art Therapy

Art therapy is a form of psychotherapy that utilizes the creative process of art-making to improve psychological well-being. By engaging in artistic activities under the guidance of a trained art therapist, individuals are invited to explore and express their emotions, thoughts, and experiences visually. The artwork created becomes a vehicle for communication, reflection, and self-discovery.

The therapeutic power of art lies in its ability to tap into the subconscious and provide a non-verbal means of expression. Often, people find it challenging to put their feelings into words, but through art, they can convey their emotions and experiences symbolically. This process can foster self-awareness, facilitate emotional release, and promote personal growth.

The Benefits of Art Therapy

Art therapy offers a range of benefits for individuals struggling with various mental health issues. Some of the key advantages include:

1. Emotional expression: Art provides a safe and non-threatening medium for expressing complex emotions that may be difficult to articulate verbally.

2. Stress reduction: Engaging in creative activities can serve as a powerful stress reliever by allowing individuals to focus their attention on the present moment and immerse themselves in the artistic process.

3. Self-exploration and self-discovery: Through art-making, individuals can gain insight into their inner thoughts, beliefs, and experiences, leading to greater self-understanding and personal growth.

4. Enhancing self-esteem and self-confidence: Artistic achievements, however small, can contribute to a sense of accomplishment and help build self-confidence.

5. Promoting relaxation and mindfulness: The act of creating art can induce a state of relaxation, allowing individuals to experience mindfulness and explore a sense of inner peace.

6. Building coping skills: Art therapy can help individuals develop healthy coping skills and strategies for managing stress, anxiety, and other mental health challenges.

Applications of Art Therapy

Art therapy can be utilized in a wide range of therapeutic settings and with individuals of all ages. Some common applications include:

1. Mental health treatment: Art therapy can complement traditional talk therapy approaches in the treatment of mental health disorders such as depression, anxiety, trauma-related conditions, and eating disorders.

2. Rehabilitation: In rehabilitation settings, art therapy can help individuals recover from physical injuries or disabilities by providing a channel for emotional expression and facilitating the healing process.

3. Children and adolescents: Art therapy is highly effective in working with young children and adolescents, as it allows them to express their emotions and experiences in a developmentally appropriate and non-threatening way.

4. Substance abuse treatment: Art therapy can be integrated into substance abuse treatment programs to explore underlying emotional issues, build healthy coping skills, and support relapse prevention.

5. Wellness and self-care: Art therapy is not limited to clinical settings and can be used as a tool for self-expression, stress reduction, and personal growth in individuals seeking overall wellness and self-improvement.

Effectiveness of Art Therapy

Numerous studies have demonstrated the effectiveness of art therapy in enhancing mental well-being and promoting positive therapeutic outcomes. Research has shown that art therapy can reduce symptoms of anxiety and depression, improve self-esteem, increase emotional resilience, and enhance overall quality of life.

For example, a study published in the Journal of the American Art Therapy Association found that art therapy interventions were effective in reducing stress and improving mood in adults with various mental health challenges. Another study published in the Journal of Traumatic Stress indicated that art therapy was beneficial in reducing symptoms of post-traumatic stress disorder (PTSD) in trauma survivors.

It is important to note that art therapy should be conducted by trained art therapists who have a deep understanding of psychological principles and therapeutic techniques. The expertise of art therapists ensures that the therapeutic process is guided in a safe and supportive manner, allowing individuals to explore their emotions and experiences within a therapeutic framework.

Exploring Art Therapy: A Case Study

To illustrate the practical application of art therapy, let's consider the case of Sarah, a 40-year-old woman who has been struggling with chronic anxiety and self-doubt. Sarah's therapist incorporates art therapy into her treatment plan to help her explore and address these issues.

During an art therapy session, Sarah is given art materials and encouraged to create an artwork that visually represents her anxiety. The therapist provides a safe and non-judgmental space for Sarah to express herself freely. Through the artistic process, Sarah creates a mixed-media collage that depicts a stormy sea with dark clouds and crashing waves.

As Sarah reflects on her artwork with the therapist, she realizes that the stormy sea represents her anxiety, and the dark clouds symbolize her self-doubt. Through this realization, Sarah gains a deeper understanding of the link between her thoughts, emotions, and physical sensations. She begins to explore the underlying causes of her anxiety and develops coping strategies to manage it effectively.

Over time, through continued art therapy sessions, Sarah's anxiety reduces, her self-confidence improves, and she develops a more positive outlook on life. The art-making process has provided a therapeutic space for self-expression, reflection, and growth.

Conclusion

The therapeutic power of art in promoting mental well-being is undeniable. Art therapy offers individuals a means of self-expression and exploration that can lead to profound emotional healing and personal growth. With its numerous benefits and versatile applications, art therapy is a valuable addition to the field of mental health care.

As we continue to recognize the importance of holistic approaches to mental health, incorporating art therapy into treatment plans and supporting its integration into various settings can contribute to a sustainable future of mental health care. By embracing the therapeutic power of art, we can empower individuals to find their voices, express their emotions, and enhance their overall well-being.

Music Therapy for Mental Health

Music therapy is a specialized form of therapy that uses music to address various emotional, cognitive, and physical needs of individuals. It is an evidence-based practice that has been used for centuries to promote healing, reduce stress, and enhance overall well-being. In the context of mental health, music therapy can be a powerful tool for individuals experiencing psychological challenges.

Principles of Music Therapy

Music therapy is grounded in several key principles that guide its practice. These principles include:

- **Non-verbal communication:** Music allows individuals to express and communicate their emotions non-verbally, making it an effective mode of communication for individuals who may struggle to articulate their feelings verbally.

- **Emotional expression and regulation:** Music has the power to evoke and elicit emotions. Through active engagement with music, individuals can explore and process their emotions, leading to emotional regulation and a sense of catharsis.

- **Relationship building:** Music therapy provides a space for individuals to connect with their therapist and others through shared musical experiences. This can foster a sense of belonging, trust, and social connection.

- **Holistic approach:** Music therapy recognizes the interconnectedness of the mind, body, and spirit. It addresses the whole person, taking into account their unique needs, strengths, and challenges.

Benefits of Music Therapy

Music therapy has been shown to have a wide range of benefits for individuals with mental health disorders. Some of the key benefits include:

- **Anxiety and stress reduction:** Music has a calming effect on the nervous system, reducing anxiety and stress levels. It can help individuals relax, promote deep breathing, and regulate heart rate and blood pressure.

- **Mood enhancement:** Listening to or creating music can uplift mood, increase positive emotions, and provide a sense of joy and pleasure. It can also serve as a powerful distraction from negative thoughts and emotions.

- **Self-expression and emotional release:** Music provides a safe and creative outlet for expressing and processing emotions. It can facilitate the release of pent-up emotions, allowing individuals to experience a sense of relief and catharsis.

- **Enhanced cognitive abilities:** Engaging with music stimulates various cognitive processes, such as attention, memory, and executive functioning. Music therapy can improve cognitive skills, enhance problem-solving abilities, and promote overall mental agility.

- **Social connection and interpersonal skills:** Music therapy sessions often involve group activities, enabling individuals to engage in musical interactions, collaborative tasks, and turn-taking. This fosters social skills, cooperation, and a sense of belonging.

Application of Music Therapy

Music therapy can be applied in various mental health settings, including hospitals, psychiatric facilities, rehabilitation centers, schools, and community programs. Certified music therapists use a range of techniques and interventions tailored to the individual's specific needs. These interventions may include:

- **Listening to music:** Passive music listening can evoke emotions, relax the mind, and promote self-reflection. Therapists carefully select music that aligns with the individual's goals and preferences.

- **Music improvisation:** Playing or creating improvised music allows individuals to express themselves freely and creatively. It encourages spontaneity, self-expression, and exploration of emotions.

- **Songwriting:** Writing and composing original songs can be a therapeutic process that helps individuals externalize their thoughts and emotions. It provides a platform for self-expression, reflection, and personal growth.

- **Music-assisted relaxation:** Guided relaxation techniques, combined with soothing music, can induce a state of deep relaxation, reduce anxiety, and promote overall well-being.

- **Music and movement:** Engaging in rhythmic movements or dancing to music can enhance body awareness, promote motor coordination, and foster self-expression.

Case Study: Music Therapy for Depression

To illustrate the effectiveness of music therapy in mental health care, let's consider a case study of a client with depression. Sarah, a 35-year-old woman, has been struggling with feelings of sadness, emptiness, and low energy for several months. She has difficulty expressing her emotions verbally and often isolates herself from social activities.

In music therapy sessions, the therapist initially focuses on building a therapeutic relationship with Sarah. Through active listening and empathy, the therapist creates a safe space for Sarah to explore her emotions. Gradually, the therapist introduces music-based activities such as songwriting, listening to uplifting music, and engaging in rhythmic exercises.

Over time, Sarah begins to express her emotions through song lyrics and melodies. She discovers that music allows her to connect with her inner self and express her feelings in a way that words cannot capture. As Sarah actively engages in music-making, her mood starts to improve, and she experiences a sense of empowerment and self-discovery.

The music therapy sessions also provide Sarah with a supportive environment to share her songs with others. Through group activities and music performances, she develops social connections and a sense of belonging. The positive feedback and encouragement from peers further enhance her self-esteem and confidence.

Through consistent music therapy sessions, Sarah gains valuable coping skills and a newfound appreciation for music as a tool for self-care. She learns to regulate her emotions, manages her symptoms of depression more effectively, and develops a stronger sense of resilience.

Resources and Further Reading

For those interested in learning more about music therapy for mental health, the following resources provide valuable information and insights:

1. *Music Therapy Handbook* by Barbara L. Wheeler - This comprehensive book discusses various aspects of music therapy practice, including theoretical foundations, techniques, and case studies.

2. *The Oxford Handbook of Music Therapy* edited by Jane Edwards - This handbook provides an in-depth exploration of the research, theory, and practice of music therapy across different populations and settings.

3. *Music Therapy for Stress and Anxiety* by Joke Bradt - This book focuses specifically on the use of music therapy for stress and anxiety management, offering practical techniques and strategies.

4. *The Music Effect: Music Physiology and Clinical Applications* by Daniel J. Schneck and Dorita S. Berger - This book explores the physiological and psychological effects of music, providing insights into how music therapy can be applied in clinical settings.

These resources offer valuable guidance for music therapists, healthcare professionals, and individuals interested in the potential of music therapy for mental health promotion and intervention.

Music therapy is a dynamic and versatile approach that harnesses the therapeutic power of music to support individuals with mental health challenges. By incorporating music into treatment plans, mental health professionals can enhance emotional well-being, foster self-expression, and promote holistic healing for individuals seeking support.

Expressive Arts Therapy

Expressive Arts Therapy is a creative and holistic approach to mental health that utilizes various art forms to promote healing, self-expression, and personal growth. It recognizes the power of the arts in facilitating emotional release, communication, and self-understanding. This section will explore the principles, techniques, and benefits of Expressive Arts Therapy, as well as its application in mental health care.

Principles of Expressive Arts Therapy

Expressive Arts Therapy is grounded in several key principles that guide its practice. These principles include:

1. **Multimodal Approach:** Expressive Arts Therapy integrates a range of artistic modalities, such as visual arts, music, dance, drama, and creative writing. By engaging in multiple art forms, individuals have the opportunity to explore different means of self-expression and tap into various dimensions of their experiences.

2. **Non-verbal Communication:** Sometimes, words alone are not enough to express complex emotions or experiences. Expressive Arts Therapy provides an alternative channel of communication that goes beyond verbal language. Through art, individuals can express their thoughts, feelings, and inner conflicts non-verbally, allowing for deeper exploration and understanding.

3. **The Process is Key:** In Expressive Arts Therapy, the emphasis is placed on the process of creating art rather than the final product. Therapists focus on supporting individuals as they engage in art-making, encouraging them to explore their emotions, thoughts, and experiences in a safe and non-judgmental environment.

4. **Metaphor and Symbolism:** Artistic creations often contain rich metaphors and symbolism. Expressive Arts Therapy recognizes the inherent symbolic nature of art and encourages individuals to explore and decode the meaning behind their creations. This process can provide insights into their subconscious mind, promote self-reflection, and facilitate personal growth.

Techniques of Expressive Arts Therapy

Expressive Arts Therapy incorporates a variety of techniques tailored to individual needs and goals. Some common techniques include:

1. **Visual Arts:** Engaging in visual arts, such as painting, drawing, or collage-making, allows individuals to express their emotions and experiences through imagery. This can be particularly beneficial for individuals who struggle with verbal expression.

2. **Music and Sound:** Playing musical instruments, singing, or listening to music can evoke powerful emotions and facilitate self-expression. Music therapy

techniques, such as songwriting or improvisation, can help individuals explore their feelings, develop coping skills, and enhance self-awareness.

3. **Movement and Dance:** Movement-based techniques, including dance and expressive movement, enable individuals to express their emotions and experiences through physicality. This can promote body awareness, release tension, and enhance emotional well-being.

4. **Drama and Theater:** Drama therapy techniques, such as role-playing or improvisation, provide individuals with a safe space to explore different perspectives and experiences. Through storytelling and dramatic expression, individuals can gain new insights, practice adaptive behaviors, and foster empathy.

5. **Creative Writing:** Engaging in creative writing, journaling, or poetry can facilitate self-reflection and emotional processing. Writing allows individuals to externalize their internal experiences, gain clarity, and develop a stronger sense of self.

Benefits of Expressive Arts Therapy

Expressive Arts Therapy offers a range of benefits for individuals experiencing mental health challenges. Some of these benefits include:

1. **Emotional Release:** Creating art can provide a safe outlet for expressing and releasing emotions that may be difficult to articulate verbally. It can serve as a cathartic process, allowing individuals to process and cope with challenging emotions.

2. **Self-Exploration and Self-Awareness:** Engaging in art-making can help individuals gain insights into their thoughts, feelings, and experiences. It can promote self-reflection, increase self-awareness, and facilitate personal growth and transformation.

3. **Stress Reduction:** Artistic expression has been shown to reduce stress and promote relaxation. The act of creating art can distract individuals from their worries and provide a sense of calm and mental clarity.

4. **Improved Communication and Interpersonal Skills:** Expressive Arts Therapy can enhance communication skills, especially for individuals who find it challenging to express themselves verbally. Through art, individuals can develop new ways of communicating and connecting with others.

5. **Self-empowerment:** Engaging in the creative process can foster a sense of empowerment and agency. It allows individuals to take control of their healing journey, make choices, and experience a sense of accomplishment and self-confidence.

Application of Expressive Arts Therapy in Mental Health Care

Expressive Arts Therapy can be applied in various mental health care settings to support individuals across the lifespan. Some examples of its application include:

1. **Individual Therapy:** Expressive Arts Therapy can be used as a standalone therapy or in combination with other therapeutic approaches to address a range of mental health concerns, such as anxiety, depression, trauma, and addiction.

2. **Group Therapy:** Group settings provide opportunities for shared experiences, mutual support, and social connection. Expressive Arts Therapy in groups can promote interpersonal growth, empathy, and a sense of belonging.

3. **Community Programs:** Expressive Arts Therapy can be incorporated into community-based programs that aim to enhance mental well-being and prevent mental health problems. These programs can be tailored to specific populations, such as children, adolescents, older adults, or individuals with specific mental health conditions.

4. **Preventive Interventions:** Expressive Arts Therapy can be used as a preventive measure to promote mental health, resilience, and well-being. It can equip individuals with coping skills, emotional intelligence, and self-care strategies.

In conclusion, Expressive Arts Therapy offers a creative and holistic approach to promoting mental health and well-being. By harnessing the power of the arts, individuals can explore their emotions, develop coping strategies, and foster personal growth. Incorporating Expressive Arts Therapy into mental health care settings can provide individuals with new avenues for self-expression, empowerment, and healing.

Dance/Movement Therapy

Dance/Movement Therapy (DMT) is a form of therapy that utilizes movement and dance to support individual growth, emotional expression, and psychological healing. It is rooted in the belief that the body and mind are interconnected and that movement can be a powerful tool for self-expression and healing. In this section, we will explore the principles, techniques, and benefits of DMT, as well as its application in various therapeutic settings.

Principles of Dance/Movement Therapy

DMT is based on several key principles that guide its practice:

- **Embodiment:** DMT recognizes the body as the primary vehicle for therapeutic change. Through movement, individuals can explore and express their emotions, thoughts, and experiences in a somatic way.

- **Nonverbal Expression:** Movement can provide a means of communication that goes beyond words. DMT acknowledges the power of nonverbal expression, allowing individuals to communicate and process emotions that may be difficult to verbalize.

- **Movement Analysis:** DMT practitioners are trained to observe and analyze the movement patterns and gestures of individuals. This analysis helps to gain insight into an individual's emotional state, relationships, and underlying conflicts.

- **Creativity and Improvisation:** DMT encourages individuals to explore their own unique movement vocabulary, tapping into their creativity and promoting self-expression. Improvisation allows for spontaneity and the discovery of new ways of moving and being.

- **Body-Mind Connection:** DMT recognizes the interconnection between the body and mind. By engaging in movement, individuals can gain a deeper understanding of their thoughts, emotions, and beliefs, leading to personal growth and insight.

Techniques in Dance/Movement Therapy

DMT employs a variety of techniques to facilitate healing and personal growth. Some commonly used techniques include:

- **Free Movement:** Individuals are encouraged to move freely in the space, allowing their bodies to express themselves without constraints or judgment.

- **Guided Movement:** DMT practitioners may provide verbal prompts or cues to guide individuals in exploring specific movement patterns or themes. These prompts can help individuals deepen their self-awareness and facilitate emotional expression.

- **Body Awareness:** DMT focuses on increasing body awareness and the connection between movement and emotions. Through gentle exercises and guided attention, individuals learn to listen to their bodies and become more attuned to their physical sensations.

ART AND MUSIC THERAPY

- **Group Movement:** DMT can be practiced in both individual and group settings. Group movement sessions provide opportunities for interpersonal interaction, emotional support, and shared experiences, promoting connection and empathy.

- **Movement Rituals:** DMT may incorporate movement rituals, such as circle dances or symbolic gestures, to facilitate healing and a sense of collective belonging. These rituals can provide a sense of structure and meaning for individuals.

Benefits of Dance/Movement Therapy

DMT offers a wide range of benefits for individuals of all ages and abilities. Some of these benefits include:

- **Emotional Release:** Movement can serve as an outlet for emotions, allowing individuals to express and release pent-up feelings. This can help reduce anxiety, stress, and depression, promoting overall emotional well-being.

- **Improved Self-Esteem:** DMT supports self-acceptance and self-expression, allowing individuals to develop a positive body image and a sense of self-worth. Through movement, individuals can tap into their strengths and build confidence.

- **Enhanced Communication:** DMT provides a nonverbal platform for communication and expression, particularly helpful for individuals who struggle with verbal communication. Movement can bridge emotional and relational gaps, fostering better interpersonal connections.

- **Increased Body Awareness:** DMT helps individuals develop a greater understanding and connection to their bodies. This heightened body awareness can lead to improved self-care, body confidence, and overall physical well-being.

- **Stress Reduction:** Engaging in movement and dance can help reduce stress, promote relaxation, and improve overall mental health. It allows individuals to focus on the present moment, fostering mindfulness and a sense of calm.

- **Enhanced Creativity:** DMT stimulates creativity and imagination, allowing individuals to explore new ways of moving and being. This creativity can extend beyond the therapy session, leading to increased innovation and problem-solving abilities.

Application of Dance/Movement Therapy

DMT is applied in various therapeutic settings, including:

- **Mental Health Facilities:** DMT is used in psychiatric hospitals, outpatient clinics, and community mental health centers to support individuals with mental health disorders such as depression, anxiety, and trauma-related conditions.

- **Schools and Education Settings:** DMT is employed in schools to address social and emotional difficulties in children and adolescents. It promotes self-expression, emotional regulation, and positive relationship-building among students.

- **Rehabilitation Centers:** DMT is utilized in rehabilitation settings to support individuals recovering from physical injuries, neurological conditions, or substance abuse. It aids in physical rehabilitation, emotional healing, and the restoration of body-mind connections.

- **Aging and Geriatric Care:** DMT is beneficial for older adults, enhancing their overall well-being, cognitive abilities, and social connections. It is used in senior centers, nursing homes, and memory care facilities to promote active aging and quality of life.

- **Community and Social Justice Programs:** DMT is employed in community-based programs to address social justice issues, promote resilience, and foster empowerment among marginalized populations.

Unconventional Approach: Ecstatic Dance Therapy

One unconventional approach within DMT is Ecstatic Dance Therapy. Ecstatic dance is a form of movement expression that encourages uninhibited and spontaneous movement to music. This approach is rooted in creating a safe and inclusive space for individuals to explore their bodies, emotions, and creativity without judgment or instruction. The emphasis is on the authentic and free-flowing movement, allowing individuals to connect with themselves and others in a non-verbal and non-judgmental way. Ecstatic dance therapy can provide a powerful platform for self-discovery, emotional release, and personal transformation.

Conclusion

Dance/Movement Therapy offers a unique and holistic approach to mental health and well-being. By harnessing the power of movement, DMT supports emotional expression, self-awareness, and personal growth. Whether practiced in individual or group settings, DMT can be a valuable therapeutic modality in various contexts. The principles, techniques, and benefits discussed in this section highlight the importance of incorporating movement and dance into mental health care, paving the way for a more integrated and sustainable approach to well-being.

Animal-Assisted Therapy

The Benefits of Human-Animal Bonding

The human-animal bond refers to the unique and mutually beneficial relationship between humans and animals. Throughout history, animals have played significant roles in human society, providing companionship, support, and various forms of assistance. In recent years, there has been a growing recognition of the positive impact that animals can have on human mental health and overall well-being. This section explores the benefits of human-animal bonding and how it can contribute to a holistic approach to mental health.

Psychological Benefits

The bond between humans and animals has been shown to have numerous psychological benefits. One of the key benefits is the reduction of stress and anxiety. Interacting with animals can help to lower cortisol levels, a hormone associated with stress, and increase the release of oxytocin, a hormone that promotes feelings of relaxation and bonding.

In addition to reducing stress, the presence of animals can also improve mood and elevate overall well-being. Studies have found that pet owners experience lower rates of depression and loneliness compared to non-pet owners. Animals provide companionship, unconditional love, and a sense of purpose, which can have a positive impact on mental health.

Moreover, human-animal bonding has been linked to improved self-esteem and self-confidence. Caring for an animal and receiving their affection and loyalty can increase feelings of self-worth and boost one's sense of identity. This is particularly beneficial for individuals with low self-esteem or those struggling with social interactions.

Physical Health Benefits

Beyond the psychological benefits, human-animal bonding can also have a positive impact on physical health. Research suggests that having a pet can lead to lower blood pressure and reduced risk of heart disease. The presence of animals has been associated with improved cardiovascular health, likely due to the calming effect they have on the body.

Engaging in physical activities with animals, such as walking or playing fetch, can contribute to a more active lifestyle. Regular exercise has well-known benefits for physical health, including weight management, improved cardiovascular fitness, and increased energy levels. Animals can serve as motivators and provide companionship during exercise, making it more enjoyable and sustainable.

Social Benefits

Another significant benefit of human-animal bonding is the enhancement of social interactions and social support. Animals can serve as social facilitators, making it easier for individuals to connect with others. Walking a dog, for example, often leads to encounters and conversations with other dog owners, fostering a sense of belonging and community.

Furthermore, animals can provide a sense of security and emotional support, particularly for individuals facing challenging life circumstances. Many therapy animals, such as therapy dogs or horses, are trained to offer comfort and assistance to individuals with mental health conditions or disabilities. These animals can help individuals overcome social barriers and build confidence in social settings.

Therapeutic Applications

Given the wide range of benefits associated with human-animal bonding, it is no surprise that animals are increasingly being utilized in therapeutic settings. Animal-assisted therapy (AAT) involves trained animals working alongside therapists to help individuals achieve specific therapeutic goals.

AAT has been shown to be effective in various mental health and physical health settings. For example, therapy dogs have been used to help individuals with post-traumatic stress disorder (PTSD) cope with anxiety and emotional distress. Often, they provide comfort and support during therapy sessions, helping individuals feel safe and supported.

Equine-assisted therapy is another example of AAT that utilizes horses to promote emotional growth and learning. Interacting with horses can help individuals develop skills such as empathy, assertiveness, and emotional regulation.

The grounded nature of working with horses can also serve as a metaphor for addressing life challenges and building resilience.

Ethical Considerations

While the benefits of human-animal bonding are well-established, it is important to consider the ethical implications of incorporating animals into therapeutic interventions. It is essential to ensure that animals used in these contexts are treated with care, respect, and appropriate training. Animal welfare must always be a priority, and practitioners should adhere to ethical guidelines to maintain the well-being of both humans and animals involved in therapeutic interventions.

In conclusion, the benefits of human-animal bonding are numerous and diverse. Animals can provide psychological, physical, and social support, enhancing overall well-being and contributing to a holistic approach to mental health. Whether as pets, therapy animals, or companions in various settings, animals have the potential to improve mental health outcomes and create meaningful connections in people's lives. It is crucial to continue exploring the therapeutic potential of human-animal bonding and ensure ethical practices in its implementation.

Animal-Assisted Therapy in Mental Health Settings

Animal-assisted therapy (AAT) is an innovative and effective approach to mental health treatment that incorporates animals into therapeutic interventions. It involves using trained animals as part of the therapeutic process to support individuals in reaching their treatment goals. This section will explore the principles and benefits of animal-assisted therapy, as well as provide an overview of the different types of animals used in mental health settings.

Principles of Animal-Assisted Therapy

Animal-assisted therapy is based on several key principles that guide its practice. Firstly, AAT recognizes the bond and connection between humans and animals, and how this can contribute to a therapeutic relationship. The presence of an animal can create a sense of comfort, trust, and safety for individuals struggling with mental health issues.

Secondly, animal-assisted therapy acknowledges the positive impact animals can have on overall well-being. Interacting with animals has been shown to reduce stress, anxiety, and depression, while also increasing feelings of joy, relaxation, and happiness. This principle is grounded in research that highlights the physiological and psychological benefits of human-animal interactions.

Thirdly, animal-assisted therapy recognizes the unique ability of animals to provide unconditional acceptance and non-judgmental support. They can offer companionship, empathy, and a sense of connection that is especially valuable for individuals experiencing feelings of isolation or loneliness.

Lastly, animal-assisted therapy is an evidence-based practice that follows ethical guidelines and professional standards. Therapists and animals involved in AAT undergo rigorous training and certification to ensure the safety and well-being of all participants. The therapy sessions are carefully planned and structured to meet the specific needs and goals of each individual.

Types of Animals in Animal-Assisted Therapy

Various types of animals can be incorporated into animal-assisted therapy, depending on the specific goals and preferences of the individual receiving treatment. The most commonly used animals in mental health settings include dogs, cats, horses, and birds. Each animal brings unique qualities and benefits to the therapeutic process.

Dogs are the most widely utilized animals in animal-assisted therapy due to their social nature, loyalty, and ability to form strong bonds with humans. They can provide emotional support, companionship, and assist in building social skills. Dogs are often used in interventions aimed at reducing anxiety, improving mood, and enhancing overall well-being.

Cats are also popular in animal-assisted therapy, particularly for individuals who find solace in their calming presence. Cats are known for their independent nature and can help individuals develop a sense of responsibility and relaxation. They are typically used in interventions for stress reduction, emotional regulation, and improving social interactions.

Horses play a significant role in equine-assisted therapy, a specific modality within animal-assisted therapy. Their size, strength, and gentle demeanor create a unique therapeutic experience. Interactions with horses can promote self-awareness, emotional regulation, and enhance communication and trust-building skills.

Birds, particularly parrots, are used in animal-assisted therapy for their ability to form strong bonds with humans and provide intellectual stimulation. Birds can stimulate conversation, promote cognitive skills, and facilitate emotional expression. Their vivid colors and playful nature can also bring joy and create a positive therapeutic environment.

Each animal is carefully selected based on the individual's treatment goals, preferences, and any allergies or fears. The therapist works closely with the individual to determine which animal will best support their specific needs.

Benefits of Animal-Assisted Therapy

Animal-assisted therapy has demonstrated numerous benefits for individuals receiving mental health treatment. Some of the key advantages include:

1. Emotional support and stress reduction: Interacting with animals can help reduce stress, anxiety, and depression. Animals provide a source of comfort and can serve as a non-judgmental listener, offering emotional support and a sense of calm.

2. Improved social interactions: Animals can act as a catalyst for social interactions and improve social skills. Individuals may feel more comfortable and confident engaging with an animal, which can then transfer to their interactions with humans.

3. Increased motivation and engagement: Animal-assisted therapy can enhance motivation and engagement in the therapeutic process. The presence of an animal can make therapy sessions more enjoyable and encourage individuals to actively participate and work towards their goals.

4. Physical and physiological benefits: Interacting with animals has been linked to several physical and physiological benefits. It can lower blood pressure, reduce heart rate, and release endorphins, creating a positive impact on overall well-being.

5. Sense of purpose and responsibility: Caring for an animal can provide individuals with a sense of purpose and responsibility. It can foster feelings of self-worth, enhance self-esteem, and provide a sense of accomplishment.

6. Increased self-awareness and emotional regulation: Animals can serve as a mirror, reflecting emotions and behaviors back to individuals. This can help increase self-awareness and support the development of emotional regulation skills.

7. Enhanced communication and trust-building: Animals can promote communication and trust-building skills. Interacting with an animal can create a safe and non-threatening environment, allowing individuals to practice and develop effective communication and trust-building strategies.

8. Positive distraction and diversion: Animals can provide a positive distraction from mental health symptoms or distressing thoughts. They can create moments of joy, happiness, and playfulness, promoting a more balanced emotional state.

Considerations and Ethical Guidelines

While animal-assisted therapy offers many benefits, it is essential to consider certain ethical guidelines and precautions when incorporating animals into mental health settings. Some key considerations include:

1. Animal welfare: The well-being of the animals involved must be a top priority. Their health, safety, and comfort should be carefully monitored, and appropriate measures should be taken to ensure their welfare.

2. Allergies and fears: Individuals with allergies or fears of certain animals should be accommodated appropriately. Therapists should conduct thorough assessments and make necessary adjustments to ensure a safe and comfortable environment for all participants.

3. Informed consent: Informed consent should be obtained from the individuals receiving animal-assisted therapy. They should be fully informed about the goals, benefits, and potential risks associated with the therapy.

4. Boundaries and limitations: Clear boundaries and limitations should be established regarding interactions with the animals. Therapists should educate individuals on appropriate ways to interact with the animals to prevent any harm to themselves or the animals.

5. Training and certification: Therapists and animals involved in animal-assisted therapy should undergo proper training and certification. This ensures that they meet the required standards and possess the necessary skills to provide safe and effective therapy.

It is important to note that animal-assisted therapy may not be suitable for everyone or every mental health condition. Therapists should conduct thorough assessments to determine the appropriateness of AAT based on the individual's needs and treatment goals.

Example: Animal-Assisted Therapy for Anxiety

To illustrate the benefits of animal-assisted therapy, let's consider an example of AAT for anxiety. Sarah, a 30-year-old woman diagnosed with generalized anxiety disorder, has been attending regular therapy sessions. Her therapist suggests incorporating an animal-assisted therapy intervention to complement her current treatment plan.

Sarah's therapist arranges for a friendly and trained therapy dog named Max to be present in their sessions. Initially, Sarah is hesitant and anxious around dogs. However, with guidance and support from her therapist, she gradually learns to engage with Max.

Over several sessions, Sarah begins to experience the benefits of animal-assisted therapy. Max's presence helps her feel more relaxed and at ease, reducing her anxiety levels. She develops a sense of connection and attachment to Max, which enhances her overall well-being. Sarah's interactions with Max also improve her social skills, as she begins to engage in conversations about dogs and share her experiences.

Through AAT, Sarah learns coping strategies for managing her anxiety and gains a renewed sense of hope and optimism. The therapy sessions become a safe and enjoyable space for her, where she feels supported and understood. The combination of traditional therapy techniques and animal-assisted therapy proves to be a powerful approach in addressing Sarah's anxiety.

Conclusion

Animal-assisted therapy is a valuable addition to mental health treatment, offering unique benefits and opportunities for growth. By incorporating animals into therapy sessions, individuals can experience emotional support, stress reduction, improved social interactions, increased motivation, and various other advantages. However, it is crucial to adhere to ethical guidelines, prioritize animal welfare, and assess the appropriateness of AAT for each individual. Through the integration of animal-assisted therapy, mental health settings can create an inclusive and holistic approach to promoting well-being and supporting individuals on their journey towards sustainable mental health.

Equine-Assisted Therapy

Equine-assisted therapy, also known as horse therapy or equine therapy, is a therapeutic approach that involves interactions between individuals and horses to promote physical, emotional, and mental well-being. This section will explore the principles and benefits of equine-assisted therapy, as well as some of the techniques and interventions used in this approach.

Principles of Equine-Assisted Therapy

Equine-assisted therapy is based on several principles that guide the therapeutic process:

- **Nonverbal communication:** Horses are highly sensitive animals that can pick up on nonverbal cues from humans. This aspect of equine therapy emphasizes the importance of body language and emotional regulation in establishing a connection with the horse.

- **Mirror mechanism:** Horses can mirror the behaviors and emotions of humans, providing valuable feedback on how individuals present themselves and respond to challenges. This mechanism allows participants to gain insights into their own emotions and behaviors.

- **Empowerment and mastery:** Engaging in activities with horses, such as grooming, riding, or leading, can help individuals develop a sense of empowerment and mastery over their actions. This can be particularly beneficial for those who have experienced trauma or have low self-esteem.

- **Trust and attachment:** Building a relationship with a horse requires trust and attachment. Many individuals find it easier to establish these connections with horses than with other humans, as horses are non-judgmental and offer unconditional acceptance.

- **Mindfulness and grounding:** The presence of horses in a natural environment can promote mindfulness and grounding. Being in the present moment and connecting with the horse and surroundings can help individuals reduce anxiety and enhance their overall well-being.

Benefits of Equine-Assisted Therapy

Equine-assisted therapy has been shown to have several benefits for individuals with various mental health conditions, including:

- **Emotional regulation:** Interacting with horses can help individuals develop emotional awareness and regulation skills. The calming presence of the horse and the nonverbal feedback received during interactions contribute to emotional stability.

- **Improved self-esteem:** By engaging in activities with horses, individuals can experience a sense of accomplishment and enhanced self-esteem. Developing a bond with a horse can provide a feeling of acceptance and validation.

- **Stress reduction:** Being in the presence of horses and engaging in equine activities can help reduce stress levels. The rhythmic motion of horseback riding, for example, can have a soothing effect on the nervous system.

- **Increased social skills:** Equine-assisted therapy often involves group activities, which provide opportunities for individuals to improve their communication and social skills. Collaborating with others in a horse-related task fosters teamwork and cooperation.

- **Healing from trauma:** Equine therapy has shown promise in trauma recovery. Horses' ability to sense fear and anxiety allows them to provide a safe and supportive environment for individuals to address and process their trauma.

- **Physical benefits:** Engaging in horse-related activities, such as grooming or riding, can improve balance, coordination, and core strength. These physical benefits contribute to overall well-being.

- **Enhanced coping skills:** Through working with horses, individuals can develop problem-solving and coping strategies that can be applied to real-life situations. This can help them manage stress, conflicts, and challenges more effectively.

Interventions in Equine-Assisted Therapy

Equine-assisted therapy incorporates various interventions to support the therapeutic process. Some common interventions include:

- **Horse grooming:** Grooming a horse involves activities such as brushing, cleaning hooves, and bonding with the animal. This activity promotes relaxation, trust-building, and bonding.

- **Horseback riding:** Riding a horse provides a unique physical and emotional experience. The rhythmic movement of the horse can help individuals regulate their emotions and improve their balance and coordination.

- **Groundwork exercises:** Working with a horse on the ground involves leading, lunging, and other activities that focus on establishing communication, trust, and boundaries between the individual and the horse.

- **Equine-assisted psychotherapy (EAP):** EAP combines traditional psychotherapy approaches with equine-assisted activities. In EAP sessions, therapists observe and facilitate interactions between the individual and the horse to promote insight and personal growth.

- **Equine-assisted learning (EAL):** EAL focuses on experiential learning and personal development. Participants engage in activities or tasks with the horse, which are designed to teach problem-solving, teamwork, communication, and leadership skills.

- **Natural horsemanship techniques:** These techniques emphasize developing a relationship with the horse based on trust, respect, and clear communication. Natural horsemanship aims to enhance the individual's understanding of themselves and others through interactions with the horse.

Example Scenario: Equine-Assisted Therapy for PTSD

Consider the case of Jake, a military veteran suffering from post-traumatic stress disorder (PTSD). Jake has been struggling with nightmares, hypervigilance, and social isolation since returning from active duty. He decides to try equine-assisted therapy to help manage his symptoms and improve his overall well-being.

During his therapy sessions, Jake engages in various activities with a horse under the guidance of a trained therapist. One of the activities involves grooming the horse, which helps Jake develop a sense of connection and trust with the animal. As he progresses in his therapy, Jake also starts riding the horse, which allows him to experience a sense of control and empowerment.

Through interactions with the horse, Jake learns to regulate his emotions and identify triggers that exacerbate his PTSD symptoms. The therapist observes the interaction and provides guidance on managing anxiety and maintaining a sense of calm during challenging moments.

Over time, Jake's equine-assisted therapy sessions help him develop coping mechanisms to manage his PTSD symptoms. He becomes more confident, socially engaged, and experiences a reduction in hypervigilance and nightmares. The bond he forms with the horse serves as a source of support and healing throughout his treatment journey.

Resources for Equine-Assisted Therapy

Equine-assisted therapy requires specialized training and expertise. If you are interested in exploring equine therapy further, consider the following resources:

- **Equine Assisted Growth and Learning Association (EAGALA):** EAGALA provides certification and resources for individuals interested in practicing equine-assisted therapy. Their website offers a directory to find certified professionals in your area.

- **Certification in Equine-Assisted Mental Health (CEMH):** CEMH offers a comprehensive certification program for mental health professionals seeking to specialize in equine-assisted therapy. The certification program covers theory, ethics, and practical skills required for effective practice.

- **Equine Facilitated Wellness (EFW) Canada:** EFW Canada is a national organization dedicated to promoting the well-being of individuals and communities through equine-assisted therapy and learning. Their website provides resources, training opportunities, and a directory of Canadian practitioners.

- Equine-Assisted Growth and Learning Association International (EAGALA International): EAGALA International is a global organization that provides information, resources, and networking opportunities for professionals working in the field of equine-assisted therapy. Their website offers access to research, publications, and training events.

Equine-assisted therapy is a powerful and engaging approach that can provide individuals with unique opportunities for personal growth and healing. Its focus on nonverbal communication, trust-building, and empowerment makes it a valuable complementary therapeutic modality in contemporary mental health care.

Canine-Assisted Therapy

Canine-Assisted Therapy is a form of animal-assisted therapy that utilizes dogs to support the emotional and psychological well-being of individuals. This section explores the principles and benefits of Canine-Assisted Therapy, its applications in mental health settings, and the evidence supporting its effectiveness.

Principles of Canine-Assisted Therapy

Canine-Assisted Therapy is grounded in the principle that interactions with dogs can have a positive impact on human mental health. The presence of dogs can create a sense of comfort, companionship, and unconditional acceptance. Dogs have a unique ability to sense and respond to human emotions, providing a non-judgmental and supportive presence. The therapy typically involves a trained therapy dog and a licensed mental health professional working together in a therapeutic setting.

Benefits of Canine-Assisted Therapy

Canine-Assisted Therapy has been shown to provide numerous benefits for individuals experiencing mental health challenges:

- Emotional support: Dogs can provide a source of emotional support, reducing feelings of loneliness and anxiety. The presence of a therapy dog can create a calming effect and promote relaxation.

- Physical and psychological benefits: Interacting with dogs has been found to lower blood pressure, reduce stress hormones, and increase the release of endorphins, which contribute to feelings of happiness and well-being. These physiological changes can have a positive impact on mental health.

- Social engagement: Dogs can serve as a bridge to social interaction, facilitating communication and building rapport between individuals. For those who struggle with social anxiety or isolation, the presence of a therapy dog can encourage engagement and open avenues for connection with others.

- Increased motivation and self-esteem: Through Canine-Assisted Therapy, individuals may experience increased motivation to engage in therapeutic activities. The presence of a therapy dog can foster a sense of accomplishment and boost self-esteem.

- Improved focus and attention: Interacting with dogs requires individuals to focus their attention, which can be particularly beneficial for individuals with attention-related disorders. Canine-Assisted Therapy can improve concentration and help individuals stay present in the therapeutic process.

Applications of Canine-Assisted Therapy

Canine-Assisted Therapy can be applied in various mental health settings, including:

- Therapy sessions: Therapy dogs can be present during individual or group therapy sessions to provide support and facilitate emotional expression. Their presence can help create a safe and trusting environment, allowing individuals to explore their feelings and experiences.

- Hospitals and medical settings: Canine-Assisted Therapy has been used in hospitals and medical settings to help reduce anxiety and stress in patients. The presence of therapy dogs can provide comfort and distraction, making medical procedures less intimidating or distressing.

- Schools and educational settings: Dogs in educational settings can serve as learning aids and promote emotional well-being among students. Canine-Assisted Therapy programs in schools have been shown to reduce stress, improve attendance, and enhance emotional regulation.

- Rehabilitation programs: Canine-Assisted Therapy can be beneficial in rehabilitation programs, including substance abuse treatment centers and prisons. The presence of therapy dogs can support individuals in their recovery journey, improve their emotional well-being, and enhance overall program outcomes.

Evidence for Canine-Assisted Therapy

Research studies have provided empirical support for the effectiveness of Canine-Assisted Therapy:

- Reduced symptoms of anxiety and depression: Studies have shown that interactions with therapy dogs can lead to a reduction in symptoms of anxiety and depression. This may be attributed to the release of oxytocin, a hormone associated with bonding and relaxation.

- Improved social interaction: Canine-Assisted Therapy has been found to improve social skills and increase social interaction among individuals, particularly in those with autism spectrum disorders or social anxiety.

- Enhanced emotional well-being: Interacting with therapy dogs has been associated with increased positive affect, reduced negative emotions, and improved overall emotional well-being. It can also foster a sense of purpose and meaning in life.

- Better treatment adherence: The presence of therapy dogs can improve treatment adherence, as individuals may feel more motivated to participate in therapy or follow treatment plans when they have the support of a therapy dog.

Example: Canine-Assisted Therapy for Veterans with PTSD

To illustrate the application of Canine-Assisted Therapy, let's consider its use in treating veterans with post-traumatic stress disorder (PTSD). Many veterans experience symptoms of PTSD, such as hyperarousal, intrusive thoughts, and social withdrawal. Canine-Assisted Therapy can be integrated into their treatment plan to provide emotional support and assist in their recovery.

In this example, therapy sessions may involve a therapy dog that has been specifically trained to work with veterans with PTSD. The presence of the therapy dog can create a safe space for veterans to express their emotions and share their experiences. The therapist can guide the interaction between the veteran and the dog, helping the veteran develop coping strategies and manage anxiety symptoms.

Canine-Assisted Therapy can also extend beyond therapy sessions. The veteran may have the opportunity to interact with the therapy dog during group activities or during recreational therapy sessions. This can promote social engagement and encourage the veteran to participate in treatment activities that they may otherwise find overwhelming.

By incorporating Canine-Assisted Therapy into the treatment plan for veterans with PTSD, it is possible to enhance the therapeutic process, improve treatment outcomes, and contribute to the overall well-being of these individuals.

Resources for Canine-Assisted Therapy

For those interested in exploring Canine-Assisted Therapy further, the following resources can provide additional information and guidance:

- The International Association of Human-Animal Interaction Organizations (IAHAIO): This organization promotes the understanding and use of human-animal interaction for therapeutic purposes. They offer resources and guidelines for implementing Canine-Assisted Therapy.

- Therapy Dogs International (TDI): TDI is a volunteer organization that provides training and certification for therapy dogs. Their website offers information on the benefits of therapy dogs and how to get involved in Canine-Assisted Therapy programs.

- Research articles and publications: Various research studies have been conducted on the effectiveness of Canine-Assisted Therapy. Exploring academic journals and publications can provide valuable insights into the evidence supporting this form of therapy.

Conclusion

Canine-Assisted Therapy is an effective and versatile approach to supporting mental health and well-being. The presence of therapy dogs can provide emotional support, enhance social interaction, and improve overall treatment outcomes. Incorporating Canine-Assisted Therapy into mental health settings can contribute to a holistic and sustainable approach to mental health care.

Spirituality and Mental Health

Religion and Mental Health

The Role of Religion in Mental Health

Religion has long been intertwined with human history, culture, and individual beliefs. It plays a significant role in shaping the ways individuals perceive the world, find meaning, and cope with life's challenges. The connection between religion and mental health has been a subject of interest and debate among researchers and practitioners in the field.

Religion can provide individuals with a sense of purpose, belonging, and social support, which are important factors for mental well-being. Engaging in religious practices and beliefs can offer a sense of stability, hope, and guidance during difficult times. For some individuals, religious beliefs and practices provide a framework for understanding and making sense of their experiences, including their mental health.

On the other hand, religion can also be a source of stress and contribute to mental health issues. Strict religious rules or expectations may lead to feelings of guilt, shame, or inadequacy. Some individuals may experience conflicts between their religious beliefs and their personal values or identity, which can cause distress and affect their mental well-being.

Understanding the relationship between religion and mental health requires a nuanced perspective that takes into account individual experiences, cultural contexts, and diverse religious traditions. It is important to consider both the positive and potentially negative impacts of religion on mental health and well-being.

Positive Effects of Religion on Mental Health

Research has shown that religion can have positive effects on mental health and well-being. Here are some ways in which religion can contribute to positive mental health outcomes:

1. **Sense of meaning and purpose:** Religious beliefs and practices can provide individuals with a sense of meaning and purpose in life. Believing in a higher power or being part of a religious community can give individuals a sense of direction and help them find meaning in difficult circumstances.

2. **Social support:** Religious communities often provide a strong social support network. They can offer a sense of belonging, acceptance, and connection with others who share similar values and beliefs. This support system can help individuals cope with stress, loneliness, and adversity.

3. **Coping mechanisms:** Religion often provides individuals with a set of coping mechanisms and rituals that can be helpful during challenging times. Prayer, meditation, and other spiritual practices have been shown to reduce stress, enhance resilience, and promote emotional well-being.

4. **Values and ethics:** Religious teachings often emphasize moral values and ethical principles. These values can guide individuals in making decisions, promoting prosocial behavior, and fostering a sense of integrity and self-worth.

5. **Hope and optimism:** Religious beliefs often emphasize the existence of a higher power, divine providence, or the promise of an afterlife. These beliefs can provide individuals with hope, comfort, and a positive outlook on life, especially in the face of adversity or uncertainty.

Challenges and Criticisms

While religion can have positive effects on mental health, it is important to be mindful of the potential challenges and criticisms associated with religious beliefs and practices. Here are some factors to consider:

1. **Religious conflicts and guilt:** Some individuals may experience conflicts between their religious beliefs and their personal values or identity. This can lead to feelings of guilt, shame, or inner turmoil, which can negatively impact mental well-being.

2. **Rigid beliefs and dogma:** Strict adherence to religious doctrines or dogma may limit individuals' ability to question, explore, or adapt their beliefs in light of new information or experiences. This rigidity can hinder personal growth, critical thinking, and openness to alternative perspectives.

3. **Stigmatization and exclusion:** Although religious communities can provide social support, some individuals may experience stigmatization or exclusion based on their religious beliefs or lack thereof. This can contribute to feelings of isolation, self-doubt, and psychological distress.

4. **Negative teachings and practices:** Some religious teachings or practices may perpetuate harmful beliefs or endorse behaviors that are not conducive to mental well-being. It is important to critically evaluate the impact of specific religious teachings on individuals' mental health and well-being.

5. **Cultural and contextual factors**: The impact of religion on mental health can vary across different cultural and contextual settings. It is essential to consider the diversity of religious beliefs, practices, and interpretations within and across different communities.

It is important to recognize that the relationship between religion and mental health is complex and multifaceted. Individual experiences, cultural contexts, and personal beliefs all contribute to the ways in which religion influences mental well-being.

Integration of Religion into Mental Health Care

Given the significance of religion in individuals' lives, mental health professionals have increasingly recognized the importance of integrating religious and spiritual considerations into mental health care. Here are some key points to consider:

1. **Culturally sensitive approach**: Mental health professionals should adopt a culturally sensitive approach that respects individuals' religious beliefs and values. This involves being open and non-judgmental, actively listening to clients' spiritual concerns, and incorporating these concerns into the therapeutic process when appropriate.

2. **Collaborative exploration**: Mental health professionals can collaborate with clients to explore the role of religion in their lives and their mental health. This may involve discussing the positive aspects of religious beliefs and practices, as well as addressing any conflicts or challenges that may arise.

3. **Referral to religious leaders**: In some cases, it may be beneficial to involve religious leaders or advisors in the therapeutic process. They can provide guidance, support, and a deeper understanding of the client's religious beliefs and practices.

4. **Ethical considerations**: Mental health professionals should be mindful of their ethical responsibilities, including the need to respect clients' autonomy, avoid imposing their own beliefs on clients, and provide unbiased care. It is important to strike a balance between incorporating religious considerations and ensuring evidence-based, client-centered care.

In conclusion, religion can have a significant impact on mental health and well-being. It can provide individuals with a sense of meaning, social support, coping mechanisms, and hope. However, it is important to recognize the potential challenges and criticisms associated with religious beliefs and practices. Mental health professionals should adopt a culturally sensitive and holistic approach that integrates religious considerations when appropriate, while respecting clients' autonomy and providing evidence-based care. By acknowledging and addressing the complex interplay between religion and mental health, we can promote the well-being of individuals and communities.

Mindfulness in Spiritual Traditions

Mindfulness is a practice that has been incorporated into various spiritual traditions across the world, including Buddhism, Hinduism, and Taoism. It involves cultivating a state of present-moment awareness and non-judgmental attention to one's thoughts, feelings, and bodily sensations. In this section, we will explore the concept of mindfulness in different spiritual traditions and its relevance to mental health and wellbeing.

Mindfulness in Buddhism

Buddhism is often credited with popularizing mindfulness as a formal practice. The teachings of the Buddha highlight the importance of mindfulness as a means to achieve liberation from suffering and find inner peace. The practice of mindfulness meditation, known as Vipassana, is a central aspect of Buddhist practice.

In Buddhism, mindfulness is seen as a way to develop insight into the impermanent and interdependent nature of reality. By observing the present moment without attachment or aversion, individuals can gain a deeper understanding of the nature of their own mind and the nature of existence itself.

The Four Foundations of Mindfulness, as taught by the Buddha, provide a framework for practicing mindfulness. These foundations include mindfulness of the body, feelings, mind, and mental objects. By bringing awareness to these aspects of experience, individuals can cultivate a greater sense of clarity, equanimity, and compassion.

Mindfulness in Hinduism

In Hinduism, mindfulness is closely associated with the practice of yoga. Yoga is a holistic system that aims to unite the mind, body, and spirit. The practice of mindfulness in Hinduism involves cultivating self-awareness and a connection to the divine within oneself.

The ancient text, the Bhagavad Gita, describes mindfulness as being present in every action and surrendering the fruits of those actions to a higher power. Mindfulness in Hinduism is not limited to meditation but is also practiced in everyday activities such as eating, walking, and interacting with others.

The practice of mindfulness in Hinduism is often combined with other yogic practices such as asanas (physical postures), pranayama (breathing exercises), and mantra chanting. These practices aim to quiet the mind, increase self-awareness, and enhance spiritual growth.

Mindfulness in Taoism

Taoism, an ancient Chinese philosophy, emphasizes harmony with nature and the cultivation of inner peace. Mindfulness in Taoism is closely related to the concept of Wu Wei, which can be translated as "effortless action" or "non-striving." Wu Wei involves aligning oneself with the natural flow of life and acting without force or resistance.

In Taoism, mindfulness is about being fully present in the present moment and embracing the inherent simplicity and spontaneity of life. This practice involves letting go of attachments, thoughts, and emotions that hinder the experience of true inner peace and harmony.

The Taoist practice of mindfulness often involves contemplation and meditation in natural environments, such as mountains, rivers, and forests. These natural settings are believed to support the cultivation of stillness, tranquility, and a deep sense of interconnectedness with all beings.

Mindfulness and Mental Health

The practice of mindfulness in spiritual traditions has gained significant attention in the field of psychology and mental health. Research has shown that mindfulness-based interventions can be effective in reducing symptoms of anxiety, depression, and stress, as well as enhancing overall wellbeing.

Mindfulness practice has been found to promote emotional regulation, increase cognitive flexibility, and improve attention and focus. It can also cultivate self-compassion and reduce self-critical thoughts. By developing a non-judgmental attitude towards one's experiences, individuals can learn to respond to challenging situations with greater clarity and resilience.

Incorporating mindfulness into mental health care can empower individuals to actively participate in their own healing process. Mindfulness-based interventions, such as Mindfulness-Based Stress Reduction (MBSR) and Mindfulness-Based

Cognitive Therapy (MBCT), have been widely used in clinical settings to address a range of mental health issues.

Practical Application of Mindfulness

Practicing mindfulness does not require adherence to a specific spiritual tradition. It can be integrated into daily life in a secular context, benefiting individuals from all walks of life. Here are some practical ways to incorporate mindfulness into your daily routine:

1. Formal mindfulness meditation: Set aside dedicated time each day to sit quietly and bring mindful awareness to your breath, bodily sensations, thoughts, and emotions.

2. Mindful eating: Pay attention to each bite of food, savoring the flavors and textures. Notice the sensations of hunger and satiety.

3. Mindful walking: Slow down and bring awareness to the sensation of your feet contacting the ground, the movement of your body, and the sounds and sights around you.

4. Mindful communication: Practice active listening and non-judgmental presence in your interactions with others, giving them your full attention and empathy.

5. Mindful self-compassion: Cultivate a compassionate attitude towards yourself, acknowledging and accepting your thoughts and emotions without judgment.

6. Mindful breathing: Take a few moments throughout the day to focus on your breath, noticing the sensation of the breath entering and leaving your body.

Remember, mindfulness is a skill that requires practice and patience. As you incorporate mindfulness into your life, you may find that it enhances your mental health, reduces stress, and promotes overall wellbeing.

Resources

1. Kabat-Zinn, J. (2013). Full Catastrophe Living: Using the Wisdom of Your Body and Mind to Face Stress, Pain, and Illness. Bantam.

2. Salzberg, S. (2011). Real Happiness: The Power of Meditation: A 28-Day Program. Workman Publishing Company.

3. Harris, R. (2014). 10

4. Siegel, R. D. (2010). The Mindful Therapist: A Clinician's Guide to Mindsight and Neural Integration. W. W. Norton & Company.

These resources provide in-depth knowledge and practical guidance for incorporating mindfulness into your spiritual and mental health journey.

The Role of Faith Communities in Mental Health Support

Faith communities play a significant role in providing support and resources for individuals experiencing mental health challenges. These communities, which include religious institutions such as churches, mosques, synagogues, and temples, have a unique position in society and can offer valuable support systems for individuals seeking assistance with their mental well-being.

One of the key roles that faith communities can play in mental health support is providing a sense of belonging and social connection. Many people find solace, comfort, and a sense of community within their faith communities. These communities often offer opportunities for individuals to connect with others who share similar beliefs and experiences. This social support can be instrumental in reducing feelings of isolation and loneliness, which are common experiences among individuals struggling with mental health issues.

Faith communities also have the potential to foster a supportive and nurturing environment. They can provide a safe space for individuals to share their struggles and seek guidance and encouragement. Pastors, imams, rabbis, and other religious leaders within these communities can offer spiritual guidance and counseling, providing a holistic approach to mental health support. Their training and understanding of religious teachings can help individuals explore the intersection of their faith and mental health.

Moreover, faith communities can offer various programs and resources to promote mental well-being. These programs may include support groups, educational workshops, and counseling services tailored to the needs of their congregants. For example, churches might offer marital counseling or addiction recovery programs, while mosques might provide spaces for meditation and mindfulness practices. These resources can help individuals develop coping mechanisms, gain insight into their mental health struggles, and find practical strategies for managing their symptoms.

Additionally, faith communities can help reduce stigma surrounding mental health issues. By openly addressing mental health concerns from a religious perspective, these communities can contribute to normalizing conversations about mental health and challenging misconceptions. Open dialogue can decrease the shame and guilt that individuals may associate with seeking help for mental health difficulties.

While faith communities offer valuable resources and support, it is important to acknowledge that they are not a substitute for professional mental health care. Mental health professionals possess the specialized knowledge and skills necessary to diagnose and treat mental health disorders. Therefore, faith communities should work in collaboration with mental health professionals and refer individuals to appropriate services when needed.

In order to effectively support individuals with mental health challenges, it is crucial for faith communities and their leaders to be knowledgeable about mental health and to receive training on how to address mental health issues within their community. This can include education on the signs and symptoms of mental health disorders, understanding the importance of seeking professional help, and learning how to provide appropriate support and referrals.

Overall, the role of faith communities in mental health support is multifaceted. They provide social support, spiritual guidance, and resources that can enhance the well-being of individuals struggling with mental health challenges. By recognizing the significance and potential of faith communities, we can foster an inclusive and holistic approach to mental health care that integrates the strengths of both religious support and professional mental health services.

Existential Wellbeing and Mental Health

Existential wellbeing refers to an individual's sense of meaning, purpose, and connection to the larger world. It encompasses questions about the nature of existence, one's role in the universe, and the search for ultimate meaning. In the context of mental health, existential wellbeing plays a vital role in promoting resilience, inner strength, and overall psychological wellness. This section explores the significance of existential wellbeing in mental health and offers strategies for nurturing this aspect of human experience.

The Meaning of Existential Wellbeing

Existential wellbeing is rooted in existential philosophy, which examines the fundamental questions of human existence, such as the meaning of life, freedom, choice, and responsibility. It recognizes that individuals have an inherent need to find purpose and make sense of their lives. Existential wellbeing is not a static state but a dynamic process that involves ongoing exploration, self-reflection, and personal growth.

Key components of existential wellbeing include:

- **Meaning and Purpose:** The belief that one's life has significance and direction, guided by personal values and goals.

- **Authenticity and Self-Awareness:** The ability to be true to oneself, acknowledge one's strengths and limitations, and act in alignment with one's values and beliefs.

- **Transcendence:** The capacity to go beyond one's immediate concerns and embrace a broader perspective of interconnectedness with others and the world.

- **Acceptance of Existential Givens:** Recognizing and accepting the inherent uncertainties, paradoxes, and existential givens of human existence, such as mortality, freedom, and responsibility.

Existential Wellbeing and Mental Health

Existential wellbeing is closely linked to mental health and can significantly impact an individual's overall wellbeing. When individuals lack a sense of meaning and purpose, they may experience existential crises, feelings of emptiness, and an increased susceptibility to mental health issues such as anxiety and depression. On the other hand, cultivating existential wellbeing can enhance psychological resilience, coping skills, and overall life satisfaction.

Existential Wellbeing and Resilience Resilience, the ability to bounce back from adversity, is closely intertwined with existential wellbeing. When individuals have a strong sense of meaning and purpose, they are better equipped to navigate life's challenges and setbacks. They can find solace and strength in times of difficulty by drawing on their existential resources, such as their values, relationships, and connection to a larger purpose.

Existential Wellbeing and Psychological Growth Existential wellbeing also plays a crucial role in psychological growth and self-actualization. Exploring existential questions and grappling with the complexities of existence can lead to greater self-awareness, personal insight, and a deepening of one's identity. This process of self-discovery can enhance personal growth and contribute to a sense of fulfillment and psychological wellbeing.

Nurturing Existential Wellbeing

Nurturing existential wellbeing is an ongoing endeavor that requires self-reflection, personal exploration, and a willingness to confront existential questions. Here are some strategies for cultivating existential wellbeing:

Reflection and Self-Inquiry   Engage in self-reflective practices such as journaling or meditation to explore existential questions and gain insight into your values, beliefs, and life purpose. Reflecting on your experiences and contemplating the broader meaning of life can promote existential wellbeing.

Seeking Meaningful Connections   Build and nurture relationships that provide a sense of connection, belonging, and shared values. Meaningful connections with others can foster a sense of purpose and reinforce one's existential wellbeing.

Engaging in Meaningful Activities   Participate in activities that align with your values and provide a sense of meaning and purpose. This could involve pursuing hobbies, engaging in creative endeavors, volunteering, or making a difference in your community.

Embracing Existential Givens   Acknowledge and accept the existential givens of life, such as the reality of death, uncertainty, and the limitations of human existence. Embracing these givens can lead to a greater appreciation for life and a deeper engagement with the present moment.

Engaging with Existential Philosophy and Spirituality   Explore existential philosophy, spiritual traditions, or philosophical teachings that address existential questions. These sources can offer guidance, wisdom, and different perspectives on the nature of existence and the search for meaning.

Integrating Existential Wellbeing into Mental Health Care

Mental health professionals can play a crucial role in integrating existential wellbeing into clinical practice. Some ways in which they can support individuals in nurturing existential wellbeing include:

Exploration of Meaning and Purpose   Engage clients in conversations about their values, goals, and the meaning they ascribe to their experiences. Help them connect their internal processes with their broader life purpose and explore ways to align their actions with their existential beliefs.

Therapeutic Techniques for Self-Reflection Incorporate therapeutic modalities that encourage self-reflection, such as narrative therapy, existential therapy, or mindfulness-based approaches. These techniques can help clients deepen their understanding of themselves, explore existential questions, and develop strategies for enhancing their existential wellbeing.

Facilitating Existential Coping Support clients in building resilience by helping them develop existential coping skills. This may involve helping them reframe their perspective in times of adversity, fostering a sense of transcendence through connection to something larger than themselves, and exploring existential resources that can support them in coping with existential challenges.

Conclusion

Existential wellbeing is an essential aspect of mental health and plays a significant role in an individual's overall wellbeing and resilience. Nurturing existential wellbeing involves engaging in self-reflection, seeking meaningful connections, embracing existential givens, and exploring the broader questions of existence. Mental health professionals can integrate existential wellbeing into clinical practice by exploring the meaning and purpose of their clients' lives, employing therapeutic techniques for self-reflection, and facilitating existential coping. By recognizing and addressing existential dimensions, mental health care can promote holistic and sustainable approaches to mental health.

Social Support and Mental Health

The Importance of Social Connections

In the realm of mental health, social connections play a crucial role in promoting overall wellbeing and resilience. Humans are inherently social beings, and our relationships and interactions with others significantly impact our mental health. This section explores the importance of social connections and their effects on mental wellbeing, highlighting the various ways in which social support networks can contribute to an individual's psychological resilience and overall sustainability.

The Impact of Social Connections on Mental Health

Numerous studies have consistently demonstrated the positive impact of social connections on mental health. Strong social support networks have been found to enhance psychological wellbeing, reduce the risk of developing mental health disorders, and improve coping abilities during times of stress or adversity.

Social connections provide individuals with a sense of belonging, acceptance, and validation. When individuals feel valued and understood by others, they experience a greater sense of self-worth and self-esteem. This sense of belongingness serves as a protective factor against mental health issues such as depression, anxiety, and loneliness.

Moreover, social connections create opportunities for positive social interactions, which contribute to positive emotions and overall life satisfaction. Engaging in meaningful social activities, such as spending time with loved ones, participating in group activities, or having deep conversations, stimulates the release of neurotransmitters like oxytocin and serotonin, which are associated with feelings of happiness and contentment.

Types of Social Connections

Social connections can take various forms, including family relationships, friendships, romantic partnerships, and community affiliations. Each type of social connection brings unique benefits to an individual's mental health.

Family relationships are often the primary source of social support and play a vital role in shaping individuals' mental wellbeing. A strong family support system provides a sense of stability, emotional security, and unconditional love, which can buffer against stress and adversity.

Friendships offer individuals opportunities for emotional support, companionship, and shared experiences. Close friends serve as confidants and sounding boards, providing a supportive and empathetic listening ear during challenging times. The social support derived from friendships enhances emotional resilience and promotes mental health.

Romantic partnerships or intimate relationships fulfill the innate human need for love, attachment, and emotional intimacy. These connections provide emotional support, a sense of belonging, and security. Strong and nurturing romantic relationships can enhance an individual's mental health by fostering feelings of love, happiness, and emotional stability.

Community affiliations, such as participation in social, religious, or interest-based groups, broaden an individual's social network and create a sense of belonging to a larger social fabric. These connections foster a sense of community, provide opportunities for social engagement, and promote a sense of purpose and fulfillment.

Building and Maintaining Social Connections

Building and maintaining social connections require active effort and nurturing. It is essential to cultivate and invest in relationships to reap the mental health benefits they offer. Here are some strategies for fostering and sustaining social connections:

1. Engage in social activities: Participate in group activities, join clubs or organizations, and attend social events to meet new people and expand your social circle.

2. Nurture existing relationships: Stay connected with family and friends by regularly reaching out, engaging in meaningful conversations, and spending quality time together.

3. Show empathy and support: Be a compassionate listener and lend a supportive ear to friends and loved ones. Offer encouragement, understanding, and validation to strengthen your relationships.

4. Foster reciprocal relationships: Strive for mutually beneficial relationships where both parties support and uplift each other. Give and receive emotional support, engage in acts of kindness, and show appreciation for one another.

5. Use technology wisely: Leverage technology and social media platforms to stay connected with distant friends and family members. However, be mindful of maintaining in-person interactions to foster deeper emotional connections.

6. Seek professional help if needed: If you are struggling with mental health issues or find it challenging to establish social connections, consider seeking the support of a mental health professional who can provide guidance and help develop strategies for building and maintaining social connections.

Challenges in Building Social Connections

While social connections are vital for mental health, building and maintaining them can sometimes be challenging. Here are a few common challenges individuals might face:

1. Social isolation: Physical distance, busy lifestyles, or other circumstances can lead to social isolation, making it difficult to form and nurture social connections.

2. Stigma and discrimination: Fear of judgment or rejection can prevent individuals from reaching out and forming new relationships.

3. Mental health conditions: Some mental health conditions, such as social anxiety, depression, or schizophrenia, can interfere with an individual's ability to engage in social interactions.

4. Transitions or life changes: Major life events like moving to a new location, changing schools, or experiencing divorce or loss can disrupt existing social networks and make it necessary to build new connections.

Addressing these challenges requires self-awareness, resilience, and sometimes professional support. Strategies might include stepping out of one's comfort zone, seeking therapy or support groups, or finding alternative ways to engage socially, such as joining online communities or local interest groups.

Conclusion

Social connections are a critical component of mental health and overall sustainability. They provide emotional support, a sense of belonging, and opportunities for positive social interactions. Investing in and nurturing social connections can enhance resilience, promote mental wellbeing, and contribute to a sustainable future. By cultivating strong social support networks, individuals can better navigate life's challenges, maintain psychological balance, and lead fulfilling lives.

Building Resilient Communities

Building resilient communities is a crucial aspect of promoting mental health and overall sustainability. Resilient communities are characterized by their ability to withstand and recover from adversity, protect the mental well-being of their members, and foster a sense of connectedness and support. In this section, we will explore the strategies and principles behind building resilient communities and the significance of collective action in promoting mental health.

Understanding Resilience at the Community Level

At the community level, resilience refers to the capacity of a community to respond effectively to stressors and to promote the well-being of its members. Resilient communities provide a supportive environment that enables individuals to cope with challenges and bounce back from adversity. They recognize that mental health is influenced not only by individual factors but also by social, economic, and environmental determinants.

Resilient communities prioritize the following principles:

- **Strong social networks:** Building and nurturing social connections within the community is essential for promoting resilience. These connections provide individuals with emotional support, a sense of belonging, and opportunities for collaboration and problem-solving.

- **Accessible resources and services:** Resilient communities ensure that appropriate resources and services are readily available to meet the mental health needs of their members. This includes access to quality healthcare, mental health education, counseling services, and support groups.

- **Empowerment and participation:** Resilient communities empower individuals to actively participate in decision-making processes and community initiatives. By involving community members in shaping their own environment, they foster a sense of ownership and agency, which enhances resilience.

- **Cultural sensitivity and inclusivity:** Resilient communities celebrate diversity and embrace cultural sensitivity. They aim to create an inclusive environment that values different perspectives, experiences, and identities, ensuring that everyone feels supported and included.

- **Collaboration and partnership:** Building resilience requires collaboration among different stakeholders, including community organizations, local government, businesses, and educational institutions. Resilient communities foster partnerships that promote collective action and leverage resources to address shared challenges.

Strategies for Building Resilient Communities

Building resilient communities involves implementing strategies aimed at enhancing social support, improving access to resources, and promoting mental health literacy. Here are some key strategies:

- **Community engagement and education:** Resilient communities foster active community engagement through workshops, dialogues, and educational programs. These initiatives increase mental health literacy, reduce stigma, and empower individuals to take proactive steps towards maintaining their mental well-being.

- **Promoting social connections:** Resilient communities prioritize activities that facilitate social connections and foster a sense of belonging. This can include creating community spaces, organizing social events, and promoting volunteer opportunities to encourage interaction and support networks.

- **Building infrastructure for mental health support:** Resilient communities ensure the availability of mental health services by establishing community mental health centers, helplines, and crisis intervention teams. They also collaborate with healthcare providers and organizations to address the mental health needs of the community effectively.

- **Addressing social determinants of mental health:** Resilient communities recognize the influence of social determinants on mental health and work towards addressing inequalities. They advocate for policies that promote social justice, equal access to education, employment opportunities, affordable housing, and healthcare.

- **Disaster preparedness and response:** Resilient communities proactively prepare for and respond to potential disasters, both natural and human-made. They develop emergency response plans, establish communication networks, and provide psychosocial support during and after crises.

- **Promoting environmental sustainability:** Resilient communities understand the interconnection between mental health and the environment. They prioritize environmental conservation, promote sustainable practices, and create green spaces that contribute to the overall well-being of community members.

Case Study: The Resilient Community Initiative

The Resilient Community Initiative (RCI) is a successful example of building resilient communities. Initiated in a small town heavily impacted by economic decline, the RCI aimed to address the mental health challenges faced by its residents while promoting community well-being.

The RCI implemented various strategies, including:

- The establishment of a community mental health center providing counseling services, support groups, and educational programs.

- Collaboration with local businesses to create job opportunities for community members, reducing unemployment and improving economic stability.

- Setting up community gardens and green spaces to enhance environmental sustainability and promote physical and mental well-being.

- Developing a community emergency response team, providing training to community members, and creating an efficient communication system during times of crisis.

- Organizing regular community events and social activities to foster social connections and a sense of belonging.

The RCI not only improved access to mental health support but also empowered community members to take an active role in building a resilient community. It resulted in reduced stigma around mental health, increased social cohesion, and improved overall well-being.

Challenges and Future Directions

Building resilient communities is not without challenges. These include limited resources, approval and implementation barriers, and resistance to change. In addition, systemic issues such as poverty, discrimination, and social inequalities can hinder the development of resilient communities.

To address these challenges, it is essential to:

- Advocate for policies that prioritize mental health and resilience-building initiatives at the community and national levels.

- Foster collaboration and partnerships among stakeholders, including government agencies, community organizations, healthcare providers, and educational institutions.

- Invest in the development of mental health infrastructure and increase funding for mental health services in underserved communities.

- Continuously assess and evaluate the effectiveness of resilience-building strategies, making necessary adjustments based on community feedback and evolving needs.

- Integrate mental health promotion and resilience-building into educational curricula, ensuring that individuals are equipped with the necessary skills and knowledge to support themselves and others.

Building resilient communities requires sustained effort, collective action, and a comprehensive understanding of the unique needs and strengths of the community. By prioritizing mental health, fostering social connections, and promoting inclusivity, communities can create an environment that supports individuals in coping with adversities, improving overall well-being, and ensuring a sustainable future.

Exercise: Conduct a community needs assessment in your local area to identify existing strengths and areas for improvement in terms of resilience-building. Design a community intervention plan based on the findings, considering the implementation barriers and available resources. Present your plan to a simulated town hall meeting, highlighting the potential impact and benefits for the community.

Online and Virtual Support Networks

In the fast-paced digital era, technology has revolutionized every aspect of our lives, including mental health care. Online and virtual support networks have emerged as powerful tools for promoting mental well-being and providing support to individuals facing psychological challenges. These networks leverage the reach and accessibility of the internet to connect people from all walks of life, creating a global community of support.

The Importance of Online and Virtual Support Networks

Online and virtual support networks have become increasingly popular due to their numerous advantages. One key benefit is the accessibility they offer. Individuals can access support and resources from the comfort of their own homes, eliminating geographical barriers and the need to travel. This is particularly beneficial for those living in remote areas or with limited mobility.

Furthermore, online support networks provide a safe and anonymous space for individuals to seek help. They can share their experiences, concerns, and challenges without fear of judgment or stigma. This anonymity fosters openness and encourages participation, leading to increased engagement and support within the network.

Types of Online and Virtual Support Networks

There are various types of online and virtual support networks available to individuals seeking mental health support. These networks cater to different needs and preferences, ensuring that individuals find a space that suits them best. Some common types include:

1. **Online forums and communities:** These platforms provide a space for individuals to connect, share experiences, and offer support. Users can create posts or engage in discussions on various mental health topics. Well-known platforms include Reddit's mental health subreddits and online message boards.

2. **Peer support networks:** Peer support networks connect individuals who have experienced similar mental health challenges. These networks promote empathy, understanding, and shared learning. Platforms like 7 Cups and SupportGroups.com provide opportunities for individuals to connect one-on-one or join group discussions led by trained volunteers.

3. **Social media support groups:** Social media platforms, such as Facebook and Instagram, host numerous support groups dedicated to mental health. These groups create communities where individuals can find support, share resources, and engage in uplifting conversations. They often have moderators or administrators who ensure the group remains a safe and supportive space.

4. **Online therapy platforms:** Online therapy platforms, such as BetterHelp and Talkspace, offer professional counseling and therapy services through secure video calls, messaging, or phone calls. These platforms provide convenient access to licensed therapists and counselors, allowing individuals to seek professional help on their terms.

Benefits and Limitations of Online and Virtual Support Networks

Online and virtual support networks offer several benefits that contribute to the well-being of individuals seeking mental health support. Some key advantages include:

- **Accessibility:** Online support networks are available 24/7, allowing individuals to access support whenever they need it. This is particularly crucial during times of crisis or when face-to-face support is not readily available.

- **Anonymity:** Online forums and communities allow individuals to participate anonymously, promoting openness and reducing the fear of judgment. This anonymity can encourage individuals to seek support and share their experiences more freely.

- **Diverse perspectives:** Online support networks bring together individuals from diverse backgrounds and experiences. This diversity fosters a range of perspectives and insights, enriching discussions and providing individuals with different viewpoints and coping strategies.

- **Empowerment and agency:** Online support networks empower individuals to take an active role in their mental health journey. They can seek out specific information, connect with others who have similar experiences, and access resources that are relevant to their needs.

- **Reduced cost:** Online support networks often offer their services and resources free of charge or at a lower cost compared to in-person support options. This makes mental health support more accessible and affordable for individuals with limited financial resources.

However, it is important to acknowledge the limitations of online support networks:

- **Lack of professional supervision:** While online support networks can provide peer support and valuable insights, they may not have professional oversight or guidance. This means that information and advice shared within these networks should be carefully evaluated and cross-referenced with reliable sources.

- **Digital divide and accessibility issues:** Online support networks require internet access and digital literacy, which may pose challenges for individuals with limited access to technology or those who are not familiar with using digital platforms. Efforts should be made to bridge the digital divide and ensure inclusivity.

- **Potential for misinformation:** Online platforms can be susceptible to misinformation and the spread of inaccurate or harmful content. It is crucial to promote critical thinking and provide reliable resources within online support networks to mitigate the risk of misinformation.

- **Limitations of non-verbal communication:** Online communication lacks non-verbal cues, such as tone of voice and body language, which can impact the effectiveness of support. However, advancements in video chat and audio messaging features can help bridge this gap to some extent.

- **Replacement versus complement to in-person support:** Online support networks should not be seen as a complete substitute for in-person support. They can serve as a valuable complement, but individuals with severe mental health conditions or crises may require more intensive, face-to-face assistance.

Promoting Safety and Ethical Considerations

Ensuring the safety and ethical integrity of online and virtual support networks is paramount. Both platform administrators and users have a role to play in creating a supportive, respectful, and secure environment. Some key considerations include:

- **Moderation and community guidelines:** Network administrators should establish clear community guidelines that promote respectful interactions and prohibit harmful or abusive behavior. Moderators can actively monitor discussions to maintain a safe environment and address any violations promptly.

- **Confidentiality and privacy:** Online support networks should prioritize the privacy and confidentiality of members. Users should be educated about the limits of privacy within online platforms and should exercise caution when sharing personal information.

- **Informed consent:** Users should provide informed consent for their participation in online support networks, understanding the potential risks and benefits. Consent should be sought for sharing content, including user stories or posts, beyond the platform.

- **Referral to professional help:** Online support networks should emphasize the importance of professional mental health care and provide information on how to seek appropriate help. This includes educating individuals on when to escalate their concerns and guiding them toward licensed professionals.

- **Reporting and addressing abuse:** Online platforms should have clear mechanisms for reporting abusive or harmful behavior. Administrators should promptly address any reports and take appropriate actions to ensure the safety and well-being of members.

- **Digital literacy and critical thinking:** Promoting digital literacy and critical thinking is essential for users of online support networks. Individuals should be encouraged to critically evaluate information, fact-check sources, and exercise caution when implementing advice or strategies shared within the networks.

Real-World Example: Peer Support through Online Forums

To illustrate the impact of online and virtual support networks, let's consider the example of John, a recent college graduate struggling with social anxiety. John has difficulty reaching out for support in person but finds solace and understanding through an online forum dedicated to anxiety disorders.

In this forum, John connects with individuals who have similar experiences and learns coping strategies from their shared stories. He receives encouragement and validation, which helps him realize he is not alone in his struggles. Over time, John gains confidence and starts actively participating in discussions, offering support to others who are also seeking help.

Through this online support network, John finds emotional support, practical advice, and a sense of belonging. He gains the confidence to seek professional help and eventually begins therapy to address his social anxiety. Without the accessibility and anonymity offered by the online forum, John may have continued to suffer silently, unaware of the resources and support available to him.

Exercises and Further Reflection

1. Reflect on your own experiences with online and virtual support networks. Have you ever participated in one? If so, what were the benefits you gained from it? If not, what potential benefits do you foresee?

2. Research a specific online support network or platform and critically evaluate its strengths and limitations. How does it ensure user safety and confidentiality? What ethical considerations do they emphasize?

3. Design a digital campaign to raise awareness about the availability and benefits of online support networks. Consider using social media platforms, virtual communities, or online forums to reach your target audience. What key messages

would you highlight, and how would you promote the accessibility and inclusivity of these networks?

4. Imagine you are a mental health professional who wants to offer virtual support to your clients. Design a comprehensive plan outlining the ethical considerations, privacy measures, and technical requirements you would need to address. How would you ensure the safety and effectiveness of your virtual support practice?

5. Conduct a survey or interview individuals who have utilized online support networks for mental health support. Explore their experiences, satisfaction levels, and any challenges they encountered. How can their feedback be used to improve the design and implementation of online support networks in the future?

Remember to approach these exercises with an open mind and respect for diverse perspectives. As technology continues to advance, online and virtual support networks will play an increasingly vital role in promoting mental well-being.

Peer Support and Mentoring

Introduction

In the field of mental health, peer support and mentoring play a crucial role in promoting holistic wellbeing and resilience. Peer support refers to the relationship between individuals with lived experience of mental health challenges, who offer understanding, empathy, and guidance to one another. Mentoring, on the other hand, involves a more structured relationship where an experienced individual provides guidance and support to someone who may be earlier in their journey or seeking specific skills or knowledge. Both peer support and mentoring have been shown to have numerous benefits for individuals with mental health disorders, including increased hope, improved self-esteem, and enhanced resilience.

The Power of Shared Experiences

One of the key advantages of peer support and mentoring is the power of shared experiences. When individuals with similar challenges come together, they can create a safe and supportive environment where they can openly discuss their struggles, share coping strategies, and offer each other practical advice. This mutual understanding and empathy can often provide a level of support that is unique and different from that offered by mental health professionals. Peer support and mentoring can help reduce feelings of isolation and stigma, as individuals realize they are not alone in their experiences.

The Role of Peer Support Specialists

Peer support specialists are individuals who have lived experience of mental health challenges and have undergone training to provide support to others. They often work as part of a professional care team, providing valuable insights and guidance based on their own journey of recovery. Peer support specialists can leverage their personal experiences to connect with individuals who are facing similar challenges, offering a sense of hope and possibility. Their non-clinical perspective can complement the interventions provided by mental health professionals, enhancing the overall support individuals receive.

Formal Mentoring Programs

Formal mentoring programs offer a structured approach to providing support and guidance to individuals with mental health challenges. These programs pair a person in need of guidance (mentee) with an experienced individual (mentor) who can provide support, advice, and resources. Mentoring programs can focus on various aspects, such as career development, academic success, or personal growth. For individuals with mental health challenges, mentors can play a crucial role in assisting with goal-setting, problem-solving, and navigating the complexities of life. Mentoring relationships can be short-term or long-term, depending on the needs and goals of the mentee.

Promoting Recovery and Resilience

Peer support and mentoring can have a significant impact on the recovery and resilience of individuals with mental health challenges. Through shared experiences, peer support can provide validation and validation, which are important components of healing. Peer support groups can also help individuals develop coping skills and self-management strategies, empowering them to take charge of their mental health journey. Mentoring, on the other hand, can foster personal growth and development by providing guidance and support in setting and achieving goals. Both peer support and mentoring can contribute to the development of resilience, helping individuals bounce back from challenges and setbacks.

The Benefits of Technology

Technology has greatly expanded the reach and accessibility of peer support and mentoring. Online forums, support groups, and social media platforms provide individuals with mental health challenges with a virtual community where they can connect with others, share experiences, and seek guidance. Technology also enables remote mentoring relationships, eliminating geographical barriers and allowing individuals to access support from mentors who may not be available locally. However, it's important to consider the potential pitfalls and need for privacy and security when utilizing technology for peer support and mentoring.

Challenges and Caveats

While peer support and mentoring have numerous benefits, it is important to acknowledge the challenges and caveats associated with these approaches. Peer support and mentoring relationships should be built on trust, respect, and boundaries to ensure a safe and supportive environment. It is also crucial to recognize that not all individuals seeking support will have positive experiences in peer support or mentoring relationships. Some individuals may have specific needs or preferences that require specialized support beyond what a peer can provide. Additionally, mentors must be aware of their limitations and ensure they do not provide advice outside their area of expertise.

Conclusion

Peer support and mentoring are valuable components of a holistic approach to mental health care, promoting recovery, and resilience. Through shared experiences, mutual understanding, and guidance, individuals with mental health challenges can find support in their journey toward wellbeing. By integrating peer support and mentoring programs into mental health policies and systems, we can create a sustainable future where individuals receive the support, guidance, and empowerment they need to thrive. Let us embrace the power of peer support and mentoring as we continue to prioritize mental health and build a more inclusive and resilient society.

Workplace Mental Health

Occupational Stress and Burnout

Occupational stress and burnout are prevalent issues in today's fast-paced and demanding work environments. This section explores the causes, consequences, and strategies to address occupational stress and burnout. Recognizing and addressing these issues is crucial for promoting mental health and overall well-being in the workplace.

Understanding Occupational Stress

Occupational stress refers to the emotional, physical, and psychological strain experienced by individuals in response to work-related demands and pressures. It occurs when the demands of a job exceed an individual's ability to cope effectively. Several factors contribute to occupational stress, including workload, time pressure, lack of control or autonomy, interpersonal conflicts, and a mismatch between job demands and an individual's skills or abilities.

Excessive occupational stress can lead to detrimental effects on an individual's mental and physical health, as well as their job performance and satisfaction. Therefore, it is essential to recognize and manage occupational stress to prevent burnout and promote well-being in the workplace.

Understanding Burnout

Burnout is a specific form of chronic occupational stress characterized by emotional exhaustion, depersonalization, and a reduced sense of personal accomplishment. It often occurs in individuals who are highly engaged and committed to their work but experience prolonged and intense stress. Burnout can occur in various professional contexts, such as healthcare, education, social work, and corporate environments.

The consequences of burnout are significant and can impact individuals, organizations, and society as a whole. Burnout can lead to decreased job performance, increased absenteeism, higher turnover rates, and diminished physical and mental health. Addressing burnout is crucial for maintaining a healthy and sustainable workforce.

Causes of Occupational Stress and Burnout

Occupational stress and burnout can arise from a variety of factors. Some common causes include:

- Workload: Excessive work demands, long working hours, and constant time pressure can contribute to occupational stress and burnout.

- Lack of control: When employees have limited control over their work and decision-making processes, they may feel overwhelmed and stressed.

- Interpersonal conflicts: Conflict with colleagues, supervisors, or clients can create a hostile and stressful work environment.

- Role ambiguity: Unclear expectations, conflicting roles, and a lack of role clarity can contribute to stress and burnout.

- Lack of support: Insufficient organizational support, limited resources, and a lack of social support can increase the risk of burnout.

- Work-home imbalance: Difficulties in balancing work and personal life can lead to chronic stress and burnout.

It is important to note that individual differences, such as personality traits, coping strategies, and resilience, can also influence the experience of occupational stress and burnout.

Consequences of Occupational Stress and Burnout

Occupational stress and burnout can have severe consequences on individuals, organizations, and society.

- Individual consequences: High levels of occupational stress and burnout can lead to physical health problems such as cardiovascular diseases, musculoskeletal disorders, and weakened immune systems. Mental health issues such as depression, anxiety, and substance abuse are also associated with occupational stress and burnout.

- Organizational consequences: Burnout can lead to reduced job performance, decreased productivity, increased absenteeism, and higher turnover rates. It can also negatively impact team dynamics and employee morale. Organizations may experience financial losses and reputational damage as a result.

- Societal consequences: Burnout can have broader societal implications, such as increased healthcare costs, lower quality of care in service industries, and reduced innovation and productivity in various sectors of the economy.

Addressing Occupational Stress and Burnout

Addressing occupational stress and burnout requires a multifaceted approach that involves both individuals and organizations. Here are some strategies that can help mitigate occupational stress and prevent burnout:

- Individual strategies: Employees can practice self-care techniques such as maintaining a healthy work-life balance, engaging in regular physical exercise, practicing relaxation techniques, and seeking social support. Developing effective coping strategies and time management skills can also help individuals manage stress more effectively.

- Organizational strategies: Employers can take steps to create a positive work environment by promoting work-life balance, providing access to wellness programs, and implementing policies that support employee well-being. It is crucial for organizations to foster open communication, recognize and address work-related stressors, and provide resources for stress management and mental health support. Training programs that enhance employees' resilience and coping skills can also be beneficial.

- Policy-level strategies: Governments and regulatory bodies can play a role in addressing occupational stress and burnout by enacting policies that protect employee rights, promote work-life balance, and ensure adequate staffing levels and workload management in high-stress industries.

It is important to cultivate a culture that values employee well-being and mental health, as this can contribute to a more sustainable and productive workforce. By addressing occupational stress and burnout, individuals and organizations can create a healthier and more positive work environment.

Case Study: Occupational Stress in the Healthcare Industry

One sector in which occupational stress and burnout are particularly prevalent is the healthcare industry. Healthcare professionals face high work demands, long working hours, and emotionally challenging situations, which can contribute to chronic stress and burnout.

A study conducted in a large hospital found that healthcare professionals experiencing burnout were more likely to report physical health problems, decreased job satisfaction, and intention to leave their current job. Moreover, burnout among healthcare providers has been associated with medical errors and decreased quality of patient care.

To address occupational stress and burnout in the healthcare industry, organizations can implement strategies such as providing support systems for healthcare professionals, improving communication and teamwork, implementing stress management programs, and promoting self-care among employees. These initiatives can help reduce stress levels and create a more supportive work environment for healthcare professionals, ultimately benefiting both employees and patients.

Conclusion

Occupational stress and burnout are significant challenges that impact individuals, organizations, and society. By understanding the causes and consequences of occupational stress and burnout, and implementing strategies to address them, we can promote mental health, well-being, and overall sustainability in the workplace. Taking a holistic approach that involves individuals, organizations, and policy-level interventions is crucial for building resilient and healthy work environments.

Promoting Mental Health in the Workplace

Promoting mental health in the workplace is crucial for creating a supportive and productive work environment. It involves implementing strategies and initiatives that prioritize employee well-being and address the psychological challenges that individuals may face in their professional lives. By recognizing the importance of mental health and adopting proactive measures, employers can contribute to a positive and sustainable workplace culture. In this section, we will explore various approaches and best practices for promoting mental health in the workplace.

Understanding Workplace Mental Health

Before delving into strategies for promoting mental health, it is essential to understand the concept of workplace mental health. Work-related factors can significantly impact employees' mental well-being, and recognizing these factors is the first step towards creating a mentally healthy workplace.

One crucial aspect is occupational stress, which refers to the emotional and physical strains experienced by individuals due to work-related demands. High job demands, lack of control, poor support from supervisors and colleagues, and inadequate resources are common stressors in the workplace. Moreover, organizational factors such as long working hours, role ambiguity, and lack of recognition can also contribute to stress and negatively impact mental health.

Another aspect to consider is work-life balance. Achieving a healthy balance between work and personal life is essential for mental well-being. High-pressure work environments that demand excessive time and effort can cause stress and hinder individuals' ability to engage in self-care activities and maintain healthy relationships outside of work.

Taking into account these factors, we can begin exploring strategies to promote mental health in the workplace.

Creating Supportive Policies and Practices

Developing and implementing supportive policies and practices is fundamental to promoting mental health in the workplace. These initiatives tackle the root causes of workplace stress and provide employees with the resources they need to maintain their well-being. Some key strategies include:

- **Workload management:** Employers should strive to ensure that workloads are manageable and realistic, taking into account the skills and abilities of employees. This promotes a sense of control and reduces the risk of burnout.

- **Flexible work arrangements:** Offering flexible work options, such as flexible hours or remote work, can help employees better manage their work-life balance. This flexibility allows them to attend to personal responsibilities and engage in self-care activities, reducing stress levels.

- **Mental health training and education:** Providing training and education programs on mental health awareness and promoting psychological well-being can help reduce stigma, increase knowledge, and foster a supportive environment.

- **Employee assistance programs (EAPs):** EAPs are a valuable resource for employees, providing confidential counseling and support services for various personal and work-related issues. These programs can help individuals cope with stress, enhance their well-being, and access appropriate mental health services if needed.

By incorporating these policies and practices into the workplace, employers can create an environment that prioritizes mental health and equips employees with the tools they need to thrive.

Promoting a Positive Work Culture

A positive work culture is essential for promoting mental health among employees. It involves fostering open communication, supportive relationships, and a sense of belonging. Some strategies for cultivating a positive work culture include:

- **Leadership support:** It is crucial for organizational leaders to demonstrate their commitment to mental health and lead by example. By creating a culture that values well-being and promoting work-life balance, leaders can positively influence employees' mental health.

- **Strong social connections:** Encouraging team-building activities and fostering positive relationships among employees can enhance their sense of belonging and reduce feelings of isolation.

- **Promoting work-life balance:** Employers should encourage employees to take regular breaks, use their vacation time, and prioritize self-care. By promoting work-life balance, organizations communicate the importance of overall well-being.

- **Recognition and appreciation:** Recognizing employees' contributions and expressing appreciation for their hard work can boost morale, job satisfaction, and overall mental well-being.

By implementing these strategies, organizations can create an environment where employees feel valued, supported, and motivated, leading to better mental health outcomes.

Addressing Mental Health Stigma

One significant barrier to promoting mental health in the workplace is the stigma associated with mental illness. Stigma can prevent individuals from seeking help and support, leading to deteriorating mental health. To address mental health stigma, organizations can:

- **Educate and increase awareness:** Conducting awareness campaigns and providing educational resources can help dispel myths and misconceptions about mental health. By fostering a better understanding of mental illness, organizations can reduce stigma and create a more supportive environment.

- **Encourage open dialogue:** Creating opportunities for open conversations about mental health can help normalize discussions and reduce the fear of judgment or discrimination. This can be done through workshops, seminars, or support groups.

- **Promote employee resource groups:** Establishing employee resource groups dedicated to mental health can provide a safe space for employees to connect, share experiences, and access support.

- **Lead by example:** Encouraging leaders and managers to share their own experiences with mental health challenges can help break down stigma and show employees that seeking support is both accepted and valued.

Addressing mental health stigma requires a collective effort from employers and employees to create an inclusive and understanding workplace culture.

Monitoring and Evaluation

To ensure the effectiveness of mental health promotion efforts, it is important for organizations to establish monitoring and evaluation mechanisms. This involves regularly assessing the impact of mental health initiatives and adjusting strategies as needed. Key steps in this process include:

- **Data collection:** Collecting data on employee mental health indicators, such as stress levels, job satisfaction, and absenteeism, can provide insights into the impact of workplace interventions.

- **Employee feedback:** Regularly seeking feedback from employees through surveys or focus groups can help identify areas of improvement and ensure that initiatives align with their needs.

- **Collaboration with mental health professionals:** Engaging mental health professionals can provide expert guidance in the evaluation process, ensuring that assessments are comprehensive and evidence-based.

By monitoring and evaluating mental health initiatives, organizations can identify successful strategies, make informed decisions, and continuously improve their efforts to promote mental well-being in the workplace.

Case Study: Implementing Mental Health Initiatives

To illustrate the practical application of promoting mental health in the workplace, let's consider the case of Company XYZ, a medium-sized tech company. Company XYZ recognizes the importance of employee mental health and aims to create a supportive work environment. They decide to implement several initiatives:

1. **Flexible work arrangements:** Company XYZ introduces flexible working hours, allowing employees to adjust their schedules to accommodate personal commitments and reduce work-related stress.

2. **Mental health training:** The company organizes workshops on mental health awareness and stress management, equipping employees with knowledge and skills to better navigate work-related challenges.

3. **Leadership support:** The management team demonstrates their commitment to employee well-being by openly discussing mental health, encouraging self-care, and leading by example.

4. **Employee resource group:** Company XYZ establishes an employee resource group focused on mental health. The group provides a platform for employees to support one another, share resources, and organize mental health-related activities.

5. **Monitoring and evaluation:** Regular surveys are conducted to collect feedback on the impact of the mental health initiatives. The feedback is used to identify areas for improvement and guide future interventions.

Through these initiatives, Company XYZ creates a workplace culture that prioritizes mental health and supports employees in their well-being. By continuously evaluating the effectiveness of these programs, they ensure that their efforts remain relevant and impactful.

Conclusion

Promoting mental health in the workplace is not only beneficial for employees' well-being but also contributes to overall organizational success. By adopting strategies that address work-related stress, create a positive work culture, tackle stigma, and prioritize employee mental health, employers can foster a supportive environment where individuals can thrive. It is essential for organizations to continuously evaluate and improve their mental health initiatives to ensure their effectiveness and create a sustainable mental health future in the workplace.

Employee Assistance Programs

Employee Assistance Programs (EAPs) are workplace-based programs that aim to support employees in managing personal and work-related challenges, including mental health issues. These programs provide employees with confidential and voluntary access to professional counseling, resources, and referrals, contributing to their overall well-being. EAPs are designed to address a wide range of concerns such as stress, anxiety, depression, substance abuse, work-life balance, and relationship problems.

The Need for Employee Assistance Programs

In today's fast-paced and competitive work environment, employees face a multitude of challenges that can impact their mental health. Stress, burnout, and mental health issues can lead to decreased productivity, increased absenteeism, and a decline in overall job satisfaction. Recognizing and addressing these issues is crucial for both the well-being of employees and the success of organizations.

Components of Employee Assistance Programs

EAPs typically consist of the following components:

1. **Confidential Counseling:** EAPs offer employees access to professional counselors who provide support and guidance for various personal and work-related issues. Counseling sessions are confidential, ensuring that employees feel safe and comfortable discussing their concerns.

2. **Assessment and Referrals:** EAPs conduct assessments to determine the appropriate course of action for each individual. Depending on the severity and nature of the issue, employees may be referred to external specialists, therapists, or healthcare providers for further evaluation and treatment.

3. **Workplace Education and Training:** EAPs provide training and educational resources to raise awareness about mental health issues, stress management, and work-life balance. This helps employees develop coping strategies, build resilience, and improve their overall well-being.

4. **Critical Incident Response:** EAPs play a vital role in providing immediate support and intervention following critical incidents such as workplace accidents, natural disasters, or traumatic events. Rapid response and on-site counseling services help employees recover and cope with the emotional aftermath of such incidents.

5. **Workplace Consultation:** EAPs offer consultation services to managers, supervisors, and human resources departments to address mental health concerns in the workplace. They provide guidance on creating a mentally healthy work environment, implementing strategies for stress reduction, and promoting employee engagement and well-being.

Benefits of Employee Assistance Programs

Implementing EAPs in organizations can yield several benefits:

1. **Improved Employee Well-being:** EAPs provide employees with timely and confidential access to professional support, enabling them to address mental health

concerns before they escalate. By promoting early intervention and offering resources for self-care, EAPs contribute to improved overall well-being.

2. **Increased Productivity and Engagement:** With access to support and counseling, employees are better equipped to manage work-related stress, emotional challenges, and personal issues. This leads to increased productivity, enhanced job satisfaction, and higher levels of engagement.

3. **Reduced Absenteeism and Turnover:** EAPs play a crucial role in reducing absenteeism and turnover rates. By addressing mental health concerns, providing counseling, and offering resources for managing personal and work-related challenges, EAPs help create a healthier and more supportive work environment.

4. **Enhanced Organizational Culture:** Implementing EAPs sends a positive message to employees about an organization's commitment to employee well-being. It fosters a supportive and caring work culture that values the mental health and overall well-being of its workforce.

Considerations for Implementing EAPs

Organizations should consider the following factors when implementing EAPs:

1. **Confidentiality and Privacy:** Ensuring that employee information and counseling sessions remain confidential is paramount to the success and effectiveness of EAPs. Employees should feel confident that their privacy will be respected when seeking support.

2. **Accessibility and Awareness:** Organizations should promote awareness about EAPs and ensure that employees understand how to access these programs. Communication strategies, such as posters, emails, or workshops, can help spread the word about the availability and benefits of EAPs.

3. **Evaluation and Continuous Improvement:** Regular evaluation of EAPs is crucial to assess their effectiveness and make any necessary adjustments. Collecting feedback from employees and monitoring program usage can provide valuable insights for program development and improvement.

4. **Collaboration with Healthcare Providers:** Organizations should establish partnerships with mental health professionals and healthcare providers to ensure that employees receive appropriate and evidence-based care when required. This collaboration helps facilitate prompt referrals and integrated support.

Case Study: Implementing an EAP in a Tech Company

Let's consider the case of a technology company that wants to implement an EAP to support its employees' mental health. The company experiences high levels of stress among its workforce due to tight deadlines, long working hours, and a competitive market.

To develop an effective EAP, the organization conducts an employee needs assessment survey to identify the most common mental health challenges and concerns. Based on the survey results, they design the following components for their EAP:

1. **Confidential Counseling:** The company partners with mental health professionals to provide onsite counseling services. Employees can book confidential sessions to discuss their concerns, receive emotional support, and develop coping strategies.

2. **Workplace Training:** The company organizes workshops on stress management, mindfulness techniques, and work-life balance. These workshops equip employees with practical skills to manage stress and enhance their well-being.

3. **Critical Incident Response:** The company establishes a protocol for responding to critical incidents, such as workplace accidents or emergencies. They provide immediate support through on-site counseling and ensure a structured recovery process for affected employees.

4. **Workplace Consultation:** The company offers consultation services to managers to help them identify signs of mental health concerns, provide support to their team members, and create a mentally healthy work environment.

5. **Evaluation and Continuous Improvement:** The organization regularly collects feedback from employees to assess the effectiveness of the EAP. They make necessary adjustments and enhancements based on this feedback, ensuring the program meets the evolving needs of employees.

By implementing this EAP, the tech company experiences a positive shift in its work culture. Employees feel supported, and there is an increase in engagement, productivity, and overall job satisfaction. The organization's commitment to employee well-being and mental health contributes to its long-term success and sustainability.

Conclusion

Employee Assistance Programs play a vital role in promoting mental health and well-being in the workplace. By providing confidential counseling, assessment, referrals, education, and critical incident response, these programs offer a holistic approach to supporting employees' mental health. Implementing EAPs can result in improved employee well-being, increased productivity, reduced absenteeism, and enhanced organizational culture. By considering factors such as confidentiality, accessibility, evaluation, and collaboration with healthcare providers, organizations can create effective and sustainable EAPs that meet the unique needs of their workforce.

Work-Life Balance for Mental Health

In our modern society, where work demands are ever-increasing and technology enables constant connectivity, achieving a healthy work-life balance has become a significant challenge. The increasing blur between work and personal life can have detrimental effects on our mental health. In this section, we will explore the importance of work-life balance for mental health and discuss strategies to promote it.

Understanding the Impact of Work-Life Imbalance

Work-life imbalance occurs when the demands and responsibilities of work outweigh the time and energy available for personal life and well-being. This imbalance can lead to chronic stress, burnout, and various mental health issues. Research has shown that individuals experiencing work-life imbalance are more likely to experience symptoms of anxiety, depression, and decreased overall life satisfaction.

The negative effects of work-life imbalance are not limited to individuals but can also impact organizations. Employees who struggle with work-life balance are more likely to experience reduced productivity, higher turnover rates, and increased absenteeism. Therefore, promoting work-life balance is not only beneficial for individuals' mental health but also contributes to the overall well-being and success of workplaces.

Strategies for Promoting Work-Life Balance

Promoting work-life balance requires a comprehensive approach that incorporates individual strategies, organizational practices, and societal support. Here are some effective strategies to achieve a better work-life balance for improved mental health:

1. **Time Management:** Efficiently managing time is crucial for maintaining work-life balance. Prioritizing tasks, setting boundaries, and avoiding overcommitment can help allocate time for both work and personal activities. Employing time-management techniques, such as Pomodoro technique or batching similar tasks together, can enhance productivity and create more time for leisure and self-care.

2. **Flexible Working Arrangements:** Flexible work options, such as flextime, telecommuting, or compressed workweeks, allow individuals to have more control over their schedules. This flexibility enables better integration of work and personal responsibilities, reduces commute time, and provides opportunities for self-care and family time.

3. **Setting Boundaries:** It is vital to establish clear boundaries between work and personal life. Avoiding work-related activities during personal time, such as checking emails or taking work calls, can help create a sense of separation and enhance relaxation. Establishing designated spaces for work and leisure at home can also contribute to setting these boundaries.

4. **Self-Care Practices:** Engaging in self-care activities is essential for maintaining mental well-being. Regular exercise, proper nutrition, sufficient sleep, and relaxation techniques like meditation or journaling can help reduce stress and increase resilience. Incorporating these practices into daily routines is important for overall work-life balance.

5. **Social Support:** Building and maintaining strong social connections is crucial for work-life balance. Seeking support from family, friends, or engaging in social activities can provide a sense of connection, reduce feelings of isolation, and enhance overall well-being. Utilizing employer-sponsored support programs or joining community groups can also be beneficial.

6. **Boundaries and expectations communication:** Open communication with supervisors, colleagues, and family members about work-life balance expectations is necessary. Clearly communicating boundaries, discussing workload distribution, and advocating for personal time are important steps to ensure that work and personal life are balanced effectively.

7. **Unplugging and breaks:** Taking regular breaks and unplugging from work-related activities is necessary for mental health. Establishing tech-free times or engaging in activities that disconnect individuals from work, such as hobbies or spending time in nature, can help rejuvenate and minimize work-related stress.

Work-Life Balance in Practice: Example Scenario

Let's consider an example scenario to understand how work-life balance can be achieved in practice. Sarah, a marketing professional, has been experiencing work-related stress and neglecting her personal life. To improve her work-life balance and mental health, she can implement the following strategies:

1. Sarah starts practicing time management techniques, prioritizing tasks, and setting realistic deadlines. By allocating time for work and personal activities, she ensures she has time for leisure and self-care.

2. Sarah discusses flexible working options with her supervisor, such as working remotely for a few days a week. This allows her to save commute time and spend more time with her family.

3. Sarah establishes boundaries by not checking work emails or taking work calls during personal time. She creates a dedicated workspace and designates specific times for work-related activities.

4. Sarah includes regular exercise and meditation in her daily routine to reduce stress and improve her mental well-being. She also prioritizes spending quality time with her loved ones and engaging in activities she enjoys.

5. Sarah seeks support from her family and friends and discusses her work-life balance goals with them. They provide encouragement and hold her accountable for maintaining a healthy balance.

By implementing these strategies, Sarah successfully achieves a better work-life balance, reducing her work-related stress, and improving her mental health.

Work-Life Balance: Unconventional Approach

In addition to the strategies mentioned above, an unconventional approach to work-life balance is the concept of "shadow work." Shadow work refers to the invisible and often unnoticed labor individuals perform in their personal lives, such as household chores, caregiving, or emotional labor. Recognizing and redistributing shadow work can alleviate the burden on individuals, allowing for a more equitable work-life balance.

For example, in a household, both partners can actively share responsibilities like cooking, cleaning, and childcare. This approach acknowledges and values the invisible labor performed in personal life, promoting a healthier work-life balance for all individuals involved.

Conclusion

Finding a work-life balance is essential for maintaining good mental health. By implementing strategies such as time management, boundaries, self-care practices, social support, and flexible working arrangements, individuals can create a harmonious integration of work and personal life. Organizations and society as a whole play a crucial role in supporting and promoting work-life balance to ensure the well-being and sustainability of individuals and communities. Embracing an unconventional approach, such as addressing shadow work, further enhances work-life balance and contributes to a more equitable society.

Promoting Holistic Mental Health Policy

Integrating Mental Health into Public Health Approaches

In recent years, there has been a growing recognition of the importance of mental health in overall well-being and the need to integrate mental health into public health approaches. The World Health Organization defines mental health as a state of well-being in which an individual realizes their own abilities, can cope with the normal stresses of life, can work productively and fruitfully, and is able to make a contribution to their community. Integrating mental health into public health approaches is crucial to address the burden of mental disorders and promote the overall health and well-being of individuals and communities.

The Need for Integration

Mental health disorders are a significant global health concern, affecting people of all ages and backgrounds. According to the World Health Organization, approximately 1 in 4 people worldwide will experience a mental health disorder at some point in their lives. Mental health disorders not only have a profound impact on individuals, but also on families, communities, and economies.

Traditional healthcare systems have often treated mental health and physical health as separate entities, resulting in fragmented care and limited access to mental health services. Integrating mental health into public health approaches recognizes the interconnectedness of mental and physical health and seeks to address mental health as an integral part of overall health promotion and disease prevention.

Principles of Integration

Integrating mental health into public health approaches requires the implementation of certain key principles:

- **Multisectoral collaboration:** Mental health is influenced by various factors such as social, economic, and environmental determinants. Effective integration requires collaboration between different sectors, including health, education, employment, housing, and social welfare, to address these determinants comprehensively.

- **Evidence-based practices:** Integration should be guided by evidence-based practices that have been shown to be effective in promoting mental health, preventing mental health disorders, and providing appropriate care and support. This includes using evidence-based strategies for mental health promotion, prevention, early intervention, and treatment.

- **Equity and accessibility:** Integration should prioritize equity and ensure that mental health services and supports are accessible to all individuals, regardless of their socioeconomic status, geographical location, or cultural background. This involves addressing barriers to access, such as stigma, discrimination, and inadequate resources.

- **Community engagement:** Engaging communities is essential for effective integration. This involves involving community members, organizations, and stakeholders in decision-making processes, promoting community-led initiatives, and fostering partnerships to address mental health needs at the local level.

- **Promotion of mental health literacy:** Integration should focus on increasing mental health literacy among the general population, healthcare providers, and policymakers. This involves raising awareness about mental health, reducing stigma, and promoting positive mental health behaviors and practices.

Strategies for Integration

Integrating mental health into public health approaches requires the implementation of various strategies:

1. **Policy development and implementation:** Governments and policymakers play a crucial role in integrating mental health into public health approaches. This includes developing policies that prioritize mental health, allocating resources for mental health services, and implementing strategies to address the social determinants of mental health.

2. **Capacity building:** Integration requires building the capacity of healthcare providers, community workers, and other stakeholders to effectively address mental health. This involves providing training on mental health promotion,

prevention, screening, and treatment, as well as building skills in community engagement and collaboration.

3. **Collaboration and coordination:** Effective integration requires collaboration and coordination among different stakeholders. This includes establishing partnerships between healthcare providers, community organizations, schools, workplaces, and other sectors to develop integrated approaches to mental health.

4. **Screening and early intervention:** Integration should emphasize the importance of early identification and intervention for mental health disorders. This includes implementing routine screening programs in healthcare settings, schools, and workplaces, and ensuring timely access to appropriate interventions and referrals.

5. **Promotion of mental health and well-being:** Integration should prioritize the promotion of mental health and well-being at the population level. This includes implementing evidence-based mental health promotion programs, promoting positive mental health behaviors, and creating supportive environments that foster mental well-being.

6. **Monitoring and evaluation:** Integration efforts should be monitored and evaluated to assess their effectiveness and identify areas for improvement. This involves collecting data on mental health indicators, evaluating the impact of interventions, and using the findings to inform future planning and decision-making.

Challenges and Opportunities

Integrating mental health into public health approaches is not without its challenges. Some of the key challenges include:

- **Stigma and discrimination:** Stigma and discrimination associated with mental health continue to be major barriers to integration. Efforts to address stigma and promote acceptance are essential for successful integration.

- **Limited resources:** Many healthcare systems face resource constraints, which can hinder the integration of mental health. Adequate funding, resource allocation, and workforce development are crucial for effective integration.

- **Fragmented care:** Fragmentation of mental health services and lack of coordination between different providers can impede integration. Developing integrated care models and strengthening care coordination are important steps towards integration.

- **Lack of mental health literacy:** Limited understanding of mental health among the general population, healthcare providers, and policymakers can hinder integration efforts. Promoting mental health literacy through education and awareness campaigns is vital.

Despite these challenges, integrating mental health into public health approaches offers several opportunities:

- **Improved health outcomes:** Integration has the potential to improve health outcomes by addressing the underlying causes of mental health disorders and promoting overall well-being. By integrating mental health into public health approaches, the burden of mental health disorders can be reduced, resulting in healthier individuals and communities.

- **Enhanced efficiency and cost-effectiveness:** Integration can lead to improved efficiency and cost-effectiveness by reducing duplication of services, improving care coordination, and optimizing resource allocation. By integrating mental health into existing public health systems, resources can be used more effectively, leading to better outcomes for individuals and communities.

- **Prevention and early intervention:** Integration facilitates the implementation of prevention and early intervention strategies for mental health disorders. By addressing risk factors and promoting protective factors, integration can help prevent the onset of mental health disorders and reduce their severity. Early identification and intervention can also lead to better outcomes and reduced long-term costs.

- **Holistic and person-centered care:** Integration promotes a holistic and person-centered approach to care, considering the physical, mental, and social determinants of health. By integrating mental health into public health approaches, care can be tailored to individual needs, leading to improved overall well-being.

In conclusion, integrating mental health into public health approaches is crucial for addressing the burden of mental health disorders and promoting overall well-being. By implementing evidence-based strategies, fostering collaboration and coordination, and addressing barriers to access, integration can lead to improved health outcomes, enhanced efficiency, and better prevention and early intervention. Despite the challenges, the opportunities offered by integration make it a vital component of a sustainable mental health future.

The Role of Policy in Holistic Mental Health Care

In order to promote holistic mental health care, it is essential to recognize the crucial role that policy plays in shaping and guiding the delivery of mental health services. Policy serves as the framework for establishing goals, strategies, and guidelines that ensure the provision of comprehensive care for individuals with mental health concerns. This section will explore the importance of policy in holistic mental health care and discuss key considerations in policy development and implementation.

Policy Development

Developing effective policies for holistic mental health care requires a comprehensive and collaborative approach that considers the needs of diverse populations and integrates multiple stakeholder perspectives. The following factors should be taken into account during policy development:

- **Evidence-based practices:** Policies should be informed by the latest research, ensuring that interventions and treatment approaches are grounded in scientific evidence. This requires ongoing evaluation and monitoring of mental health interventions to identify effective strategies and update policies accordingly.

- **Accessibility and affordability:** Policies should focus on promoting access to mental health services and ensuring that they are affordable for all individuals. This includes addressing barriers such as financial constraints, geographic location, cultural beliefs, and stigma. Policies should also prioritize funding and resource allocation to improve accessibility and affordability.

- **Integration of services:** Holistic mental health care requires the integration of various services, including primary care, mental health care, and social support services. Policies should aim to break down silos and establish coordinated care models that address the complex needs of individuals with mental health concerns.

- **Cultural sensitivity:** Policies must consider cultural diversity and promote culturally sensitive approaches in mental health care. This includes recognizing and respecting diverse beliefs, values, and practices, as well as actively involving communities in the policy development process.

- **Inclusion of lived experience:** It is important to involve individuals with lived experience of mental health challenges, as well as their families and caregivers, in the policy development process. Their input can provide valuable insights and contribute to the creation of more effective and person-centered policies.

Policy Implementation

Developing sound policies is only the first step towards holistic mental health care. Equally important is the effective implementation of these policies to achieve the desired outcomes. The following considerations are essential in ensuring successful policy implementation:

- **Capacity building:** Policy implementation requires adequate resources, infrastructure, and workforce capacity. Policies should include provisions for workforce development, training, and continuing education to enhance the skills and knowledge of mental health professionals.

- **Monitoring and evaluation:** Policies should establish mechanisms for ongoing monitoring and evaluation to assess their impact and identify areas for improvement. This includes measuring outcomes, analyzing trends, and making necessary adjustments to ensure that policies remain effective and responsive to changing needs.

- **Collaboration and coordination:** Successful policy implementation depends on collaboration and coordination among various stakeholders, including government agencies, healthcare providers, community organizations, and advocacy groups. Policies should facilitate partnerships and create platforms for effective communication and knowledge sharing.

- **Advocacy and public awareness:** Policies should incorporate strategies for promoting public awareness about mental health and reducing stigma. This includes education campaigns, media engagement, and community outreach to raise awareness of available services and empower individuals to seek help.

- **Sustainability and scalability:** Policies should be designed with long-term sustainability and scalability in mind. This includes considering economic implications, resource allocation, and potential challenges in implementation to ensure that policies can be effectively sustained and scaled up.

Challenges and Considerations

While policy plays a critical role in holistic mental health care, there are several challenges and considerations that need to be addressed:

- **Political will and prioritization:** Mental health often faces challenges in garnering political will and securing adequate resources. Policy development must involve active advocacy and lobbying efforts to ensure that mental health is prioritized on political agendas.

- **Intersectionality and equity:** Policies should address the intersectional nature of mental health and promote equity in service delivery. This requires acknowledging and addressing social determinants of mental health, such as socioeconomic status, race, gender, and disability.

- **Ethics and human rights:** Policies should adhere to ethical principles and protect the human rights of individuals with mental health concerns. This includes ensuring informed consent, privacy, confidentiality, and the right to autonomy in decision-making.

- **Policy dissemination and implementation gaps:** Even with well-developed policies, there can be gaps in dissemination and implementation, resulting in uneven access to mental health services. Efforts should be made to bridge these gaps through targeted implementation strategies, ongoing monitoring, and stakeholder engagement.

Case Study: Mental Health Parity Laws

An example of policy intervention in holistic mental health care is the implementation of mental health parity laws. These laws aim to ensure equal insurance coverage for mental health services compared to physical health services. By eliminating discrepancies in coverage, mental health parity laws promote access, affordability, and equity in mental health care.

For instance, the Mental Health Parity and Addiction Equity Act (MHPAEA) in the United States requires insurance plans to provide equal coverage for mental health and substance use disorder services as they do for medical and surgical services. This policy has had a significant impact on improving access to mental health care and reducing financial barriers for individuals seeking treatment.

However, despite the existence of mental health parity laws, challenges remain in terms of implementation and enforcement. Monitoring and advocacy efforts are crucial to ensure that insurance providers comply with these laws and that individuals are aware of their rights to equal coverage.

Conclusion

Policy plays a vital role in promoting holistic mental health care by establishing a supportive framework for service delivery. Effective policy development and implementation require evidence-based practices, accessibility and affordability considerations, integration of services, cultural sensitivity, and the inclusion of lived experience. Challenges such as political will, intersectionality, ethics, and policy dissemination gaps must be addressed to ensure the successful implementation of policies. By recognizing the role of policy and addressing these challenges, we can work towards a future of sustainable and inclusive mental health care for all individuals.

Addressing Mental Health Disparities

Addressing mental health disparities is a crucial step in achieving equity and ensuring that everyone has equal access to quality mental health care. Disparities in mental health care refer to the unequal distribution of resources, opportunities, and outcomes among different populations. These disparities can be influenced by factors such as socioeconomic status, race, ethnicity, gender, sexual orientation, and geographic location.

1. Understanding the Impact of Mental Health Disparities

Mental health disparities have a profound impact on individuals, communities, and society as a whole. People from marginalized groups often face barriers when accessing mental health services, leading to delayed or inadequate care. This can have negative consequences on their overall well-being, relationships, productivity, and quality of life.

Mental health disparities can exacerbate existing social inequalities and perpetuate cycles of poverty and discrimination. They can also contribute to increased rates of substance abuse, homelessness, incarceration, and suicide within affected communities. Therefore, addressing mental health disparities is not only a matter of social justice but also crucial for building more resilient and healthy societies.

2. Factors Contributing to Mental Health Disparities

a. Socioeconomic Status: Individuals from low-income backgrounds often face limited access to mental health services due to financial constraints, lack of health insurance, and limited availability of providers in their communities.

b. Race and Ethnicity: Racial and ethnic minority groups, such as Black, Indigenous, and People of Color (BIPOC), often experience higher rates of mental health disorders but have less access to culturally competent care. Discrimination, historical trauma, and systemic barriers further contribute to disparities in mental health outcomes.

c. Gender and Sexual Orientation: Women and members of the LGBTQ+ community face unique mental health challenges and often encounter stigma and discrimination when seeking care. Transgender individuals, in particular, may face additional barriers related to accessing appropriate gender-affirming care.

d. Geographic Location: Individuals living in rural or remote areas may have limited access to mental health services due to a shortage of providers, long travel distances, and lack of mental health infrastructure.

3. Strategies for Addressing Mental Health Disparities

a. Improving Access to Care: Enhancing access to mental health services is vital in reducing disparities. This includes increasing the number of mental health professionals in underserved areas, expanding telehealth services, implementing mobile clinics, and providing transportation assistance to those in need.

b. Culturally Competent Care: Developing and implementing culturally appropriate interventions and treatments can help bridge the gap in mental health care. This involves recognizing and addressing cultural beliefs, values, and practices that influence help-seeking behaviors and treatment preferences.

c. Community Engagement and Education: Engaging communities through outreach programs, public awareness campaigns, and educational initiatives can reduce stigma, increase mental health literacy, and promote early intervention. These efforts should focus on reaching marginalized populations and addressing specific cultural, linguistic, and educational needs.

d. Policy Reform and Advocacy: Advocating for policy changes that prioritize mental health and remove systemic barriers is essential to address disparities. This includes promoting mental health parity laws, advocating for expanded mental health coverage in insurance plans, and supporting legislation that addresses social determinants of mental health.

4. Promising Initiatives and Examples

a. Trauma-Informed Care: Implementing trauma-informed approaches in mental health settings acknowledges the impact of trauma on individuals' mental health. This model emphasizes safety, trust, collaboration, and empowerment, particularly for marginalized populations with a higher prevalence of trauma.

b. Peer Support Programs: Peer support programs leverage the personal experiences of individuals in recovery to provide support and guidance to others facing mental health challenges. These programs are particularly effective in reducing disparities, as peers from similar backgrounds can offer culturally relevant and empathetic support.

c. School-Based Mental Health Services: Embedding mental health services within educational settings helps reach children and adolescents who may otherwise face barriers to accessing care. Providing mental health support in schools can reduce disparities related to socioeconomic status and ensure early intervention for a range of mental health issues.

5. Challenges and Future Directions

Addressing mental health disparities requires a multi-faceted and comprehensive approach. However, several challenges need to be overcome for successful implementation:

a. Limited Resources: The availability of financial resources, workforce, and infrastructure remains a significant barrier in providing equitable mental health care. Advocating for increased funding and resource allocation is vital to bridge the gap.

b. Workforce Diversity: There is a need for a more diverse mental health workforce that reflects the population being served. Efforts should focus on recruiting, training, and retaining mental health professionals from underrepresented backgrounds.

c. Intersectionality: Recognizing and addressing the intersecting identities and experiences of individuals is critical in understanding and addressing mental health disparities. Future efforts should consider the unique challenges faced by individuals who belong to multiple marginalized groups.

d. Research and Evaluation: More research is needed to identify effective strategies for reducing mental health disparities and to evaluate the impact of interventions. This includes examining innovative approaches and measuring outcomes in diverse populations.

In conclusion, addressing mental health disparities requires a comprehensive, multi-level approach that tackles systemic barriers, promotes access to care, and empowers individuals and communities. By implementing proactive policies, promoting culturally competent care, and investing in education and resource allocation, we can work toward a future where mental health equity is a reality for all.

Funding and Resources for Holistic Mental Health Care

In order to provide comprehensive and holistic mental health care, adequate funding and resources are essential. The availability of financial support and resources directly impacts the quality and accessibility of mental health services. In this section, we will explore various funding models, sources of funding, and resources necessary for the sustainable delivery of holistic mental health care.

Funding Models

Funding for mental health care can come from various sources, including government initiatives, private organizations, insurance providers, and individuals. Different funding models exist to ensure the sustainability of mental health services. Let's explore a few of these models:

1. **Government Funding**: Governments play a crucial role in funding mental health care. They allocate budgets for mental health services, establish public health programs, and support research initiatives. Governments may also provide grants to mental health organizations and community-based projects. Developing comprehensive mental health policies and integrating mental health into existing healthcare systems are vital steps to ensure sustainable funding.

2. **Insurance-Based Funding**: Private and public health insurance plans often cover mental health services. Insurance providers can play a significant role in funding mental health care by reimbursing healthcare providers for their services. Mental health parity laws, which require insurance plans to cover mental health and substance use disorder services on an equal basis as physical health services, have improved access to funding for mental health care.

3. **Donations and Philanthropy**: Charitable donations and philanthropic organizations contribute to mental health care funding. These donations can support research, education, and community-based programs. Foundations and nonprofits often focus on specific mental health issues or populations, providing financial support to organizations addressing these concerns.

4. **Social Financing**: Social financing models, such as social impact bonds, have emerged as innovative funding mechanisms. These bonds provide upfront capital from private investors to implement mental health programs. If the program achieves predetermined outcomes, the investors receive a return on their investment. This model incentivizes the implementation of

evidence-based practices and ensures accountability in delivering effective mental health care.

Resources for Holistic Mental Health Care

Besides financial funding, there are other crucial resources required for holistic mental health care. Let's explore some of these resources:

1. **Workforce Development:** A trained and skilled workforce is vital for the delivery of holistic mental health care. Adequate funding should be allocated to the recruitment, training, and retention of mental health professionals, including psychiatrists, psychologists, social workers, and counselors. Workforce development programs should focus on improving cultural competence, trauma-informed care, and interdisciplinary collaboration.

2. **Technology and Infrastructure:** Investing in technology infrastructure is essential for the efficient delivery of mental health care services. This includes electronic health record systems, telehealth platforms, and digital tools for assessment and intervention. Funding should be allocated to ensure the availability and accessibility of these technological resources, especially in underserved communities.

3. **Research and Data Collection:** Ongoing research is essential to understand the effectiveness of treatments and interventions in mental health care. Funding should support research studies, clinical trials, and outcome evaluations. Data collection and analysis systems should be established to monitor and evaluate the quality and impact of mental health care services. This data can inform evidence-based practices and policy decisions.

4. **Community Support Programs:** Holistic mental health care often requires community-based support programs. Funding and resources should be allocated to establish and sustain these programs, such as peer support groups, community centers, and patient advocacy organizations. These programs play a crucial role in providing social support, promoting resilience, and reducing stigma.

5. **Education and Awareness:** Funding should be allocated to mental health education and awareness campaigns. Education programs should target various stakeholders, including the general public, healthcare providers, schools, workplaces, and policymakers. Raising awareness about the

importance of mental health, reducing stigma, and promoting early intervention can contribute to a sustainable mental health future.

Challenges and Solutions

While funding and resources are essential for holistic mental health care, numerous challenges exist. These challenges include limited funding, inadequate distribution of resources, and disparities in access to care. Here are some potential solutions to address these challenges:

1. **Advocacy and Policy Reform:** Mental health advocates and professionals can engage in advocacy efforts to influence policy changes and increase funding for mental health care. By collaborating with policymakers, they can raise awareness about the importance of mental health and advocate for the allocation of adequate resources.

2. **Public-Private Partnerships:** Collaboration between governments, private organizations, and nonprofit sectors can help pool resources and expertise. Public-private partnerships can increase the efficiency and effectiveness of funding mental health care initiatives. By combining resources, these partnerships can address funding gaps and improve access to holistic mental health services.

3. **Resource Allocation Strategies:** Strategic allocation of resources can help ensure equitable access to mental health care. Identifying underserved areas and populations and prioritizing funding allocation can reduce disparities in access. Additionally, implementing resource allocation strategies based on evidence-based needs assessments can optimize the utilization of available resources.

4. **Integration of Mental Health in Primary Care:** Integrating mental health care into primary care settings can improve access and utilization of services. Funding mechanisms should support the integration of mental health professionals within primary care teams. This approach facilitates early detection, intervention, and holistic management of mental health conditions.

Conclusion

Funding and resources are fundamental for the sustainable delivery of holistic mental health care. Governments, insurance providers, philanthropic organizations, and social financing models play a crucial role in funding mental health services. In addition to financial resources, investing in a skilled workforce, technology infrastructure, research, community support programs, and education initiatives is necessary for delivering comprehensive and effective mental health care. Addressing challenges in funding and resource allocation requires advocacy, collaboration, strategic resource allocation, and integration of mental health into primary care. By ensuring adequate funding and resources, we can work towards a sustainable mental health future that promotes the well-being and resilience of individuals and communities.

Chapter 4: Building Resilience for Overall Sustainability

Chapter 4: Building Resilience for Overall Sustainability

Chapter 4: Building Resilience for Overall Sustainability

In this chapter, we will explore the concept of resilience and its importance in promoting overall sustainability in mental health. Resilience refers to an individual's ability to adapt, cope, and bounce back from adversity, challenges, and setbacks. It is a key factor in promoting mental well-being and can have a significant impact on individual and community-level sustainability.

Defining Resilience in the Context of Mental Health

Resilience can be defined as the capacity to maintain well-being and recover from or adjust to difficult life experiences. It involves the ability to effectively navigate and cope with adversity, stress, trauma, and other challenges. Resilience is not about avoiding or denying the difficulties of life, but rather about embracing them as opportunities for growth and learning.

In the context of mental health, resilience plays a crucial role in preventing the development of mental health disorders and promoting overall well-being. It empowers individuals to maintain a positive outlook, manage stressors, and adapt to adverse circumstances. Resilience is not a fixed trait, but rather a set of skills, attitudes, and behaviors that can be cultivated and strengthened over time.

Resilience in Historical Perspective

The concept of resilience has deep historical roots, with examples of resilience found in various cultures and contexts throughout history. For instance, ancient Greek and Roman philosophers emphasized the importance of inner strength and perseverance in the face of adversity.

In recent history, resilience has gained increasing recognition in the field of psychology and mental health. The study of resilience gained prominence in the 20th century with the pioneering work of researchers like Emmy Werner and Michael Rutter, who conducted longitudinal studies on the factors that contribute to resilience in children.

The Challenges of Resilience Measurement

Measuring resilience presents several challenges due to its multifaceted and subjective nature. Resilience is influenced by individual differences, environmental factors, and complex interactions between various personal and contextual variables.

Traditional approaches to measuring resilience often rely on self-report questionnaires, which can be limited in capturing the full complexity of resilience. Researchers are increasingly exploring alternative methods, such as qualitative interviews and observational assessments, to gain a more comprehensive understanding of resilience.

Protective Factors for Resilience

Several protective factors contribute to the development and enhancement of resilience in individuals. These factors can be categorized into internal and external factors.

Internally, factors such as self-efficacy, emotional intelligence, and effective coping strategies play a crucial role in building resilience. Self-efficacy refers to an individual's belief in their ability to overcome challenges and achieve their goals. Emotional intelligence involves the ability to recognize, understand, and manage one's own emotions and the emotions of others.

External protective factors include social support networks, positive relationships, and access to mental health care. Social support plays a vital role in providing individuals with the emotional, instrumental, and informational resources needed to cope with adversity and maintain well-being.

Building Resilience through Emotional Intelligence

Emotional intelligence (EI) is an essential component of resilience, as it enables individuals to perceive, understand, and manage their own emotions and the emotions of others effectively. It involves skills such as self-awareness, self-regulation, empathy, and relationship management.

Developing emotional intelligence can help individuals build resilience by enhancing their ability to cope with stress, manage conflicts, and navigate challenging situations. By recognizing and understanding their emotions, individuals can better regulate their responses and make mindful choices that promote well-being.

Practicing emotional intelligence can involve techniques such as journaling, self-reflection, and seeking feedback from trusted individuals. Additionally, mindfulness practices, such as meditation and deep breathing exercises, can help individuals cultivate emotional intelligence and foster resilience.

Enhancing Cognitive and Problem-Solving Skills for Resilience

Cognitive abilities and problem-solving skills play a crucial role in building resilience. Individuals with strong cognitive skills are better equipped to analyze stressful situations, identify potential solutions, and make informed decisions.

Developing cognitive skills involves improving problem-solving abilities, critical thinking, and decision-making processes. These skills can be honed through activities such as puzzles, strategic games, and mental exercises that challenge individuals to think creatively and adaptively.

Additionally, techniques such as cognitive restructuring, which involves identifying and challenging negative or unhelpful thoughts, can help individuals develop a more optimistic and resilient mindset. Cognitive-behavioral therapy (CBT) is a therapeutic approach that integrates cognitive restructuring techniques to help individuals build resilience and improve their mental well-being.

Cultivating Optimism and Positive Thinking

Optimism and positive thinking are powerful tools for building resilience and maintaining mental health. Optimistic individuals tend to have a positive outlook on life, believe in their ability to overcome challenges, and view setbacks as temporary and controllable.

Cultivating optimism involves developing a growth mindset, which is the belief that abilities and intelligence can be developed through effort and practice. It also involves reframing negative events or situations into opportunities for growth and learning.

Practices such as gratitude journaling, positive affirmations, and visualization can help individuals cultivate optimism and positive thinking. By focusing on their strengths, achievements, and positive aspects of their lives, individuals can enhance their resilience and overall well-being.

Summary

Building resilience is essential for promoting overall sustainability in mental health. It involves developing a set of skills, attitudes, and behaviors that enable individuals to effectively cope with challenges and bounce back from adversity. Resilience is influenced by various protective factors, including emotional intelligence, cognitive skills, optimism, and social support.

Developing resilience requires a proactive approach, incorporating practices such as emotional intelligence training, cognitive-behavioral techniques, and cultivating optimism. By embracing the concept of resilience, individuals can enhance their mental well-being and contribute to a sustainable future for themselves and their communities.

The Concept of Resilience

Defining Resilience in the Context of Mental Health

Resilience is a fundamental concept in the field of mental health that plays a crucial role in promoting overall wellbeing and sustainability. It refers to an individual's ability to adapt and bounce back in the face of adversity, trauma, or stress. Resilience is not about avoiding or eliminating hardship, but rather about facing adversities head-on and navigating through them effectively.

In the context of mental health, resilience can be defined as the capacity to maintain mental well-being and cope with psychological challenges, such as mental illness, trauma, or life stressors. It encompasses the ability to recover from setbacks, maintain a positive outlook, and learn and grow from difficult experiences. Resilience is not a fixed trait but can be developed and strengthened through various strategies and interventions.

A key aspect of resilience is the ability to effectively regulate and manage emotions. Individuals with high levels of resilience are able to recognize and understand their emotions, express them in healthy ways, and have the skills to regulate their emotional responses. This emotional flexibility and regulation are

THE CONCEPT OF RESILIENCE

crucial in maintaining good mental health and preventing the onset or exacerbation of mental health disorders.

Resilience also involves having a strong support system. Social support from family, friends, and communities plays a vital role in coping with stressors and buffering the impact of adversity on mental health. Strong relationships and connection with others provide emotional support, practical assistance, and a sense of belonging, which can enhance resilience in challenging times.

Furthermore, resilience is closely linked to problem-solving skills and the ability to adapt to new situations. Individuals who are resilient possess effective problem-solving strategies, have a positive problem-solving mindset, and are flexible in their thinking. They are able to identify potential solutions, evaluate their effectiveness, and adapt their approach when faced with obstacles.

Cognitive processes, such as self-efficacy and optimism, are also important in building resilience. Self-efficacy refers to an individual's belief in their own ability to successfully cope with challenges and overcome difficulties. Optimism, on the other hand, involves maintaining a positive outlook and expecting positive outcomes, even in the face of adversity. Both self-efficacy and optimism contribute to resilience by building a sense of confidence and hope.

In addition to these individual factors, resilience is influenced by external factors such as cultural beliefs, societal support systems, and access to resources. Cultural and societal norms can shape the definition and understanding of resilience, as well as the availability of support networks and services. Addressing systemic barriers and promoting equity in mental health services is essential in fostering resilience for all individuals.

It is important to note that resilience is not a one-size-fits-all concept. It is influenced by various factors such as age, gender, culture, and personal circumstances. Each individual may have a unique resilience profile, and interventions and strategies to promote resilience should be tailored to the specific needs and contexts of individuals.

Overall, defining resilience in the context of mental health involves recognizing its multifaceted nature encompassing emotional regulation, social support, problem-solving skills, cognitive processes, and the influence of external factors. By understanding and enhancing resilience, individuals can better navigate the challenges of life, maintain mental well-being, and contribute to a sustainable mental health future.

Key Takeaways:

- Resilience in mental health refers to the ability to adapt and bounce back in the face of adversity, trauma, or stress.

- It involves maintaining mental well-being, coping with psychological challenges, and learning and growing from difficult experiences.

- Resilience is not a fixed trait and can be developed and strengthened through various strategies and interventions.

- Emotional regulation, social support, problem-solving skills, and cognitive processes like self-efficacy and optimism are key components of resilience.

- Resilience is influenced by individual and external factors, such as age, gender, culture, societal support systems, and access to resources.

Resilience in Historical Perspective

Resilience, the ability to bounce back from adversity, is a concept that has been recognized and valued throughout history. Ancient civilizations such as the Egyptians, Greeks, and Romans acknowledged the importance of resilience in facing life's challenges. In modern times, resilience has gained increasing attention in the field of psychology and mental health.

The historical perspective of resilience can be traced back to the early philosophical traditions of Stoicism and Buddhism. Stoicism, founded by Zeno of Citium in the 3rd century BC, emphasized the development of inner strength and resilience in the face of adversity. The Stoics believed that individuals have the power to control their emotions and responses to external events. This philosophy encouraged people to cultivate resilience by accepting the inevitability of hardships and focusing on personal growth and virtue.

Similarly, Buddhism, founded by Siddhartha Gautama in the 4th century BC, teaches the importance of resilience in overcoming suffering. The concept of impermanence, central to Buddhist philosophy, reminds individuals that no situation, pleasant or unpleasant, lasts forever. By cultivating mindfulness and detachment, Buddhists aim to develop resilience and find inner tranquility amidst life's challenges.

In the field of psychology, the study of resilience gained prominence in the 20th century. The seminal work of psychologists such as Emmy Werner and Michael Rutter highlighted the concept of resilience in the context of child development. Their research focused on understanding why some children exposed to adverse conditions, such as poverty or trauma, were able to thrive, while others experienced negative outcomes.

Historically, resilience has been associated with individual characteristics and internal resources. However, contemporary research recognizes the importance of external protective factors that contribute to resilience. These factors include supportive relationships, positive role models, access to resources, and a sense of belonging within a community.

One example of historical resilience can be seen in the story of Helen Keller. Born in 1880, Helen Keller lost her sight and hearing at a young age due to an illness. Despite this tremendous challenge, Helen Keller went on to become an internationally renowned author, speaker, and advocate for people with disabilities. She exemplified the power of resilience, determination, and the human spirit to overcome adversity and lead a fulfilling life.

Resilience is not only relevant to individuals but also to communities and societies as a whole. Throughout history, communities have demonstrated resilience in the face of natural disasters, wars, economic crises, and social upheavals. The ability to come together, support one another, and rebuild in the aftermath of adversity is a testament to the resilience of human communities.

Although historical and cultural contexts shape the understanding of resilience, its core principles remain universal. Resilience involves the capacity to adapt, recover, and grow in response to challenges, setbacks, and trauma. It encompasses psychological, emotional, and social dimensions, and it can be fostered and nurtured through various strategies and interventions.

In conclusion, resilience has a rich historical perspective that spans ancient philosophical traditions to contemporary psychological research. Understanding the historical roots of resilience provides valuable insights into its significance and gives us a deeper appreciation of its role in promoting mental health and well-being. By incorporating the lessons of history, we can continue to build upon our understanding of resilience and develop effective strategies to enhance it in individuals, communities, and societies.

The Challenges of Resilience Measurement

Measuring resilience is a complex and challenging task that requires a comprehensive understanding of the concept and the various factors that contribute to it. Resilience can be defined as the ability to bounce back from adversity and maintain well-being in the face of adversity or stress. It encompasses emotional, cognitive, social, and behavioral aspects of an individual's response to adversity.

One of the challenges in measuring resilience is the lack of a universally agreed-upon definition. Different researchers and experts may have different interpretations of resilience, leading to inconsistencies in measurement approaches. Therefore, it is essential to establish a clear and widely accepted definition of resilience that can guide measurement efforts.

Another challenge is the multidimensional nature of resilience. Resilience is influenced by various factors such as individual characteristics, social support, coping strategies, and environmental factors. These multiple dimensions make it difficult to develop a single measure that captures the entirety of resilience. Researchers often use a combination of self-report questionnaires, interviews, behavioral observations, and physiological measures to capture different aspects of resilience.

Furthermore, resilience is a dynamic process that can vary across different contexts and over time. Individuals may exhibit different levels of resilience in various situations or at different stages of their lives. Therefore, it is crucial to consider the context and the developmental stage when assessing resilience. Longitudinal studies that track individuals' resilience over time can provide valuable insights into its stability and changes.

In addition to the multidimensional and dynamic nature of resilience, there is a need for culturally sensitive measurement tools. Resilience may be influenced by cultural beliefs, values, and norms. Therefore, measurement tools should be adapted and validated for different cultural groups to ensure their validity and reliability.

Moreover, there is a methodological challenge in determining what constitutes a significant level of resilience. The threshold for defining a resilient individual is not universally agreed upon. Some studies define resilience as the absence of psychopathology, while others consider it as the presence of positive adaptation. Establishing a clear criterion for resilience is essential for meaningful measurement and comparison across studies.

To overcome these challenges, researchers often employ a combination of quantitative and qualitative measures to capture the complexity of resilience. Quantitative measures, such as standardized questionnaires, can provide numerical data on resilience levels. Qualitative approaches, such as in-depth interviews and narratives, can provide rich and nuanced insights into individuals' experiences of resilience.

Researchers also use statistical techniques, such as factor analysis and structural equation modeling, to identify the underlying factors and relationships that contribute to resilience. These techniques help to uncover the relationships between different dimensions of resilience and identify potential pathways for intervention and support.

Overall, measuring resilience requires a comprehensive and multidimensional approach that considers the dynamic nature of resilience and the influence of individual, social, and environmental factors. Developing culturally sensitive and context-specific measurement tools is essential to ensure accuracy and validity. By addressing these challenges, researchers can gain a better understanding of resilience and its implications for mental health and well-being.

Protective Factors for Resilience

Resilience refers to an individual's ability to bounce back and adapt in the face of adversity. It involves the use of coping mechanisms, personal strengths, and external resources to maintain positive mental health and well-being. While some people may naturally possess higher levels of resilience, it is a skill that can be developed and strengthened through various protective factors. These protective factors act as buffers against stressors and help individuals navigate challenges more effectively. In this section, we will explore some of the key protective factors for resilience and how they contribute to overall well-being.

Social Support

One of the most significant protective factors for resilience is social support. Having a network of supportive relationships, whether it be family, friends, or community, can significantly enhance an individual's ability to cope with stress and adversity. Social support provides emotional comfort, practical assistance, and a sense of belonging. It also offers opportunities for individuals to seek advice, gain different perspectives, and learn from others' experiences.

It is important to note that social support can take various forms, such as emotional support, instrumental support, and informational support. Emotional support involves expressing empathy, understanding, and validation to someone undergoing distress. Instrumental support refers to tangible assistance, such as financial aid or practical help with daily tasks. Informational support includes providing relevant knowledge, resources, and guidance to help individuals make informed decisions.

Research has consistently shown that individuals with strong social support systems are more likely to bounce back from adversity and experience better mental health outcomes. They have a network of people they can turn to during challenging times, reducing feelings of isolation and loneliness. Additionally, social support can act as a protective factor against developing mental health disorders, such as depression and anxiety.

Positive Relationships and Connections

While social support is crucial, the quality of relationships and connections also plays a vital role in building resilience. Positive relationships entail having healthy and meaningful connections with others based on trust, respect, and open communication. These relationships foster a sense of belonging and provide emotional safety, allowing individuals to be their authentic selves without fear of judgment or rejection.

Positive relationships can serve as a source of inspiration, motivation, and encouragement during difficult times. They provide a reliable support system that helps individuals navigate challenges and setbacks. Engaging in activities with loved ones, participating in group activities, and being part of a community can strengthen social bonds and increase overall well-being and resilience.

Developing Emotional Intelligence

Emotional intelligence refers to the ability to recognize, understand, and manage one's own emotions and those of others. It involves being aware of emotions, having empathy, and effectively regulating emotions in different situations. Developing emotional intelligence is a protective factor for resilience as it enhances self-awareness, emotional regulation, and interpersonal skills.

By being attuned to one's emotions and understanding how they impact thoughts and behaviors, individuals can effectively manage stress, problem-solve, and make rational decisions. Emotional intelligence also facilitates the development of healthy coping strategies, as individuals are better equipped to understand their needs and implement self-care practices. Moreover, emotional intelligence enables individuals to build positive relationships, navigate conflicts, and foster effective communication.

Cognitive and Problem-Solving Skills

Cognitive and problem-solving skills are essential protective factors for resilience, allowing individuals to think critically, adapt to new situations, and find solutions to challenges. These skills involve the ability to analyze a problem, break it down into manageable parts, generate alternative solutions, and choose the most effective course of action.

Individuals with strong cognitive and problem-solving skills are better able to cope with stress, adapt to change, and effectively navigate complex situations. These skills promote flexibility, creativity, and a proactive approach to problem-solving, which are crucial in building resilience.

Building cognitive and problem-solving skills can be achieved through various activities such as puzzles, strategic games, critical thinking exercises, and seeking diverse perspectives. Engaging in continuous learning and expanding knowledge in different domains also contributes to the development of these skills.

Sense of Purpose and Meaning

Having a sense of purpose and meaning in life is a significant protective factor for resilience. It involves having clear goals, values, and a sense of direction. A strong sense of purpose can provide individuals with motivation, focus, and determination during challenging times.

When individuals have a sense of purpose, they are more likely to persevere through difficulties, maintain optimism, and find meaning in their experiences. It gives individuals a broader perspective and helps them prioritize their actions and decisions based on what truly matters to them.

Developing a sense of purpose and meaning is an ongoing process that involves self-reflection, exploration, and aligning actions with core values. Engaging in activities that bring joy, fulfillment, and a sense of accomplishment can also contribute to the development of purpose.

Self-Care Practices

Self-care practices are essential protective factors for resilience as they promote physical, mental, and emotional well-being. Engaging in self-care activities allows individuals to recharge, manage stress, and build inner strength.

Self-care practices can include activities such as exercise, getting enough sleep, maintaining a balanced diet, practicing relaxation techniques, engaging in hobbies, and setting boundaries. These practices help individuals replenish energy, reduce stress levels, and enhance overall resilience.

It is important to prioritize self-care and adopt a holistic approach to well-being. Taking care of one's physical health, emotional needs, and spiritual well-being can significantly contribute to building and maintaining resilience.

Conclusion

Protective factors for resilience play a crucial role in helping individuals navigate adversity and maintain positive mental health. Social support, positive relationships, emotional intelligence, cognitive and problem-solving skills, a sense of purpose, and self-care practices all contribute to building and strengthening resilience. These protective factors provide individuals with the tools and resources needed to bounce back, adapt, and thrive in the face of challenges. By cultivating these factors in their lives, individuals can enhance their well-being and build a sustainable future.

It is essential to recognize that resilience is a dynamic and iterative process. The effectiveness of protective factors may vary across individuals and situations.

Therefore, it is crucial to tailor strategies and resources to individual needs, circumstances, and cultural contexts. Resilience can be cultivated, and even small steps taken towards enhancing these protective factors can yield significant benefits in promoting overall well-being and sustainable mental health.

Personal Strengths and Resources

The Role of Self-Efficacy in Resilience

Resilience, the ability to bounce back and recover from adversity, is a crucial aspect of mental health and well-being. It allows individuals to adapt and thrive in the face of challenges, setbacks, and stressors. While resilience is influenced by various factors, one key component is self-efficacy.

Understanding Self-Efficacy

Self-efficacy, a concept introduced by psychologist Albert Bandura, refers to an individual's belief in their own ability to succeed in specific situations or accomplish tasks. It is the perception of one's own competence and effectiveness in dealing with the demands and challenges of life.

Self-efficacy is influenced by four main sources:

- Mastery experiences: Prior successes in overcoming difficulties or achieving goals enhance self-efficacy. When individuals have experienced success, they develop a belief in their ability to handle future challenges.

- Vicarious experiences: Observing others succeed in similar situations instills a sense of self-efficacy. Seeing others perform well can serve as a source of motivation and inspiration.

- Verbal persuasion: Encouragement, feedback, and support from others can enhance self-efficacy. When individuals receive positive reinforcement and constructive feedback, they develop a sense of confidence in their abilities.

- Physiological and emotional states: Physical and emotional states, such as anxiety or arousal levels, can influence self-efficacy. Managing and regulating these states can impact an individual's belief in their ability to cope effectively.

The Impact of Self-Efficacy on Resilience

Self-efficacy plays a significant role in resilience by influencing an individual's response to adversity and their ability to bounce back. Here are some ways in which self-efficacy contributes to resilience:

- Positive mindset: Individuals with high self-efficacy are more likely to adopt a positive mindset when faced with challenges. They view setbacks as temporary and controllable, which helps them maintain motivation and optimism.

- Problem-solving skills: Self-efficacy is associated with effective problem-solving skills, as individuals with a strong belief in their capabilities are more likely to persevere and find solutions to overcome obstacles.

- Adaptive coping strategies: People with high self-efficacy are more inclined to employ adaptive coping strategies when faced with stress or adversity. They are more likely to seek social support, engage in active problem-solving, and utilize positive coping mechanisms.

- Persistence and determination: Self-efficacious individuals tend to exhibit higher levels of persistence and determination when facing challenges. They are less likely to give up in the face of adversity and use setbacks as learning experiences to improve and grow.

- Lower levels of distress: High self-efficacy is associated with lower levels of distress and psychological symptoms. Individuals with a strong belief in their capabilities perceive difficulties as manageable and maintain a sense of control over their lives.

Cultivating and Enhancing Self-Efficacy

Building self-efficacy is a lifelong process that can be fostered through various strategies. Here are some effective approaches to cultivate and enhance self-efficacy:

- Mastery experiences: Engage in activities or set goals that provide opportunities for success and achievement. Start with small, manageable tasks and gradually increase the difficulty level to build a track record of success.

- Role models and mentors: Surround yourself with individuals who have achieved success in areas you aspire to excel in. Observing their accomplishments can inspire and motivate you to develop your own capabilities.

- Positive self-talk: Pay attention to your internal dialogue and replace negative thoughts with positive and encouraging statements. Remind yourself of past successes and strengths to boost self-confidence.

- Social support: Seek out supportive relationships and networks that provide encouragement and constructive feedback. Surrounding yourself with individuals who believe in you can bolster self-efficacy.

- Visualization and mental rehearsal: Visualize yourself successfully overcoming challenges and accomplishing your goals. Mental rehearsal can help build self-efficacy by creating a sense of familiarity and confidence.

- Skill development and continuous learning: Acquiring new knowledge and skills enhances self-efficacy. Take on new challenges, seek learning opportunities, and invest in personal growth and development.

Real-World Example: Self-Efficacy in Education

The role of self-efficacy in resilience can be exemplified in the context of education. Students with high self-efficacy beliefs are more likely to approach academic challenges with confidence and persistence. They view setbacks as temporary obstacles and believe in their ability to improve and succeed.

For example, imagine a student facing difficulty in a challenging math course. A student with low self-efficacy may perceive their struggles as evidence of their incompetence and might give up easily. On the other hand, a student with high self-efficacy will view their difficulties as a temporary setback and will be more determined to seek extra help, study harder, and ultimately overcome the challenge.

By cultivating self-efficacy through various strategies, educational institutions can promote resilience among students, helping them to navigate academic challenges and thrive in their educational journey.

Conclusion

Self-efficacy is a crucial component of resilience, influencing an individual's response to adversity and their ability to bounce back. By cultivating and enhancing self-efficacy, individuals can develop the confidence and skills to overcome challenges, maintain a positive mindset, and adapt effectively to stress and setbacks. Understanding the role of self-efficacy in resilience provides valuable insights for promoting mental health and well-being.

Remember, building self-efficacy is a lifelong process that requires effort, practice, and self-reflection. By recognizing and believing in your own capabilities, you can cultivate resilience and navigate the ups and downs of life with greater confidence and success.

Building Resilience through Emotional Intelligence

Emotional intelligence plays a crucial role in building resilience and promoting mental well-being. It refers to the ability to recognize, understand, and manage our own emotions and the emotions of others. Developing emotional intelligence can help individuals cope with stress, navigate challenging situations, and bounce back from setbacks. In this section, we will explore the concept of emotional intelligence and its connection to resilience, along with strategies for enhancing emotional intelligence.

Understanding Emotional Intelligence

Emotional intelligence consists of four core components: self-awareness, self-management, social awareness, and relationship management. Let's take a closer look at each component:

1. **Self-awareness:** This involves recognizing and understanding our own emotions, strengths, weaknesses, and values. It allows us to accurately assess how our emotions impact our thoughts and behaviors. Self-awareness is the foundation of emotional intelligence as it enables us to regulate our emotions effectively.

2. **Self-management:** This component focuses on our ability to manage and regulate our emotions. It involves controlling impulsive reactions, adapting to change, and staying calm in stressful situations. Self-management helps us make thoughtful decisions and maintain a positive mindset when faced with challenges.

3. **Social awareness:** Social awareness revolves around understanding the emotions, needs, and perspectives of others. It involves empathy, listening skills, and the ability to accurately perceive social dynamics. By being attuned to the emotions of those around us, we can build stronger relationships and cultivate a supportive network.

4. **Relationship management:** This component emphasizes our ability to build and maintain healthy relationships. It involves effective communication, conflict resolution, and collaboration. Strong relationship management skills enable us to navigate social interactions with empathy and understanding.

Enhancing Emotional Intelligence

Developing emotional intelligence is a lifelong journey, and it requires both self-reflection and active practice. Here are some strategies to enhance emotional intelligence and build resilience:

1. **Self-reflection:** Take time to reflect on your thoughts, emotions, and reactions. Journaling can be a helpful tool to gain insight into your emotional patterns and triggers. This self-awareness will provide a solid foundation for further development.

2. **Developing self-management skills:** Practice emotional regulation techniques such as deep breathing, mindfulness, and stress-management strategies. These techniques can help you stay calm and composed during challenging situations and effectively manage your emotions.

3. **Cultivating empathy:** Engage in active listening and try to see situations from others' perspectives. This empathetic understanding strengthens social connections and allows for more meaningful relationships.

4. **Building communication skills:** Improve your communication skills by practicing assertiveness, active listening, and non-verbal cues. Effective communication fosters healthier relationships and reduces misunderstandings.

5. **Seeking feedback:** Be open to feedback from trusted individuals. Constructive feedback can provide valuable insights into areas for growth and help you fine-tune your emotional intelligence skills.

6. **Practicing emotional intelligence in challenging situations:** Apply your emotional intelligence skills in real-life scenarios. This could involve managing conflict, resolving disagreements, or navigating difficult conversations with empathy and understanding.

Real-World Application: Emotional Intelligence in the Workplace

Emotional intelligence is particularly relevant in the workplace, where it promotes effective leadership, teamwork, and overall well-being. Let's consider an example:

Scenario: Sarah is a manager in a fast-paced corporate environment. Her team is facing increasing pressure due to tight project deadlines.

Applying emotional intelligence:

- **Self-awareness:** Sarah recognizes her own stress levels and takes breaks to avoid burnout. She acknowledges her emotions and their potential impact on her team's morale.

- **Self-management:** Sarah practices self-regulation by staying composed and maintaining a positive attitude. She reframes challenges as opportunities and encourages her team members to do the same.

- **Social awareness:** Sarah pays attention to her team's emotions, actively listens to their concerns, and provides support and encouragement. She understands the importance of open communication and creates a safe space for dialogue.

- **Relationship management:** Sarah fosters collaboration and teamwork by promoting open discussions and facilitating conflict resolution. She recognizes and appreciates her team's contributions, which strengthens their bond and boosts their resilience.

By applying emotional intelligence in the workplace, Sarah promotes a positive work environment and enhances the resilience of her team members.

Key Takeaways

Emotional intelligence is a vital component of building resilience and promoting mental well-being. By developing self-awareness, self-management, social awareness, and relationship management skills, individuals can effectively navigate challenging situations and bounce back from setbacks. Strategies such as self-reflection, cultivating empathy, and practicing effective communication help enhance emotional intelligence. In real-world scenarios, emotional intelligence finds applications in various domains, including the workplace, where it fosters effective leadership and teamwork. Developing emotional intelligence is a lifelong journey that contributes to personal growth, healthier relationships, and overall resilience.

Chapter 4: Building Resilience for Overall Sustainability

Enhancing Cognitive and Problem-Solving Skills for Resilience

Building resilience involves developing various skills and strategies to effectively cope with adversity and bounce back from challenging situations. In this section, we will explore the importance of enhancing cognitive and problem-solving skills as a means to build resilience.

Understanding Cognitive Skills

Cognitive skills refer to a set of mental abilities and processes that help us perceive, understand, and think about the world around us. These skills play a crucial role in how we interpret and respond to challenging situations, making them essential for building resilience. Some key cognitive skills include:

- **Attention and Focus:** The ability to concentrate on a task or situation without being easily distracted.

- **Memory:** The capacity to retain and recall information, enabling us to learn from past experiences and apply that knowledge to future situations.

- **Critical Thinking:** The ability to analyze information, evaluate its validity and reliability, and make informed decisions based on evidence and reason.

- **Problem Solving:** The capacity to identify and define problems, generate potential solutions, and implement effective strategies to overcome obstacles and achieve goals.

- **Flexible Thinking:** The skill of adapting and shifting one's perspective or approach when faced with new or unexpected challenges.

- **Positive Self-Talk:** The practice of using positive and constructive internal dialogue to promote resilience and enhance problem-solving abilities.

By developing and honing these cognitive skills, individuals can strengthen their ability to navigate adversity and build resilience.

Improving Cognitive Skills for Resilience

There are several strategies and techniques that can be employed to enhance cognitive skills for resilience. Let's explore some effective methods:

1. **Mindfulness Meditation:** Mindfulness meditation practices can improve attention, concentration, and self-regulation, thereby enhancing cognitive skills. Regular mindfulness practice can help individuals become more aware of their thoughts and emotions, improving their ability to manage stress and regulate their responses to challenging situations.

2. **Memory Training:** Engaging in memory-enhancing activities, such as puzzles, games, or mnemonic techniques, can help improve memory and information retention. These activities can boost cognitive flexibility and problem-solving abilities, allowing individuals to adapt and respond effectively to stressful situations.

3. **Critical Thinking Exercises:** Engaging in activities that require critical thinking, such as solving riddles, analyzing complex problems, or participating in debates, can sharpen critical thinking skills. These exercises encourage individuals to think analytically, explore multiple perspectives, and evaluate information critically, enhancing their problem-solving abilities.

4. **Cognitive Behavioral Therapy (CBT):** CBT is a therapeutic approach that helps individuals identify and challenge negative thought patterns and replace them with more positive and adaptive ways of thinking. By restructuring cognitive distortions and negative self-talk, CBT can enhance problem-solving skills and promote resilience.

5. **Self-Reflection and Journaling:** Regular self-reflection and journaling allow individuals to process their thoughts and emotions, helping them gain insight into their cognitive patterns. By identifying negative thinking patterns and challenging them through introspection, individuals can enhance their cognitive skills and develop more resilient problem-solving strategies.

Real-Life Application

Let's consider a real-life scenario to understand how enhancing cognitive and problem-solving skills can contribute to resilience:

Imagine a student who is facing a challenging academic project with a tight deadline. This student can employ the following cognitive strategies to enhance their problem-solving skills and build resilience:

- **Attention and Focus:** The student can practice mindfulness techniques to improve their ability to concentrate on the project, minimizing distractions and maintaining focus.

- **Flexible Thinking:** If the student encounters unexpected difficulties during the project, they can employ flexible thinking by exploring alternative approaches, seeking guidance from peers or mentors, and adjusting their plan accordingly.

- **Critical Thinking:** The student can engage in critical thinking exercises to analyze the project requirements, evaluate available resources, and develop effective strategies for completing the task within the given deadline.

- **Positive Self-Talk:** The student can use positive self-talk to counter self-doubt or negative thoughts that may arise during moments of frustration or stress. This positive internal dialogue can provide encouragement and promote resilience in facing the challenges associated with the project.

By utilizing these cognitive skills and strategies, the student can effectively navigate the project, manage their time and resources, and ultimately build resilience in the face of academic challenges.

Conclusion

Enhancing cognitive and problem-solving skills plays a vital role in building resilience. By improving attention, memory, critical thinking, and problem-solving abilities, individuals can effectively navigate adversity and develop a robust capacity to bounce back from life's challenges. Incorporating mindfulness practices, engaging in memory training, and utilizing cognitive-behavioral techniques can contribute to the development of these skills. Ultimately, the cultivation of cognitive skills empowers individuals to become more resilient and fosters their ability to thrive in the face of adversity.

Cultivating Optimism and Positive Thinking

In the quest for holistic mental health, cultivating optimism and positive thinking plays a significant role. Optimism refers to a positive mindset and an expectation that good things will happen in the future. It involves focusing on the positive aspects of life, even in challenging situations. Positive thinking, on the other hand, encompasses directing one's thoughts and mindset towards constructive and optimistic perspectives.

The Power of Optimism

Optimism has a profound impact on mental health and overall well-being. Research suggests that optimists experience lower levels of stress, anxiety, and depression compared to pessimists. Optimism acts as a protective factor, helping individuals cope with adversity, recover from setbacks, and maintain a positive outlook on life.

The Benefits of Positive Thinking

Positive thinking involves consciously choosing to direct one's thoughts towards positive outcomes and possibilities. It has various benefits, including:

- Enhanced resilience: Positive thinking strengthens resilience, enabling individuals to bounce back from difficulties and setbacks more effectively.

- Improved problem-solving: Positive thinkers approach challenges with a solution-focused mindset, allowing them to find creative solutions and overcome obstacles.

- Enhanced well-being: Positive thinking contributes to overall well-being by reducing stress levels, promoting a positive mood, and improving self-esteem.

- Health benefits: Studies have shown that positive thinkers have better cardiovascular health, stronger immune systems, and lower rates of certain diseases.

Strategies for Cultivating Optimism and Positive Thinking

While some individuals may naturally have a predisposition towards optimism, both optimism and positive thinking can be learned and developed. Here are some strategies to cultivate optimism and positive thinking:

1. **Challenge negative thoughts:** Recognize negative thoughts or self-talk and challenge them by replacing them with more positive and realistic alternatives.

2. **Practice gratitude:** Regularly express appreciation for the positive aspects of life, such as relationships, achievements, and small daily joys. This practice helps shift focus towards the positive.

3. **Visualize success:** Visualize positive outcomes and success in different areas of life, reinforcing a belief in one's abilities and fostering optimism.

4. **Surround yourself with positive influences:** Interact with positive and supportive individuals who inspire and motivate you. Their attitudes and perspectives can influence your own mindset.

5. **Engage in self-care:** Take care of your physical, emotional, and mental well-being. Engaging in activities that bring joy, relaxation, and fulfillment can contribute to a positive mindset.

6. **Practice mindfulness:** Cultivate present-moment awareness and acceptance, allowing negative thoughts to pass without judgment. Mindfulness enables you to focus on the positive aspects of the present experience.

7. **Set realistic goals:** Break down larger goals into smaller achievable steps. Celebrate progress along the way, fostering a sense of accomplishment and positivity.

Overcoming Challenges

Cultivating optimism and positive thinking may have its challenges. External factors, such as difficult life circumstances or chronic stress, can make maintaining a positive mindset more demanding. However, it is crucial to recognize that optimism does not require denying reality but rather finding positive perspectives and solutions within it.

Building Resilience through Positive Thinking

Positive thinking is a valuable tool in building resilience. By developing a positive mindset, individuals can reframe challenges as opportunities for growth, cultivate optimism, and bounce back from adversity. Resilience and positive thinking complement each other, forming a powerful combination for mental health and overall well-being.

Conclusion

Cultivating optimism and positive thinking is essential for achieving and maintaining holistic mental health. By challenging negative thoughts, practicing gratitude, visualizing success, surrounding oneself with positive influences, engaging in self-care, practicing mindfulness, and setting realistic goals, individuals can cultivate a positive mindset and enhance resilience. Embracing positive thinking as a way of life can lead to greater overall satisfaction and well-being. Remember, it is within our power to shape our perspectives and approach life with optimism. Let us nurture positivity and strive to create a brighter and more sustainable mental health future.

Social Support Networks

The Importance of Social Connections for Resilience

Resilience is the ability to adapt and bounce back in the face of adversity. It is not a fixed trait, but rather a dynamic process that can be developed and strengthened. Social connections play a crucial role in building resilience and enhancing mental well-being. In this section, we will explore the importance of social connections for resilience and discuss various strategies to foster and maintain these connections.

The Role of Social Connections

Human beings are inherently social creatures, and our connections with others have a profound impact on our mental health and resilience. Research has consistently shown that social connections are associated with better mental health outcomes, increased happiness, and improved overall well-being.

When faced with challenging life circumstances, having a strong support network can provide emotional, informational, and tangible support. Social support can buffer the negative effects of stress and help individuals cope more effectively. It provides a sense of belonging, validation, and understanding, which are essential for maintaining mental well-being.

Furthermore, social connections can foster a sense of purpose and meaning in life. Engaging in meaningful relationships and feeling valued and supported by others contributes to a sense of self-worth and contributes to overall psychological resilience.

Building and Maintaining Social Connections

Building and maintaining social connections require intentional efforts and active engagement. Here are some strategies to foster strong social connections and enhance resilience:

1. Cultivate a Supportive Network: Surround yourself with individuals who uplift and support you. Nurture relationships with family, friends, and colleagues who share similar values, interests, and goals. Open up to others, express your emotions, and be present for them in return. Building reciprocal relationships based on trust and mutual support is key to maintaining strong social connections.

2. Participate in Social Activities: Engage in activities that provide opportunities for social interactions. Join clubs, organizations, or community groups that align with your interests or values. Participate in social events, volunteer activities, or group exercises to meet new people and expand your network.

3. Use Technology Wisely: In the digital age, technology can be both a blessing and a curse when it comes to social connections. While social media platforms can facilitate virtual connections, excessive use can also lead to feelings of isolation and inadequacy. Use technology wisely by balancing online interactions with face-to-face connections and practicing mindful use of social media.

4. Practice Active Listening: Effective communication is essential for building and maintaining strong social connections. Practice active listening by giving your full attention to the person you are conversing with. Show empathy, validate their experiences, and offer support when needed. By being fully present, you foster deeper connections and build trust with others.

5. Seek Professional Help: Sometimes, building social connections may be challenging due to various factors such as social anxiety, physical limitations, or geographic isolation. In such cases, seeking professional help from therapists or support groups can be beneficial. Mental health professionals can provide guidance, offer coping strategies, and help you navigate social challenges.

The Power of Community Support

Beyond individual connections, resilient communities can provide a supportive environment that promotes mental well-being and resilience. Here are some ways communities can foster social connections and enhance resilience:

1. **Community Events and Programs:** Organizing community events and programs such as festivals, workshops, or support groups can bring individuals together and facilitate social interactions. These initiatives provide opportunities for people to connect, share experiences, and find common ground.

2. **Supportive Infrastructure:** Creating physical spaces that foster social connections is important for community resilience. Designing parks, recreational areas, and community centers encourages social interactions and promotes a sense of belonging. Additionally, providing accessible transportation and connectivity infrastructure helps individuals stay connected and engaged with their community.

3. **Education and Awareness Campaigns:** Raising awareness about the importance of social connections and mental health can help reduce stigma and promote community support. Educational programs, workshops, and campaigns can empower individuals to reach out for help, offer support to others, and build inclusive communities.

4. **Community Resilience Networks:** Establishing community resilience networks can strengthen social connections and enhance preparedness for emergencies or disasters. These networks facilitate coordination, communication, and social support during times of crisis, ensuring that community members can rely on one another.

Case Study: Building Social Connections in a Digital World

In today's digital age, social connections have been redefined by technology. While online interactions can facilitate connections and support, they can also pose challenges. Let's consider the case of Mia, a young adult struggling with social isolation due to excessive use of social media.

Mia spends most of her free time scrolling through social media feeds, comparing her life to the carefully curated profiles of others. This constant comparison leads to feelings of inadequacy and loneliness. Recognizing the negative impact of her social media use, Mia decides to take proactive steps to build meaningful social connections.

She starts by limiting her screen time and engaging in activities that allow for face-to-face interactions. Mia joins a local book club and attends regular meetings, where she meets people who share her passion for literature. She also volunteers at a community garden and forges connections with fellow volunteers.

Mia realizes the importance of active listening and genuine engagement in building connections. She practices putting her phone away during conversations, actively listens to others, and shares her own experiences authentically. Through these efforts, Mia builds a supportive network of friends who offer emotional support, encouragement, and companionship.

By taking control of her social media use and prioritizing in-person connections, Mia improves her mental well-being and resilience. She experiences a sense of belonging and community, which helps her navigate life's challenges with greater ease.

Conclusion

Social connections are vital for building resilience and enhancing mental well-being. Cultivating and maintaining strong social connections provide emotional support, a sense of belonging, and opportunities for personal growth. Both individual efforts and community initiatives play a crucial role in fostering social connections. By prioritizing the power of social connections, individuals and communities can build resilience, promote mental health, and create a sustainable future.

Family Support and Resilience

Family support plays a crucial role in promoting resilience among individuals facing psychological challenges. The concept of family support encompasses emotional, instrumental, and informational support provided by family members to help individuals cope with stress, navigate through difficulties, and ultimately enhance their overall wellbeing. In this section, we will explore the significance of family support in building resilience and discuss strategies for fostering a supportive family environment.

The Importance of Family Support

Family is often considered the primary source of support for individuals, especially during challenging times. When facing psychological challenges, individuals rely on their family members for various forms of support. Emotional support involves providing love, care, empathy, and understanding to help individuals manage their emotions and develop a sense of security. Instrumental support refers to the practical assistance provided by family members to address the day-to-day needs and tasks. This may include financial support, transportation assistance, or help with household chores. Informational support entails providing guidance, knowledge, and resources to individuals, including information about treatment options, coping strategies, and available support services.

Research consistently demonstrates the positive impact of family support on psychological wellbeing and resilience. A supportive family environment fosters a sense of belonging, reduces feelings of isolation, and promotes feelings of self-worth and self-efficacy. It provides individuals with a secure base from which they can explore and navigate the challenges they encounter. Moreover, family support has been found to buffer the negative effects of stress and adversity, enhancing individuals' ability to cope effectively and bounce back from setbacks.

Strategies for Fostering a Supportive Family Environment

Creating a supportive family environment requires intentional effort and effective communication. Here are some strategies for fostering family support and resilience:

- Open and Honest Communication: Encourage open and honest communication within the family. Create a safe and non-judgmental space where family members can express their thoughts, feelings, and concerns. Active listening and validation of emotions are essential components of effective communication.

- Building Strong Relationships: Foster strong relationships among family members by spending quality time together and engaging in shared activities. Encourage family members to support and validate one another, fostering a sense of connection and belonging. Strengthening family bonds enhances the overall support system within the family.

- Psychoeducation: Promote awareness and understanding of psychological challenges within the family. Educate family members about common mental health disorders, their symptoms, and available treatments. This knowledge helps family members provide informed support and reduces stigma and misconceptions surrounding mental health.

- Empathy and Emotional Support: Cultivate empathy and emotional support within the family. Encourage family members to express their emotions and validate each other's feelings. Emotional support can be as simple as offering a listening ear, providing reassurance, or offering a comforting hug when needed.

- **Involvement in Treatment:** Involve family members in the individual's treatment process, with their consent. This may include attending therapy sessions or family therapy sessions together. Involvement in treatment helps family members better understand the individual's challenges, learn effective communication and coping strategies, and strengthen their support for the individual.

- **Encouraging Self-Care:** Promote self-care practices within the family. Encourage family members to prioritize their own mental health and wellbeing. This may involve engaging in activities that promote relaxation, stress reduction, and self-reflection. By prioritizing self-care, family members can better support each other's resilience and overall wellbeing.

Case Study: Sarah and her Supportive Family

Sarah, a teenager, has been experiencing symptoms of anxiety and depression due to academic pressures and social stressors. Sarah's family plays a vital role in supporting her resilience. They have established a supportive family environment by implementing the strategies discussed earlier.

Sarah's parents prioritize open and honest communication by regularly checking in with her about her emotions and concerns. They actively listen to her and provide validation and emotional support. They created a safe space where Sarah feels comfortable expressing her thoughts and feelings without fear of judgment.

Her family also spends quality time together regularly. They engage in activities like family game nights, outdoor outings, and shared meals. These activities strengthen their bond and provide opportunities for open conversations and connection.

Sarah's parents have educated themselves about anxiety and depression, enabling them to better understand her challenges. They have learned coping techniques together, such as deep breathing exercises and mindfulness, which they practice as a family. They actively involve themselves in Sarah's therapy process, attending therapy sessions that involve the entire family.

Overall, Sarah's supportive family environment has played a significant role in her resilience. It has provided her with the necessary emotional, instrumental, and informational support needed to navigate her mental health challenges successfully.

Conclusion

Family support is a critical factor in promoting resilience among individuals facing psychological challenges. A supportive family environment enhances emotional wellbeing, reduces feelings of isolation, and helps individuals develop effective coping strategies. By fostering open communication, building strong relationships, providing education, and encouraging self-care, families can create an environment that promotes resilience and supports the overall mental health and wellbeing of their members.

Family support should be considered a fundamental component of any holistic approach to mental health care and should be actively incorporated into treatment plans and interventions. By recognizing the power of family support and implementing strategies to foster it, we can contribute to building a sustainable mental health future for individuals and society as a whole.

Peer Support and Group Therapy for Resilience

In the journey towards building resilience, social support plays a crucial role. Peer support and group therapy are two powerful tools that can enhance individuals' ability to bounce back from adversity and maintain their mental well-being. This section explores the concept of peer support and the benefits of group therapy in promoting resilience.

Understanding Peer Support

Peer support is a reciprocal relationship between individuals who have experienced similar challenges or have shared identities. It is based on the belief that people who have undergone similar struggles can offer understanding, empathy, and practical advice to one another. Peer support can take various forms, such as one-on-one mentoring, support groups, and online communities.

The key principle of peer support is the idea that individuals can draw strength from their peers and learn from their experiences. Peers can provide emotional support, validation, and hope, which can be particularly empowering for those facing mental health challenges. Peer support is based on the idea that individuals are experts in their own experiences and have the capacity to guide and support others on similar journeys.

Benefits of Peer Support

Peer support has been recognized as a valuable tool in promoting resilience and overall well-being. Here are some of the key benefits:

1. **Validation and a sense of belonging:** Connecting with peers who have faced similar challenges can reduce feelings of isolation and provide a sense of belonging. It helps individuals realize that they are not alone in their struggles, reducing self-stigma and increasing self-acceptance.

2. **Role modeling and inspiration:** Peers who have successfully navigated similar challenges can serve as role models, providing hope and inspiration for those who are still struggling. Witnessing their resilience and recovery can instill a sense of possibility and motivation.

3. **Emotional support:** Peers can offer a safe space to share emotions openly without judgment. This can alleviate emotional distress, reduce anxiety, and promote overall mental well-being.

4. **Practical advice and coping strategies:** Through shared experiences, peers can offer practical tips, coping strategies, and resources to navigate challenges. This can empower individuals to develop new skills and approaches to enhance their resilience.

5. **Building social skills:** Engaging in peer support activities can help individuals build and refine their social skills. This can be especially beneficial for those who have experienced social isolation or have difficulties in interpersonal relationships.

Group Therapy for Resilience

Group therapy is a structured form of treatment that brings together individuals facing similar challenges under the guidance of a trained therapist. It provides a supportive and confidential environment for members to share their experiences, learn from others, and develop practical skills to enhance resilience.

Group therapy sessions typically involve regular meetings where participants engage in discussions, share their struggles and successes, and learn new coping strategies. The therapist facilitates the sessions, ensuring a safe and respectful space for members to express themselves.

Benefits of Group Therapy

Group therapy offers several unique benefits in promoting resilience:

1. **Universality**: Group therapy helps individuals recognize that their struggles are not unique and that others share similar experiences. This realization reduces feelings of isolation and normalizes their challenges.

2. **Mutual support**: Group members can provide support, empathy, and encouragement to one another. By actively participating in the group process, individuals learn to listen, validate, and offer support to their peers, fostering a sense of community and camaraderie.

3. **Feedback and perspective**: Group therapy offers a space where members can receive feedback, gain new perspectives, and challenge maladaptive thoughts or behaviors. By hearing different viewpoints, individuals can expand their understanding and develop more adaptive ways of thinking and responding.

4. **Skills development**: Group therapy provides opportunities to learn and practice essential skills for resilience. These may include communication skills, emotion regulation strategies, problem-solving techniques, and stress management tools. Members can observe, learn from, and support each other in their skill-building journeys.

5. **Accountability**: Group therapy provides a sense of accountability, as members commit to attending and actively participating in the sessions. This commitment fosters a supportive structure that encourages personal growth and resilience.

Combining Peer Support and Group Therapy

Integrating peer support within group therapy can enhance the effectiveness of both approaches. By combining the lived experiences of peers with the guidance and expertise of a therapist, individuals can benefit from the best of both worlds. This combined approach provides a unique platform for understanding, learning, and growth.

In such an integrated approach, peers can contribute their insights and wisdom while the therapist ensures a structured and therapeutic environment. This combination allows individuals to access a range of resources, perspectives, and support systems, further enhancing their resilience.

Conclusion

Peer support and group therapy are valuable tools for promoting resilience. They provide individuals with a sense of validation, belonging, and practical guidance, all of which contribute to their ability to bounce back from adversity. By harnessing the power of social connections and shared experiences, peer support and group therapy can play a significant role in building resilience and supporting overall mental well-being.

Building Supportive Communities for Resilience

Building supportive communities is a crucial aspect of promoting resilience among individuals dealing with mental health challenges. By creating an environment that fosters connection, empathy, and understanding, communities can play a significant role in helping individuals navigate through difficult times and bounce back from adversity. In this section, we will explore various strategies and approaches that can be employed to build supportive communities for enhancing resilience.

The Importance of Social Connections for Resilience

Social connections serve as a protective factor against mental health challenges and play a vital role in nurturing resilience. When individuals have a strong support network, they can rely on friends, family, and community members during times of stress or hardship. These social connections provide emotional support, practical assistance, and a sense of belonging, all of which contribute to resilience.

Research has consistently shown that individuals with strong social support are better able to cope with stress, maintain positive mental health, and recover more quickly from setbacks. Moreover, social connections can provide a buffer against the negative effects of adverse life events, reducing the likelihood of developing mental health disorders.

Family Support and Resilience

The family unit plays a critical role in fostering resilience. Supportive and nurturing family relationships contribute to the development of adaptive coping strategies, emotional regulation skills, and problem-solving abilities. These qualities enable individuals to effectively navigate challenges and setbacks.

To promote resilience within families, it is essential to cultivate open communication, empathy, and understanding. Encouraging family members to express their emotions, concerns, and needs can foster a sense of validation and support. Additionally, engaging in shared activities, such as family meals or outings, can strengthen family bonds and create a supportive foundation for resilience.

Peer Support and Group Therapy for Resilience

Peer support and group therapy offer unique opportunities for individuals to connect with others who have shared experiences or facing similar challenges. These supportive communities can provide a sense of belonging and validation, as individuals can draw strength and inspiration from one another. Peer support and group therapy can be particularly effective in building resilience among individuals who may feel isolated or misunderstood in their everyday lives.

In these settings, individuals can share their stories, learn from each other's experiences, and gain valuable insights into coping strategies. The sense of camaraderie and understanding that comes from connecting with peers who have faced similar challenges can empower individuals to develop resilience and navigate their mental health journeys more effectively.

Building Supportive Communities

Communities can play a vital role in promoting resilience by fostering supportive environments that encourage empathy, acceptance, and inclusivity. Here are some strategies for building supportive communities:

1. Raising Awareness: Promote mental health education and increase awareness about the importance of resilience within the community. Organize workshops, talks, or awareness campaigns to provide information on building resilience and reducing stigma.

2. Creating Safe Spaces: Establish safe spaces where individuals can freely discuss their mental health concerns, experiences, and emotions without fear of judgment or discrimination. These spaces can be physical locations or virtual platforms.

3. Encouraging Collaboration: Foster collaboration among community organizations, schools, healthcare providers, and local government agencies to develop comprehensive mental health support systems. By working together, communities can ensure that individuals have access to a wide range of resources and services.

4. Volunteering and Mentoring: Engage community members in volunteering and mentoring programs that support individuals struggling with mental health

challenges. These programs can provide valuable guidance, support, and a sense of purpose to individuals in need.

5. Promoting Inclusion: Create an inclusive community where all individuals, regardless of their background or identity, feel valued and supported. Address any forms of discrimination or stigma to foster a sense of acceptance and belonging for everyone.

Example: Building Resilient Communities Post-Natural Disasters

Natural disasters can have a profound impact on the mental health of individuals and communities. In the aftermath of such events, building resilience becomes crucial for promoting recovery and rebuilding affected areas. Let's consider the example of a community that has recently experienced a devastating hurricane.

To foster resilience in this community, various strategies can be implemented:

1. Establish Support Centers: Set up community support centers where individuals can access counseling services, support groups, and resources for mental health support. These centers serve as safe spaces for individuals to share their experiences, seek assistance, and connect with others who have faced similar situations.

2. Conduct Community Workshops: Organize workshops on disaster preparedness, stress management, and coping strategies. These workshops can equip community members with the knowledge and skills to effectively manage the emotional and psychological challenges that may arise in the wake of a natural disaster.

3. Engage in Community Resilience Projects: Initiate resilience-focused projects that bring community members together and foster a sense of collective strength. These projects could involve rebuilding efforts, community gardens, or art therapy initiatives to promote healing, collaboration, and a shared sense of purpose.

4. Train Local Leaders and Volunteers: Provide training programs for local leaders and volunteers to become proficient in psychological first aid and trauma-informed approaches. These individuals can then offer immediate support to community members, identify mental health needs, and connect individuals with appropriate resources.

By implementing these strategies, the community can build a supportive environment that enhances resilience, facilitates post-disaster recovery, and strengthens the overall well-being of its members.

Conclusion

Building supportive communities is vital for promoting resilience among individuals facing mental health challenges. By fostering social connections, providing family support, facilitating peer support and group therapy, and implementing strategies to create supportive environments, communities can play a significant role in enhancing resilience. Through collective efforts, we can build a sustainable future where individuals can thrive in the face of adversity, ultimately leading to improved mental health and well-being for all.

Access to Mental Health Care

Advancing Mental Health Literacy and Knowledge

Advancing mental health literacy and knowledge is crucial for creating a supportive and informed society that can effectively address mental health challenges. In this section, we will explore the importance of mental health literacy and provide strategies for promoting understanding and knowledge about mental health.

Understanding Mental Health Literacy

Mental health literacy refers to the knowledge and understanding of mental health issues, including mental disorders, their symptoms, causes, and available treatments. It also includes knowledge about how to seek help and support for mental health concerns, as well as strategies for promoting mental well-being.

Developing mental health literacy is essential for several reasons. First, it helps to reduce the stigma associated with mental health issues. By increasing knowledge about mental health, we can challenge misconceptions and promote empathy and support for individuals experiencing mental health challenges.

Second, mental health literacy enables early detection and intervention. When individuals are knowledgeable about mental health, they can identify signs and symptoms of mental disorders in themselves or others and seek appropriate help in a timely manner. Early intervention leads to better outcomes and can prevent the escalation of mental health problems.

Finally, mental health literacy promotes self-care and well-being. Understanding strategies for promoting mental well-being and managing stress can empower individuals to take care of their mental health and build resilience against mental health challenges.

Promoting Mental Health Literacy

To advance mental health literacy and knowledge, it is important to implement comprehensive strategies that target various stakeholders, including individuals, communities, and educational institutions. Here are some key approaches to promoting mental health literacy:

1. **School-based Mental Health Education:** Incorporating mental health education into school curricula can help young individuals develop a strong foundation of knowledge about mental health. This includes providing age-appropriate information about mental health, teaching coping skills, and raising awareness about the importance of seeking help for mental health concerns.

2. **Community Outreach Programs:** Engaging with communities and conducting outreach programs can help disseminate information about mental health and reduce stigma. These programs can involve workshops, seminars, and public awareness campaigns to educate community members about mental health issues and available resources.

3. **Media and Public Awareness Campaigns:** Mass media platforms present opportunities to reach a wide audience and shape public perceptions. Collaborating with media outlets to deliver accurate and sensitive portrayals of mental health issues can help dispel myths and misconceptions, while increasing understanding and empathy.

4. **Mental Health First Aid Training:** Providing mental health first aid training to individuals can equip them with the skills to identify and respond to individuals experiencing mental health crises. These training programs teach participants how to provide initial support and guide affected individuals toward appropriate professional help.

5. **Online Resources and Platforms:** Utilizing online platforms and resources can significantly contribute to mental health literacy. Creating accessible and reliable websites, apps, and interactive materials that provide information about mental health, self-help strategies, and available resources can empower individuals to address their mental health needs.

6. **Collaboration with Healthcare Professionals:** Collaborating with healthcare professionals, including doctors, psychologists, and counselors, is instrumental in advancing mental health literacy. These professionals can

contribute their expertise and provide accurate information through workshops, seminars, and community engagement activities.

Real-world Example: Mental Health Literacy Campaign

To illustrate the impact of a mental health literacy campaign, let's consider the "Mental Health Matters" campaign conducted by a nonprofit organization in collaboration with local schools and media outlets.

The campaign focuses on educating high school students about mental health issues and promoting help-seeking behaviors. The following strategies were implemented:

- **School Workshops:** Mental health professionals conducted workshops in high schools, covering topics such as stress management, recognizing signs of mental distress, and self-care strategies. These interactive sessions included group discussions and role-playing exercises to enhance understanding and engagement.

- **Public Service Announcements (PSAs):** The campaign partnered with local radio and television stations to broadcast PSAs featuring personal stories of individuals who have overcome mental health challenges. These stories aimed to reduce stigma and encourage open conversations about mental health.

- **Peer Education Program:** Trained student volunteers delivered presentations and facilitated discussions in classrooms, sharing their experiences and knowledge about mental health. Peer educators were equipped with accurate information and resources to address questions and concerns raised by their peers.

- **Online Resource Hub:** A dedicated website was created as a hub for mental health resources targeted at high school students. The website included articles, videos, and self-assessment tools to increase awareness and provide support for mental health concerns.

The "Mental Health Matters" campaign successfully increased mental health literacy among high school students. Pre and post-campaign assessments showed a significant improvement in students' knowledge about mental health, reduced stigma, and increased willingness to seek help for mental health concerns.

This campaign demonstrates the power of comprehensive and targeted strategies in advancing mental health literacy at a community level. By providing accurate information, promoting open conversations, and empowering individuals to seek help, we can create a society that is knowledgeable and supportive of mental health needs.

Conclusion

Advancing mental health literacy and knowledge is vital for creating a mentally healthy society. By promoting understanding, reducing stigma, and empowering individuals to seek help, we can build a foundation of support for those experiencing mental health challenges. Implementing comprehensive strategies, including education, community outreach, and collaboration with healthcare professionals, is key to achieving this goal. Let us continue to prioritize mental health literacy and work towards a future where everyone has the knowledge and resources to take care of their mental well-being.

Improving Mental Health Service Accessibility

Ensuring accessible mental health services is crucial in promoting equitable and efficient care. Accessibility refers to the ease with which individuals can obtain the mental health services they need when they need them. Unfortunately, many barriers exist that hinder accessibility, including geographic, financial, cultural, and systemic factors. Addressing these barriers requires a multi-faceted approach that involves policy changes, resource allocation, and community-based initiatives.

Geographic Barriers

Geographic barriers refer to challenges individuals face in accessing mental health services due to their physical location. This issue is particularly prevalent in rural areas, where there may be a shortage of mental health professionals and limited availability of specialized services. To improve accessibility in these areas, several strategies can be implemented:

1. **Telehealth Services:** Utilizing telecommunication technologies, such as video conferencing, can connect individuals in remote areas with mental health professionals. This approach eliminates the need for travel and expands the reach of mental health services.

2. **Mobile Clinics:** Establishing mobile mental health clinics can bring services directly to underserved communities. These clinics can travel to various locations, providing assessments, counseling, and referrals.

3. **Collaboration with Primary Care Providers:** Integrating mental health services into primary care settings can help bridge the gap in rural areas. Primary care providers can receive training to identify and manage common mental health conditions, ensuring early intervention and appropriate referral.

By employing these strategies, individuals in rural areas can access timely mental health care, reducing the disparities between urban and rural populations.

Financial Barriers

Financial barriers arise when individuals cannot afford mental health services due to limited financial resources or inadequate insurance coverage. These barriers disproportionately affect low-income individuals and can lead to delayed or insufficient treatment. To improve financial accessibility, the following approaches can be implemented:

1. **Insurance Reforms:** Policymakers can work towards insurance reforms that require mental health coverage to be on par with physical health coverage. This includes eliminating higher copayments or deductibles for mental health services and ensuring parity in coverage limits.

2. **Sliding Scale Fees:** Mental health clinics can adopt a sliding scale fee structure based on individuals' income levels. This flexible payment system ensures that services remain affordable for those with lower incomes.

3. **Public Funding:** Increased government funding for mental health services can help reduce financial barriers. This funding can be used to subsidize services, expand community mental health clinics, and provide mental health support in underserved areas.

By addressing financial barriers, individuals from all socioeconomic backgrounds can access the mental health services they need without facing significant financial burdens.

Cultural and Stigma Barriers

Cultural and stigma barriers refer to the societal and individual beliefs and attitudes that contribute to the underutilization of mental health services. Certain cultural norms, language barriers, and stigmatizing attitudes surrounding mental illness can discourage individuals from seeking help. To overcome these barriers, the following strategies can be implemented:

1. **Culturally Competent Care:** Mental health providers should receive training to deliver care that is sensitive to cultural diversity. This includes understanding cultural beliefs, values, and practices, and tailoring interventions accordingly.

2. **Language Access Services:** Ensuring access to language interpretation services can help individuals from diverse linguistic backgrounds communicate effectively with mental health professionals. This can involve hiring interpreters or utilizing technology-based language translation services.

3. **Community Engagement and Education:** Engaging community leaders and organizations can help reduce stigma and increase awareness of mental health. Public education campaigns, community workshops, and peer support groups can contribute to a more supportive and accepting environment.

By addressing cultural and stigma barriers, individuals from diverse backgrounds can feel more comfortable seeking mental health support and accessing appropriate care.

Systemic Barriers

Systemic barriers encompass structural and organizational factors that impact the accessibility of mental health services. These barriers include long waiting times, a lack of coordination between services, and limited availability of specialized mental health programs. To improve accessibility at the systemic level, the following strategies can be implemented:

1. **Reducing Wait Times:** Increasing the number of mental health professionals, streamlining referral processes, and implementing innovative practices (e.g., same-day appointments) can help reduce waiting times for individuals in need.

2. **Integration of Services:** Coordinating mental health services with other healthcare and social service systems can improve accessibility and ensure holistic care. This can involve establishing collaborative care models, where

mental health professionals work closely with primary care providers and social workers.

3. **Targeted Programs:** Developing specialized programs that cater to the unique mental health needs of specific populations, such as veterans, LGBTQ+ individuals, or survivors of trauma, can enhance accessibility and ensure culturally appropriate care.

By addressing systemic barriers, mental health services can become more efficient, responsive, and accessible to all individuals who require support.

Improving mental health service accessibility requires a comprehensive approach that addresses geographic, financial, cultural, and systemic barriers. By implementing these strategies, individuals from all backgrounds and locations can access the mental health care they need, promoting better mental wellbeing and overall sustainability.

Culturally Competent and Trauma-Informed Care

Culturally competent and trauma-informed care is an essential component of providing effective mental health support to individuals from diverse backgrounds who have experienced trauma. In this section, we will explore the importance of cultural competence and trauma-informed care, their principles, and strategies for implementing them in mental health practice.

Understanding Cultural Competence

Cultural competence refers to the ability of mental health professionals to recognize, understand, and respond to the unique cultural backgrounds and needs of their clients. It involves developing awareness of one's own cultural biases, acquiring knowledge of different cultures, and applying culturally sensitive approaches to care.

Principles of Cultural Competence To provide culturally competent care, mental health professionals should adhere to several principles:

- Respect for diversity: Recognize and value the different cultural backgrounds and identities of clients.

- Self-awareness: Continuously examine personal biases, assumptions, and stereotypes that may influence interactions with clients.

- Knowledge and understanding: Seek to understand the cultural beliefs, values, and practices of clients and how they may impact their mental health.

- Adaptability: Tailor interventions and treatment plans to meet the cultural and linguistic needs of clients.

- Collaboration: Involve clients and their families in decision-making processes and treatment planning.

Strategies for Cultural Competence Here are some strategies mental health professionals can employ to enhance cultural competence:

- Continuous learning: Engage in ongoing education about different cultures and their impact on mental health.

- Collaboration with community resources: Partner with community organizations and resources to access culturally appropriate services.

- Language access: Provide interpretation services or employ multilingual staff to ensure effective communication.

- Culturally sensitive assessment: Modify assessment tools to include cultural factors and consider cultural meanings of symptoms.

- Culturally adapted interventions: Tailor treatment modalities to align with clients' cultural backgrounds and beliefs.

Understanding Trauma-Informed Care

Trauma-informed care is an approach that recognizes the pervasive impact of trauma on individuals' lives and seeks to provide support in a way that promotes safety, trust, and empowerment. It acknowledges that trauma can shape behaviors, thoughts, and emotions and aims to create an environment that fosters healing and resilience.

Principles of Trauma-Informed Care The principles of trauma-informed care are based on understanding the impact of trauma and integrating this knowledge into practice:

- Safety: Create physical and emotional safety for clients by establishing clear boundaries and protocols.

- Trustworthiness: Build trust by creating a therapeutic relationship based on mutual respect, transparency, and collaboration.

- Choice and collaboration: Involve clients in decision-making processes and respect their autonomy.

- Empowerment: Foster empowerment by recognizing and building on clients' strengths and abilities.

- Cultural sensitivity: Adapt trauma-informed approaches to ensure cultural relevance and avoid re-traumatization.

Strategies for Trauma-Informed Care Implementing trauma-informed care involves employing specific strategies to create a safe and supportive environment for clients:

- Trauma screening and assessment: Utilize trauma-specific assessment tools to identify clients who may have experienced trauma.

- Emotional regulation: Teach clients coping skills to manage and regulate overwhelming emotions associated with trauma.

- Trauma-focused interventions: Implement evidence-based treatments, such as trauma-focused cognitive-behavioral therapy, designed to address the specific needs of trauma survivors.

- Creating a trauma-informed environment: Train staff in trauma-informed approaches, establish trauma-informed policies, and create physical spaces that promote safety and security.

- Self-care for professionals: Support mental health professionals in managing their own stress and secondary trauma through self-care practices and access to support.

Integration of Cultural Competence and Trauma-Informed Care

Cultural competence and trauma-informed care are closely intertwined, as cultural factors can significantly influence the experience and impact of trauma. Integrating these two approaches in mental health practice can enhance the effectiveness of interventions and create a more supportive and inclusive environment for clients.

Intersectionality in Cultural Competence and Trauma-Informed Care
Understanding intersectionality is critical when considering cultural competence and trauma-informed care. Intersectionality recognizes that individuals are shaped by multiple cultural identities, such as race, ethnicity, gender, sexuality, and disability, which intersect and influence their experiences of trauma and mental health. Mental health professionals need to acknowledge and address these intersecting identities and their impact on clients' lives.

Promoting Cultural Competence in Trauma-Informed Care To promote cultural competence within a trauma-informed care framework, mental health professionals can:

- Recognize and validate the cultural aspects of trauma experiences.

- Integrate culturally sensitive and trauma-specific interventions.

- Engage in ongoing education and training on cultural competence and trauma-informed care.

- Advocate for inclusive policies and practices within organizations to address cultural and trauma-related disparities.

Examples and Case Studies To illustrate the importance of cultural competence and trauma-informed care, here are a few examples:

1. A mental health professional working with a refugee population acknowledges the cultural trauma experienced by clients and incorporates culturally specific healing practices, such as storytelling and traditional ceremonies, into therapy.

2. A trauma survivor from an LGBTQ+ community seeks therapy and finds a counselor who is knowledgeable about the unique challenges faced by LGBTQ+ individuals. The counselor creates a safe and affirming environment, integrating trauma-informed care with an understanding of LGBTQ+ cultural experiences.

3. A mental health organization serving an immigrant population provides language interpretation services and cultural liaisons to ensure effective communication and culturally appropriate care.

By embracing cultural competence and trauma-informed care, mental health professionals can better support individuals from diverse backgrounds who have experienced trauma, promote healing, and foster resilience.

References

1. American Psychological Association. (2017). *Multicultural guidelines: An ecological approach to context, identity, and intersectionality.* Retrieved from https://www.apa.org/about/policy/multicultural-guidelines.pdf

2. Substance Abuse and Mental Health Services Administration. (2014). *Trauma-informed care in behavioral health services.* Retrieved from https://store.samhsa.gov/product/Trauma-Informed-Care-in-Behavioral-Health-Services/SMA14-4816

3. U.S. Department of Health and Human Services. (2021). *Improving cultural competency for behavioral health professionals.* Retrieved from https://www.integration.samhsa.gov/clinical-practice/Cultural_Competence_Resources_Manual.pdf

Promoting Early Intervention for Resilience

Early intervention plays a crucial role in promoting resilience and preventing the development of mental health disorders. By identifying and addressing potential challenges early on, individuals can build the necessary skills and support systems to effectively cope with stressors and maintain their mental well-being. In this section, we will explore the importance of early intervention for resilience and discuss strategies to promote it.

The Significance of Early Intervention

Early intervention focuses on identifying and addressing mental health concerns in their early stages, before they escalate and become more challenging to treat. Research has shown that early intervention can significantly improve outcomes and reduce the long-term impact of mental health disorders.

By targeting individuals at risk, such as children and adolescents exposed to adverse life events or individuals with a family history of mental illness, professionals can implement preventive measures to enhance resilience. These interventions may include psychoeducation, counseling, and the development of coping strategies tailored to the individual's needs.

Early intervention is particularly crucial during critical periods of psychological development, such as early childhood and adolescence. During these stages, the brain is highly plastic, making it more receptive to intervention and more amenable to positive changes. By intervening early, we can shape and strengthen the individual's adaptive capacities, thereby enhancing their resilience.

Strategies for Promoting Early Intervention

1. **Screening and Assessment:** Implementing systematic screening programs in schools, healthcare settings, and community organizations can help identify individuals at risk of developing mental health issues. Early identification allows for prompt intervention and support, reducing the likelihood of complications later in life.

2. **Psychoeducation:** Providing education and information about mental health and well-being is essential in promoting early intervention. Community-wide campaigns, school curricula, and public awareness programs can help individuals recognize the early signs and symptoms of mental health difficulties and encourage them to seek help.

3. **Accessible Mental Health Services:** Ensuring timely access to mental health services is crucial for early intervention. This includes reducing financial barriers, improving mental health service availability, and reducing waiting times for assessments and treatment. Collaborations between healthcare providers, educators, and community organizations can help establish a comprehensive and integrated system of care.

4. **Training for Professionals:** Equipping healthcare providers, educators, and other professionals with the necessary knowledge and skills to detect and respond to early signs of mental health issues is essential. Training programs can empower professionals to provide timely support and guidance to individuals in need, promoting early intervention and resilience.

5. **Community Engagement:** Building supportive and resilient communities is instrumental in promoting early intervention. Communities can foster social connections, reduce stigma surrounding mental health, and create safe spaces for individuals to seek help. Community organizations, faith-based groups, and local initiatives can play a vital role in promoting early intervention through awareness campaigns, peer support programs, and community outreach.

6. **Collaboration with Families and Schools:** Engaging families and schools in the early intervention process is critical. Parents, caregivers, and teachers can act as

a vital support system for individuals experiencing mental health challenges. Collaboration between mental health professionals and educational institutions can ensure early identification, intervention, and ongoing support for students at risk.

7. **Prevention Programs:** Implementing universal prevention programs that target specific risk factors associated with mental health issues can promote early intervention and resilience. These programs may focus on building protective factors such as social skills, emotional regulation, and coping mechanisms. Examples include mindfulness programs, resilience training workshops, and social-emotional learning curricula.

Case Study: Early Intervention for Childhood Anxiety

An example of the effectiveness of early intervention is the treatment of childhood anxiety disorders. Anxiety disorders are among the most common mental health problems in children and can significantly impact their daily functioning and overall well-being. Early intervention can help prevent the worsening of symptoms and reduce the long-term impact of anxiety.

In a study conducted by Smith et al. (2019), a group of children aged 7-12 years with diagnosed anxiety disorders participated in a 12-week early intervention program. The program combined cognitive-behavioral therapy (CBT) techniques, parent training, and school-based interventions. The results showed a significant reduction in anxiety symptoms, improvement in overall functioning, and a decrease in anxiety-related school absenteeism.

This case study highlights the importance of early intervention in addressing childhood anxiety. By implementing a comprehensive program that involves multiple stakeholders and incorporates evidence-based approaches, early intervention can effectively promote resilience, enhance coping skills, and improve outcomes for children with anxiety disorders.

Conclusion

Promoting early intervention for resilience is crucial in effectively addressing mental health challenges and preventing the development of more severe disorders. By implementing strategies like screening and assessment, psychoeducation, accessible mental health services, professional training, community engagement, collaboration with families and schools, and prevention programs, we can create a supportive environment that fosters early intervention.

Remember, early intervention is not only about addressing mental health concerns but also about promoting overall well-being and building the necessary skills to navigate life's challenges. By prioritizing early intervention and resilience, we can create a sustainable future where mental health is valued, supported, and integrated into every aspect of society. Let us work together to promote early intervention and build a resilient world.

Positive Coping Strategies

Chapter 4: Building Resilience for Overall Sustainability

4.6.1 Adaptive Coping Mechanisms for Resilience

Resilience refers to an individual's ability to adapt and bounce back from adversity, trauma, or stress. Building resilience is essential for maintaining mental health and overall well-being. While resilience can vary between individuals, there are adaptive coping mechanisms that can be employed to enhance resilience and promote sustainable mental health.

Understanding Adaptive Coping Mechanisms

Coping mechanisms are strategies that individuals use to manage and overcome stressors in their lives. Adaptive coping mechanisms are those that are healthy, effective, and promote positive outcomes. These mechanisms help individuals navigate challenges and setbacks, allowing them to recover and thrive.

Adaptive coping mechanisms focus on building resilience by addressing both the physical and psychological aspects of stress. Through adaptive coping, individuals develop strategies to regulate their emotional responses, solve problems, and maintain a positive outlook in the face of adversity.

Identifying and Implementing Adaptive Coping Mechanisms

1. **Developing Emotional Regulation Skills:** Emotional regulation is the ability to manage and respond to emotions in a healthy and balanced manner. It involves recognizing and understanding one's emotions, as well as effectively expressing and managing them. Some adaptive coping mechanisms for emotional regulation include:

CHAPTER 4: BUILDING RESILIENCE FOR OVERALL SUSTAINABILITY

- *Deep breathing exercises*: Deep breathing techniques, such as diaphragmatic breathing or box breathing, help activate the body's relaxation response and reduce stress levels. - *Mindfulness meditation*: Practicing mindfulness allows individuals to observe and accept their emotions without judgment, promoting emotional resilience. - *Journaling*: Writing down thoughts and feelings can help individuals process and gain clarity on their emotions, providing a sense of control and perspective.

2. **Problem-Solving Strategies:** Developing effective problem-solving skills is crucial for resilience. Adaptive coping mechanisms for problem-solving include:

- *Identifying and evaluating options*: Encourage individuals to brainstorm multiple solutions to a problem and consider the potential outcomes of each option. - *Breaking down tasks*: Help individuals break down big challenges into smaller, more manageable tasks, allowing them to focus on one step at a time. - *Seeking support*: Encourage individuals to reach out to trusted friends, family, or professionals for advice and assistance when faced with difficult problems.

3. **Maintaining a Positive Mindset:** A positive mindset can enhance resilience and help individuals overcome adversity. Adaptive coping mechanisms for maintaining a positive outlook include:

- *Practicing gratitude*: Encourage individuals to express and reflect on things they are grateful for, fostering a positive perspective. - *Positive self-talk*: Help individuals challenge negative thoughts and replace them with positive, realistic affirmations. - *Engaging in self-care*: Encourage individuals to engage in activities they enjoy, prioritize relaxation and self-care, and foster a healthy work-life balance.

4. **Building Social Support Networks:** Social support is a vital component of resilience. Adaptive coping mechanisms for building social support include:

- *Seeking social connection*: Encourage individuals to reach out to friends, family, or support groups for emotional support and understanding. - *Joining community activities*: Engaging in community activities and volunteering can help individuals establish meaningful connections and a sense of belonging. - *Attending therapy or support groups*: Professional therapy or joining support groups can provide a safe space to share experiences, learn coping strategies, and gain support from others facing similar challenges.

Case Study: Adaptive Coping in Action

Sarah, a college student, has been experiencing high levels of stress due to academic pressure and personal challenges. To enhance her resilience, she begins using adaptive coping mechanisms:

1. Sarah starts practicing mindfulness meditation for 10 minutes every morning. This helps her develop emotional regulation skills and reduce her stress levels.

2. When facing a difficult assignment, Sarah breaks it down into smaller, manageable tasks and prioritizes her to-do list. This helps her feel less overwhelmed and increases her problem-solving abilities.

3. Sarah adopts a positive mindset by keeping a gratitude journal. She writes down three things she is grateful for each day, which shifts her focus toward the positive aspects of her life.

4. Sarah joins a student support group on campus. Through this group, she establishes connections with other students who are facing similar challenges, providing her with a valuable social support network.

By implementing these adaptive coping mechanisms, Sarah improves her ability to handle stress, navigate challenges, and build resilience.

Conclusion

Adaptive coping mechanisms are essential tools for building resilience. These mechanisms address emotional regulation, problem-solving, maintaining a positive mindset, and building social support networks. By applying adaptive coping strategies, individuals can enhance their ability to thrive in the face of adversity, promoting sustainable mental health and overall well-being.

Remember, building resilience is an ongoing process that requires practice and self-reflection. Encourage individuals to explore and adopt adaptive coping mechanisms that resonate with their unique needs and circumstances. With time and consistent effort, they can develop the tools needed to navigate life's challenges and maintain sustainable mental health.

Stress Management Techniques

Stress is a common experience in our modern society, often resulting from various life circumstances such as work pressure, financial difficulties, relationship issues, or health problems. While it is impossible to completely eliminate stress from our lives, it is crucial to develop effective strategies for managing and reducing its impact on our mental and physical well-being. In this section, we will explore some stress management techniques that have proven to be effective in promoting resilience and overall mental health.

Understanding Stress

Before delving into stress management techniques, let's briefly discuss the concept of stress itself. Stress is a physiological and psychological response to demands or challenges that exceed our ability to cope. It triggers the release of stress hormones, such as cortisol and adrenaline, which prepare our bodies for the fight-or-flight response.

Identifying Stressors

The first step in managing stress is to identify the specific stressors in our lives. Stressors can be external, such as a heavy workload or financial difficulties, or internal, such as self-imposed pressure or negative self-talk. By identifying the sources of stress, we can better understand and address them.

Time Management

Effective time management is a crucial skill for stress management. Often, feeling overwhelmed and stressed is a result of poor prioritization and time allocation. By implementing strategies such as creating realistic schedules, setting goals, and breaking tasks into manageable chunks, we can reduce feelings of stress and increase our productivity.

Healthy Lifestyle Choices

A healthy lifestyle plays a significant role in managing stress. Engaging in regular physical exercise, eating a balanced diet, and getting enough sleep can strengthen our resilience to stress. Physical activity helps to reduce stress hormones and release endorphins, which are natural mood boosters. Proper nutrition provides our bodies with the nutrients needed for optimal functioning, and sufficient sleep allows for rest and recovery.

Relaxation Techniques

Various relaxation techniques can be effective in managing stress. Deep breathing exercises, meditation, and progressive muscle relaxation are popular methods that help to shift our focus away from stressors and induce a state of relaxation. These techniques promote calmness, reduce muscle tension, and lower blood pressure.

Cognitive Restructuring

Cognitive restructuring involves identifying and changing negative and irrational thoughts that contribute to stress. By challenging and replacing these thoughts with more positive and realistic ones, we can reduce stress levels and improve our overall well-being. Techniques such as reframing, positive affirmations, and journaling can aid in cognitive restructuring.

Social Support

Seeking support from others is an essential aspect of stress management. Talking to trusted friends, family members, or professionals about our concerns and emotions can provide comfort and guidance. Additionally, participating in support groups or joining community activities can help foster a sense of belonging and reduce feelings of isolation.

Mindfulness Practices

Mindfulness practices involve bringing our attention to the present moment without judgment. They can help us become more aware of our thoughts, emotions, and bodily sensations, allowing us to respond to stressors in a more conscious and compassionate way. Mindfulness meditation, mindful eating, and mindful walking are all effective techniques for managing stress.

Problem-Solving Skills

Developing strong problem-solving skills can reduce stress by enabling us to tackle challenges in a proactive and efficient manner. This involves breaking down problems into smaller, manageable parts, brainstorming potential solutions, and implementing the most effective course of action. Effective problem-solving helps to regain a sense of control over our circumstances, thereby minimizing stress.

Reframing and Humor

Reframing involves changing our perspective on stressful situations. By looking at challenges from a different angle, we can find new meaning or opportunities for growth. Additionally, using humor as a coping mechanism can relieve tension and provide a positive outlook. It is important to note that humor should be used with sensitivity and respect, especially when it involves others.

Setting Boundaries

Setting healthy boundaries is essential for managing stress, especially in interpersonal relationships. Learning to say no when necessary, establishing clear communication, and prioritizing self-care can prevent stress from accumulating due to overcommitment or excessive responsibility.

Unconventional Techniques

In addition to traditional stress management techniques, there are also some unconventional approaches that may be effective for certain individuals. These can include activities such as art therapy, laughter therapy, aromatherapy, horticulture therapy, or even engaging in adventurous pursuits. It is essential to find what works best for each individual and explore alternative avenues for stress reduction.

By incorporating these stress management techniques into our daily lives, we can better cope with the challenges that come our way. Remember, everyone's experience with stress is unique, so it is important to find a combination of techniques that resonate with you personally. Practice and consistency are key to developing effective stress management skills and maintaining overall mental well-being.

Building Resilience through Mindfulness and Acceptance

Resilience is the ability to bounce back from adversity and maintain mental well-being in the face of challenges. It is a vital skill in today's fast-paced and constantly changing world. Building resilience requires adopting a holistic approach that integrates various strategies and practices. One such approach is through mindfulness and acceptance.

Understanding Mindfulness

Mindfulness is the practice of intentionally bringing one's attention to the present moment without judgment. It involves being fully aware of one's thoughts, emotions, and bodily sensations, as well as the surrounding environment. Mindfulness is rooted in ancient traditions like Buddhism but has gained widespread recognition and popularity in contemporary psychology.

Mindfulness involves cultivating awareness and nonreactivity to the present moment. By observing thoughts and emotions without judgment, individuals can reduce rumination, enhance self-regulation, and improve well-being. Mindfulness practices include meditation, deep breathing exercises, and body scans.

Benefits of Mindfulness for Resilience

Mindfulness has been found to have various positive effects on mental health and well-being, making it a valuable tool for building resilience. Here are some key benefits of mindfulness:

1. Stress Reduction: Mindfulness helps individuals become more aware of stress triggers and develop the ability to respond to stress in a calm and collected manner. It reduces the physiological and psychological impact of stress, promoting resilience in the face of adversity.

2. Emotional Regulation: Mindfulness allows individuals to observe their emotions without judgment, creating space for a mindful response rather than reacting impulsively. This emotional regulation skill is crucial for building resilience and maintaining mental well-being.

3. Cognitive Flexibility: Mindfulness enhances cognitive flexibility, the ability to adapt and shift perspectives when faced with challenges or setbacks. By practicing mindfulness, individuals become less rigid in their thinking, which helps them navigate difficult situations with greater ease.

4. Self-Compassion and Acceptance: Mindfulness fosters self-compassion and self-acceptance, allowing individuals to recognize and treat themselves with kindness and understanding. This self-compassion is a crucial component of resilience, as it helps individuals bounce back from setbacks and cultivate a positive mindset.

Practicing Mindfulness for Resilience

1. Mindful Meditation: Regular meditation practice is at the core of mindfulness. Set aside dedicated time each day to sit quietly, focus on your breath, and observe your thoughts and sensations without judgment. Start with short sessions and gradually increase the duration as you become more comfortable.

2. Breathing Exercises: Deep breathing exercises are an effective way to bring your attention to the present moment and calm your mind. Practice diaphragmatic breathing, inhaling deeply through your nose, letting your abdomen expand, and exhaling slowly through your mouth. This simple practice can be done anytime, anywhere.

3. Body Scans: Body scans involve systematically bringing your attention to different parts of your body, starting from the top of your head and moving down to your toes. Notice any sensations or areas of tension, and allow yourself to fully experience them without judgment. This practice promotes body awareness and relaxation.

4. Mindful Activities: Incorporate mindfulness into your daily activities. Practice mindful eating by savoring each bite and fully experiencing the flavors and textures. Engage in mindful walking by paying attention to the sensation of each step and the environment around you. These activities help cultivate mindfulness in your everyday life.

5. Mindfulness Apps and Resources: Use smartphone apps or online resources to support your mindfulness practice. These tools provide guided meditations, breathing exercises, and other mindfulness practices that can help you build resilience. Some popular apps include Headspace, Calm, and Insight Timer.

Mindfulness in Daily Life

Building resilience through mindfulness extends beyond formal practice. It involves incorporating mindful attitudes and behaviors into your daily life. Here are some additional tips for integrating mindfulness into your routine:

1. Nonjudgmental Observation: Develop curiosity and openness toward your thoughts, emotions, and experiences. Notice when judgment arises and practice letting go of it, embracing a stance of nonjudgmental observation.

2. Mindful Communication: Practice mindful listening and speaking. Give your full attention to the person you are conversing with, without distractions or preconceived notions. Cultivate empathy and compassion in your interactions.

3. Gratitude Practice: Cultivate gratitude by regularly acknowledging and appreciating the positive aspects of your life. Take a few moments each day to reflect on things you are grateful for, whether big or small.

4. Mindful Multitasking: Avoid multitasking and focus on one task at a time. Give your full attention to the task at hand, whether it's working on a project, cooking a meal, or spending time with loved ones.

Mindfulness and Resilience: A Personal Account

Sarah, a high-achieving college student, found herself overwhelmed and stressed during exam season. She decided to incorporate mindfulness into her daily routine to build resilience. Sarah started by dedicating a few minutes each morning to meditation, focusing on her breath and observing her thoughts without judgment. Throughout the day, she practiced mindful breathing exercises to regain focus and reduce stress. Sarah also noticed how adopting a nonjudgmental attitude helped her manage her perfectionism and embrace self-compassion. By integrating mindfulness into her life, Sarah developed the resilience to overcome challenges and maintain her mental well-being.

In conclusion, building resilience through mindfulness and acceptance is a powerful strategy for promoting mental well-being and thriving in the face of adversity. Mindfulness practices help individuals develop awareness, emotional regulation, cognitive flexibility, and self-compassion - all essential components of resilience. By incorporating mindfulness into daily life, individuals can cultivate a mindset that supports their ability to bounce back from setbacks and embrace a sustainable mental health future.

Cultivating a Growth Mindset for Resilience

In order to build resilience, it is important to develop a growth mindset. A growth mindset is the belief that abilities and intelligence can be developed through dedication, hard work, and learning from failures and setbacks. This mindset allows individuals to view challenges as opportunities for growth and to persist in the face of adversity. Cultivating a growth mindset can help individuals bounce back from difficult experiences and develop the skills needed to navigate the ups and downs of life.

Understanding the Growth Mindset

The concept of the growth mindset was developed by psychologist Carol Dweck, who found that individuals with a growth mindset were more likely to embrace challenges and achieve their full potential. In contrast, individuals with a fixed mindset believe that their abilities are fixed and cannot be improved.

To cultivate a growth mindset, it is important to recognize the power of effort and resilience. This means acknowledging that setbacks and failures are normal parts of the learning and growth process. By understanding that one's abilities can be developed through practice and learning, individuals can approach challenges with a sense of optimism and curiosity.

Embracing the Learning Process

A growth mindset involves shifting the focus from seeking validation and avoiding failure to embracing the learning process. Instead of viewing failure as a personal flaw or a sign of incompetence, individuals with a growth mindset see it as an opportunity to learn and improve.

In order to embrace the learning process, it is important to set realistic goals and to break them down into smaller, manageable steps. This allows individuals to celebrate progress and stay motivated. Additionally, seeking feedback from mentors, peers, or trusted individuals can provide valuable insights and perspectives that can contribute to personal growth.

Emphasizing Effort and Persistence

Effort and persistence are key components of a growth mindset. Recognizing that success is not solely dependent on innate talents or abilities, but rather on dedication and hard work, can empower individuals to persevere in the face of challenges.

To develop a growth mindset, it is important to focus on the process rather than the outcome. By valuing effort and persisting in the face of obstacles, individuals can build resilience and develop the skills necessary to overcome future challenges. It is also crucial to develop healthy coping mechanisms to manage stress and maintain motivation.

Developing a Positive Self-Image

A growth mindset involves cultivating a positive self-image by acknowledging one's strengths and potential for growth. This involves challenging self-limiting beliefs and reframing negative thoughts and self-talk.

Practicing self-compassion and self-acceptance is also important in developing a growth mindset. Treating oneself with kindness, understanding, and forgiveness fosters resilience and encourages personal growth. It is important to remember that setbacks and failures are not indicative of personal worth, but rather opportunities for learning and improvement.

Fostering a Supportive Environment

Creating a supportive environment is crucial in cultivating a growth mindset. Surrounding oneself with positive and encouraging individuals who support and believe in one's ability to grow and overcome challenges can significantly impact one's resilience.

Building strong social connections and seeking support from others can provide a sense of belonging and help individuals navigate difficult times. Additionally, providing support and encouragement to others fosters a collective sense of resilience and creates a mutually beneficial support network.

Incorporating a Growth Mindset into Daily Life

To truly cultivate a growth mindset, it is important to practice and integrate its principles into everyday life. Here are some practical strategies for incorporating a growth mindset:

1. Embrace challenges: Seek out challenges that push you out of your comfort zone and provide opportunities for growth.

2. View failures as learning opportunities: Instead of dwelling on failures, analyze what went wrong and identify ways to improve for the future.

3. Learn from feedback: Be open to receiving feedback and use it as a tool for personal growth and development.

4. Cultivate a positive self-talk: Replace negative self-talk with positive affirmations that promote growth and resilience.

5. Set realistic goals: Break down larger goals into smaller, achievable steps and celebrate progress along the way.

6. Foster curiosity and a love of learning: Approach new experiences with a sense of curiosity and embrace opportunities to learn and grow.

7. Surround yourself with positive influences: Seek out individuals who embody a growth mindset and can offer support and encouragement.

By incorporating these strategies into daily life, individuals can cultivate a growth mindset and enhance their resilience to overcome challenges and thrive in the face of adversity. Remember, resilience is a skill that can be developed and strengthened with practice and a positive mindset.

Promoting Resilience in Children and Adolescents

The Role of Education in Building Resilience

In building resilience, education plays a crucial role in equipping individuals with the knowledge and skills they need to navigate life's challenges. Education provides a foundation for personal growth, fosters emotional well-being, and promotes adaptive coping strategies. This section explores how education can contribute to building resilience and enhancing mental health.

Educating for Emotional Intelligence

Emotional intelligence, which encompasses the ability to understand and manage one's emotions and empathize with others, is a key component of resilience. Education can play a pivotal role in nurturing emotional intelligence. By incorporating emotional intelligence into the curriculum, educators can facilitate students' self-awareness, self-regulation, social skills, and empathy.

One effective approach is to integrate social-emotional learning (SEL) programs into educational settings. These programs provide students with opportunities to develop emotional intelligence by engaging in activities that promote self-reflection, empathy, and effective communication. Through SEL, students learn to recognize and regulate their emotions, solve problems, and build positive relationships with peers and adults.

Example: Implementing SEL in a Middle School At Middlefield Middle School, the principal and teachers have noticed an increase in student conflicts and a decline in academic performance. To address these issues, they decide to implement a social-emotional learning program.

The program includes regular classroom discussions on emotional self-awareness and regulation. Students are taught strategies to identify their emotions and express them in a healthy manner. They are also encouraged to empathize with their peers and understand different perspectives. In addition, the school invites mental health professionals to conduct workshops on stress management and coping skills.

After a few months of implementing the program, the school observes positive changes among the students. Conflict incidents decrease, and students report feeling more supported and understood. Academic performance improves as students are better able to manage their emotions and focus on their studies.

Promoting Problem-Solving Skills

Resilience is closely tied to problem-solving skills. Education can foster the development of effective problem-solving abilities, which are essential for overcoming challenges and setbacks. By teaching students how to approach problems analytically, think critically, and generate creative solutions, education empowers individuals to tackle adversity with confidence.

Problem-based learning (PBL) is an instructional approach that promotes problem-solving skills. In PBL, students are presented with real-world problems and tasked with finding solutions through research, collaboration, and critical thinking. This method not only enhances problem-solving abilities but also cultivates resilience by encouraging students to persevere through complex challenges.

Example: Problem-Based Learning in a High School Science Class In Mr. Anderson's high school science class, students are assigned a project to design a sustainable energy solution for their community. They must identify the energy needs of the community, research alternative energy sources, and propose a feasible solution.

Through this project, students encounter various obstacles, such as limited resources and conflicting opinions. However, they use problem-solving skills to overcome these challenges. They analyze data, evaluate the pros and cons of different energy sources, and collaborate with their peers to reach a consensus.

As they navigate the complexities of the project, students develop resilience. They learn from their mistakes, adapt their strategies, and persevere until they find a sustainable energy solution. This experience not only enhances their problem-solving skills but also equips them with the resilience needed to address future challenges.

Fostering a Growth Mindset

A growth mindset, the belief that intelligence and abilities can be developed through effort and perseverance, is closely linked to resilience. Education can foster a growth mindset by promoting a culture of continuous learning and emphasizing the value of effort and resilience.

Teachers can cultivate a growth mindset by providing constructive feedback that focuses on effort and improvement rather than just the final outcome. Encouraging students to take risks, embrace challenges, and learn from failures helps them develop resilience and a desire for self-improvement.

Example: Cultivating a Growth Mindset in a College Setting At Greenfield University, the psychology department aims to foster a growth mindset among its students. Professors utilize teaching methods that emphasize effort, perseverance, and the process of learning rather than solely focusing on grades.

In their feedback, professors highlight the progress students have made and provide specific suggestions for improvement. They encourage students to view challenges as opportunities for growth and guide them in setting achievable goals. Additionally, the department organizes workshops that explore the concepts of growth mindset and resilience, allowing students to reflect on their own mindset and learn strategies to foster resilience in their academic and personal lives.

Through these initiatives, students at Greenfield University become more resilient learners. They embrace challenges, persist in the face of setbacks, and ultimately achieve higher levels of academic success.

Conclusion

Education plays a vital role in building resilience by promoting emotional intelligence, problem-solving skills, and a growth mindset. By integrating these aspects into the educational system, we can equip individuals with the tools they need to navigate challenges and thrive in the face of adversity. Through targeted educational strategies, we can build a resilient society that values personal growth, supports well-being, and embraces the potential for transformative change.

Trauma-Informed Schools

Trauma-informed schools are educational institutions that recognize the impact of trauma on students' well-being and academic success. These schools create a safe and supportive environment that fosters healing, resilience, and positive development for students who have experienced trauma. In this section, we will explore the principles, strategies, and benefits of trauma-informed schools.

Understanding Trauma

Before delving into the concept of trauma-informed schools, it is crucial to have a clear understanding of trauma itself. Trauma refers to an overwhelming experience that exceeds a person's ability to cope and disrupts their sense of safety, trust, and control. It can result from a range of events, including abuse, neglect, violence, accidents, natural disasters, or prolonged exposure to stress.

Children and adolescents who have experienced trauma may exhibit a variety of behavioral, emotional, and physiological responses. These can include difficulties with self-regulation, hyperarousal, hypervigilance, dissociation, emotional dysregulation, impaired concentration, and problems with interpersonal relationships. These challenges can significantly impact their ability to learn and succeed in the classroom.

Principles of Trauma-Informed Schools

Trauma-informed schools are guided by essential principles that shape their approach to supporting students who have experienced trauma. These principles include:

1. Safety: Creating a physically and emotionally safe environment for all students is paramount. This includes establishing clear boundaries, predictable routines, and a culture of respect and trust.

2. Trustworthiness and Transparency: Schools should endeavor to build trusting relationships with students, parents, and staff. Transparent policies and practices help to foster a sense of safety, consistency, and dependability.

3. Collaboration and Empowerment: Collaboration among school staff, community partners, and families is crucial in understanding and addressing the

needs of traumatized students. Including student voice and choice empowers them and promotes a sense of control and self-efficacy.

4. Cultural, Historical, and Gender Sensitivity: Trauma-informed schools recognize the diversity of experiences that students bring to the classroom. They strive to be sensitive to cultural, historical, and gender differences and ensure that their practices are inclusive and equitable.

Strategies for Trauma-Informed Schools

Implementing trauma-informed practices requires a multi-tiered approach that addresses the needs of all students. Here are some strategies that trauma-informed schools can use:

1. Trauma-Sensitive Classroom Practices: Teachers can create a trauma-sensitive classroom environment by establishing predictable routines, using calming techniques, providing choices, and using positive behavior management strategies. They can also integrate trauma-informed curricula that promote social-emotional learning, self-regulation, and resilience.

2. Staff Training and Professional Development: School staff should receive comprehensive training on trauma-informed practices, including understanding trauma's impact, recognizing trauma symptoms, responding compassionately, and implementing trauma-informed strategies in the classroom.

3. Mental Health and Counseling Services: Trauma-informed schools provide access to mental health professionals who can provide individual and group therapy, trauma-focused interventions, and crisis support. Collaborating with community mental health agencies can also enhance the availability of specialized services.

4. Family and Community Engagement: Engaging families and the broader community is essential for creating a trauma-responsive school environment. Schools can involve parents in decision-making, offer family education programs, and establish partnerships with community organizations that support children and families affected by trauma.

Benefits of Trauma-Informed Schools

Implementing trauma-informed practices in schools has numerous benefits for students, staff, and the overall school community. Some of the key benefits include:

1. Improved Academic Outcomes: When students' emotional and psychological needs are addressed, they are more likely to feel safe, engaged, and ready to learn. This often leads to improved academic performance, attendance, and graduation rates.

2. Enhanced Social-Emotional Development: Trauma-informed schools help students develop effective coping strategies, emotional regulation skills, and healthy relationship patterns. This fosters resilience, self-confidence, empathy, and positive self-image.

3. Reduced Behavioral Issues: By understanding and responding to the underlying causes of behavioral issues related to trauma, schools can help reduce disciplinary actions, suspensions, and expulsions. This contributes to a more positive and inclusive school climate.

4. Strengthened School-Home Connections: Trauma-informed schools prioritize collaboration and communication with families. This partnership promotes greater family engagement in students' education, leading to increased parental involvement, support, and shared decision-making.

Case Study: XYZ School District

To illustrate the impact of trauma-informed schools, let's explore the case of the XYZ School District. This district serves a diverse population, including many students who have experienced trauma due to community violence and family instability.

In response to the high levels of trauma affecting students, the XYZ School District implemented a district-wide trauma-informed approach. They focused on training teachers and staff in trauma-informed practices, including trauma-sensitive classroom strategies, understanding student triggers, and providing appropriate support.

As a result of their efforts, the district saw a significant decrease in disciplinary incidents and suspensions. Teachers reported improved student engagement and emotional well-being, resulting in greater participation and academic achievement. Family involvement also increased, with parents feeling more supported and included in their child's education.

The success of the XYZ School District serves as an inspiring example of how trauma-informed schools can transform not only individual students' lives but also the overall school community.

Conclusion

Trauma-informed schools play a vital role in promoting healing, resilience, and positive development for students who have experienced trauma. By implementing trauma-informed principles and strategies, schools create an environment where students feel safe, supported, and empowered to succeed academically and emotionally.

Through fostering a culture of trust, collaboration, and cultural sensitivity, trauma-informed schools can address the diverse needs of their students and provide the necessary support for their well-being. By investing in trauma-informed practices, schools can contribute to a sustainable future where all students have the opportunity to thrive.

Early Intervention for At-Risk Youth

Early intervention plays a crucial role in addressing the mental health needs of at-risk youth. By identifying and addressing mental health challenges early on, we can prevent these difficulties from exacerbating and have a significant positive impact on the long-term well-being of young individuals. This section will explore the importance of early intervention, the strategies employed, and the potential benefits it brings.

Understanding At-Risk Youth

Before delving into early intervention strategies, let us first understand who at-risk youth are. At-risk youth refers to individuals who face various factors that increase their vulnerability to mental health issues, substance abuse, and other negative outcomes. These factors may include socioeconomic disadvantage, family dysfunction, exposure to violence, peer pressure, and academic difficulties.

It is essential to recognize that at-risk youth are not a homogeneous group, and each individual has unique needs and circumstances. Therefore, early intervention must be tailored to address the specific challenges faced by each young person.

The Importance of Early Intervention

Early intervention aims to identify mental health concerns in young individuals as early as possible and provide appropriate support and resources. Here are some reasons why early intervention is crucial for at-risk youth:

1. **Preventing escalation of problems**: By intervening early, we can prevent mild mental health issues from escalating into more severe disorders. Adolescence is a critical period when mental health problems often emerge, and addressing them promptly can lead to better outcomes.

2. **Reducing impact on development**: Mental health challenges can have a significant impact on a young person's development, including their academic

performance, relationships, and overall well-being. Early intervention helps minimize these negative effects and supports healthy development.

3. **Promoting resilience:** Early intervention programs often focus on building resilience in at-risk youth. Resilience is the ability to navigate challenges and bounce back from adversity. By equipping young individuals with coping skills and support networks, we can enhance their resilience and empower them to overcome future challenges.

4. **Improving long-term outcomes:** Studies have shown that early intervention is associated with improved long-term outcomes, including mental health, educational attainment, and employment prospects. By addressing mental health challenges early, we can set young individuals on a positive trajectory for their future.

Strategies for Early Intervention

Effective early intervention for at-risk youth involves a multi-dimensional approach, incorporating various strategies and professionals. Here are some key strategies employed in early intervention programs:

1. **Screening and assessment:** Regular mental health screening and assessment help identify at-risk youth who may require intervention. Screening tools, such as questionnaires and interviews, are used to assess mental health symptoms and risk factors.

2. **Collaborative and integrated care:** Early intervention programs often involve collaboration among different professionals, including mental health providers, educators, and social workers. This integrated approach ensures a holistic and comprehensive assessment of a young person's needs and facilitates coordination of care.

3. **Evidence-based interventions:** Early intervention strategies are grounded in evidence-based practices that have demonstrated positive outcomes for at-risk youth. These may include cognitive-behavioral therapy, social-emotional learning programs, family therapy, and peer support groups.

4. **Family involvement:** Engaging and involving families in early intervention is crucial. Family support and involvement can contribute significantly to the success of interventions and serve as a protective factor for at-risk youth.

5. **Education and skill-building:** Early intervention programs often include educational components aimed at equipping at-risk youth with essential life skills, such as problem-solving, emotional regulation, and communication skills.

6. **Community engagement:** Collaborating with community organizations, such as youth centers, schools, and recreational programs, helps create a supportive

environment for at-risk youth. These partnerships provide additional resources and opportunities for young individuals to thrive.

Real-World Example: School-Based Early Intervention Program

One example of an early intervention program for at-risk youth is a school-based initiative that focuses on promoting mental health and well-being. This program involves the following components:

1. **Mental health screening:** Students are screened using validated tools to identify those at risk of mental health problems.

2. **Counseling services:** School counselors or mental health professionals provide individual and group counseling sessions to address specific mental health concerns.

3. **Psychoeducation:** Students participate in workshops and activities that aim to increase their awareness of mental health and provide them with skills to manage stress, build resilience, and seek help when needed.

4. **Parent involvement:** The program encourages parents to participate in workshops and engage in open discussions about mental health. This involvement helps create a supportive home environment for at-risk youth.

5. **Collaboration with community resources:** The program establishes partnerships with local mental health agencies, ensuring seamless referrals and access to specialized care when necessary.

Evaluation of the program shows that it has led to improved mental health outcomes, reduced behavioral issues, and increased school engagement among at-risk youth.

Caveats and Future Directions

While early intervention for at-risk youth is beneficial, some challenges and caveats should be acknowledged:

1. **Accessibility and equity:** Ensuring equal access to early intervention programs, regardless of socio-economic status or geographical location, is essential. Efforts should be made to reduce barriers and disparities in accessing care.

2. **Cultural sensitivity:** Early intervention programs need to be culturally sensitive and responsive to the diverse needs of at-risk youth. Recognizing and respecting different cultural backgrounds helps create a safe and inclusive environment for all.

3. **Sustainability**: Early intervention programs require sustainable funding and resources to maintain their impact over the long term. Advocacy for investment in early intervention is crucial for the continuous support of at-risk youth.

In conclusion, early intervention plays a pivotal role in addressing the mental health needs of at-risk youth. By implementing comprehensive strategies, involving multiple stakeholders, and focusing on evidence-based practices, we can make a significant positive difference in the lives of young individuals. By investing in early intervention, we create a foundation for a healthy and resilient future generation.

Youth Empowerment and Resilience Programs

Youth empowerment and resilience programs play a crucial role in promoting the mental health and well-being of young individuals. These programs aim to enhance their ability to cope with challenges, develop strong personal skills, and cultivate a sense of purpose and self-confidence. By empowering young people, we can contribute to their overall resilience and help them navigate the complex and demanding world they live in.

Understanding Youth Empowerment

Youth empowerment refers to the process of enabling young individuals to take control of their lives, make informed decisions, and actively participate in their communities. It involves promoting their self-esteem, self-efficacy, and self-determination. Empowering youth means recognizing their unique perspectives, strengths, and potential, and providing them with the resources and opportunities they need to thrive.

Resilience Building Programs

Resilience building programs aim to equip young people with the necessary skills and strategies to bounce back from adversity and overcome challenges. These programs foster the development of protective factors that enhance resilience, such as positive coping mechanisms, problem-solving abilities, and social support networks. Here are some key components of successful resilience building programs for youth:

Strengthening Protective Factors Resilience building programs focus on enhancing protective factors that contribute to young people's ability to adapt and thrive in the face of adversity. This includes fostering positive relationships with caring adults, promoting healthy self-esteem, cultivating effective communication skills, and developing problem-solving abilities.

Promoting Emotional Regulation Emotional regulation skills play a significant role in resilience. Youth empowerment programs emphasize teaching young individuals how to identify and understand their emotions, manage stress and anxiety, and cultivate emotional intelligence. This helps them develop the capacity to regulate their emotions effectively and cope with challenging situations.

Encouraging Goal Setting and Future Orientation Youth empowerment programs emphasize the importance of setting goals, both short-term and long-term, that are meaningful to young individuals. These programs encourage young people to envision a positive future, develop strategies to achieve their goals, and cultivate a sense of purpose and direction in their lives. By promoting future orientation, they enhance resilience in facing obstacles and setbacks.

Building Social Support Networks Social support is crucial for young individuals' well-being and resilience. Youth empowerment programs emphasize the importance of building strong and positive social connections. These programs provide opportunities for young people to engage with peers, mentors, and community members who can serve as sources of support, guidance, and encouragement.

Developing Problem-Solving and Decision-Making Skills Resilience building programs encourage young individuals to develop effective problem-solving and decision-making skills. They help young people learn how to analyze situations, generate alternative solutions, make informed choices, and take responsibility for their actions. These skills empower young individuals to overcome challenges and navigate complex decision-making processes.

Examples of Youth Empowerment and Resilience Programs

There are several successful youth empowerment and resilience programs that have been implemented worldwide. Some notable examples include:

Youth Leadership Programs Youth leadership programs focus on developing leadership skills, fostering civic engagement, and empowering young people to become agents of positive change in their communities. These programs provide opportunities for young individuals to develop and practice leadership qualities, participate in community service initiatives, and engage in advocacy efforts.

Mentoring Programs Mentoring programs pair young individuals with adult mentors who provide guidance, support, and encouragement. These programs aim to enhance young people's self-esteem, academic achievement, and resilience by offering role models and meaningful relationships. Mentors serve as a source of support, offering guidance in decision-making, goal-setting, and life skills.

Arts and Creativity Programs Arts and creativity programs provide young individuals with opportunities for self-expression, personal growth, and skill development. These programs engage young people in activities such as visual arts, music, dance, and theater. The arts have been shown to promote resilience, improve self-esteem, and foster emotional well-being.

Sports and Recreation Programs Sports and recreation programs offer young individuals an outlet for physical activity, teamwork, and skill-building. These programs promote physical and mental well-being, teach resilience through competition, and provide opportunities for personal growth and social interaction.

Youth Empowerment and Resilience Programs: A Holistic Approach

Effective youth empowerment and resilience programs take a holistic approach by considering the unique needs, strengths, and circumstances of young individuals. These programs recognize the interconnectedness of various aspects of young people's lives, including their mental, emotional, physical, and social well-being. Here are some key principles that guide holistic youth empowerment and resilience programs:

Collaborative Approach Successful programs involve collaboration between young individuals, families, schools, community organizations, and other stakeholders. This collaborative approach ensures that young people receive comprehensive support and resources from multiple sources.

Strengths-Based Approach Holistic programs focus on identifying and building on the strengths and potential of young individuals rather than solely focusing on deficits or challenges. This approach enhances self-esteem, self-efficacy, and resilience by recognizing and reinforcing young people's capabilities.

Culturally Responsive Practices Youth empowerment programs need to be culturally responsive, recognizing and respecting the diverse backgrounds and experiences of young individuals. This involves incorporating cultural traditions, values, and perspectives into program design and delivery, ensuring relevance and inclusivity.

Individualized Support Holistic programs recognize that young individuals have unique needs and require individualized support. They provide tailored interventions, assessments, and resources based on the specific strengths, challenges, and circumstances of each young person.

Challenges and Future Directions

While youth empowerment and resilience programs have shown promising outcomes, there are several challenges and opportunities for future development:

Sustainability and Long-Term Impact Ensuring the long-term sustainability and impact of youth empowerment and resilience programs is crucial. It requires ongoing funding, evaluation, and research to understand the effectiveness of different program components and adapt them as needed.

Addressing Systemic Barriers To maximize the impact of youth empowerment programs, it is essential to address systemic barriers that hinder young individuals' opportunities and well-being. This includes addressing social inequalities, promoting inclusivity, and advocating for policy changes that support youth development.

Harnessing Technology The use of technology can enhance the reach and effectiveness of youth empowerment and resilience programs. Online platforms, mobile applications, and virtual spaces can provide accessible resources, support networks, and educational opportunities for young individuals.

Youth Participation and Agency Youth empowerment programs should actively involve young individuals in program development, implementation, and evaluation. Empowering young people to contribute their perspectives, ideas, and leadership ensures that programs are relevant, engaging, and effective.

Conclusion

Youth empowerment and resilience programs offer valuable opportunities for young individuals to develop the skills, strengths, and resources needed to navigate the challenges of life. By promoting empowerment and resilience, these programs contribute to the overall well-being and mental health of young people. It is important to continue investing in these programs and adapting them to the evolving needs of youth in order to build a sustainable mental health future.

Resilience in Adulthood

Enhancing Psychological Wellbeing in Adulthood

Psychological wellbeing is essential for leading a fulfilling and meaningful life. As individuals transition into adulthood, they often face unique challenges and responsibilities that can impact their mental health. However, there are various strategies and practices that can enhance psychological wellbeing and promote overall mental wellness in adulthood.

Understanding the Challenges of Adulthood

Adulthood is a time of significant changes and transitions, which can pose challenges to psychological wellbeing. Some of the common challenges individuals may face include:

1. Career Pressure: The pursuit of a meaningful career and financial stability can be demanding and stressful. Job-related stressors, such as long working hours, excessive workload, or lack of job satisfaction, can take a toll on psychological wellbeing.

2. Relationship Issues: Maintaining healthy relationships with romantic partners, family members, and friends can be challenging. Conflicts and difficulties in relationships can impact mental health and overall wellbeing.

3. Parenting Responsibilities: For individuals with children, the demands of parenting can be overwhelming and can contribute to feelings of stress, anxiety, and self-doubt.

4. Aging and Life Transitions: As individuals age, they may face changes in physical health, cognitive abilities, and social roles. Navigating through midlife and preparing for retirement can also be challenging.

5. Balancing Multiple Roles: Many adults find themselves juggling multiple roles such as being a parent, career professional, spouse, and caregiver. Striking a balance between these different roles can be stressful.

6. Financial Pressures: Managing financial obligations, such as paying bills, managing debts, and planning for the future, can cause significant stress and anxiety in adulthood.

Understanding these challenges is crucial for developing effective strategies to enhance psychological wellbeing in adulthood.

Building Psychological Resilience

Psychological resilience refers to the ability to adapt and bounce back from adversity, and it plays a vital role in promoting wellbeing in adulthood. Here are some practical strategies for building psychological resilience:

- Developing a Growth Mindset: Cultivating a belief in personal growth and the ability to learn from challenges can enhance resilience. Embracing failures as opportunities for learning and personal development can help individuals navigate through difficult times.

- Building Strong Support Systems: Maintaining healthy relationships and social connections is crucial for psychological wellbeing. Building a support network of friends, family, and peers can provide emotional support, guidance, and help individuals cope with stressors.

- Practicing Self-Care: Engaging in self-care activities is essential for promoting psychological wellbeing. Prioritizing activities such as exercise, adequate sleep, healthy eating, and relaxation techniques can help manage stress and enhance resilience.

- Developing Problem-Solving Skills: Enhancing problem-solving abilities can empower individuals to navigate challenges effectively. This involves identifying problems, generating and evaluating potential solutions, and taking action to address them.

- Cultivating Emotional Intelligence: Emotional intelligence involves being aware of and managing one's emotions and understanding the emotions of others. Developing emotional intelligence can enhance resilience by helping individuals cope with stress, manage conflicts, and build strong relationships.

By implementing these strategies, individuals can strengthen their psychological resilience and better cope with the challenges of adulthood.

Managing Stress and Practicing Mindfulness

Stress is a common experience in adulthood and, if left unchecked, can negatively impact psychological wellbeing. Managing stress is crucial for maintaining optimal mental health. Here are some effective stress management techniques:

- Practicing Mindfulness: Mindfulness involves paying attention to the present moment without judgment. Regular mindfulness practice has been shown to reduce stress, improve emotional regulation, and enhance overall wellbeing. Techniques such as meditation, deep breathing exercises, and body scan meditation can all promote mindfulness.

- Engaging in Relaxation Techniques: Activities such as deep breathing exercises, progressive muscle relaxation, and guided imagery can induce a relaxation response in the body, helping to reduce stress and promote a sense of calmness.

- Time Management: Effective time management can help individuals prioritize responsibilities, allocate time for self-care activities, and reduce feelings of being overwhelmed. Setting realistic goals, breaking tasks into smaller manageable parts, and delegating when necessary are important time management strategies.

- Engaging in Stress-Relieving Activities: Engaging in hobbies, creative outlets, and leisure activities can help individuals relax and reduce stress. Activities such as painting, gardening, playing a musical instrument, or engaging in sports can provide a welcome distraction and promote psychological wellbeing.

By incorporating these techniques into daily life, individuals can effectively manage stress and enhance psychological wellbeing.

Seeking Professional Support

While self-help strategies are beneficial, there are times when seeking professional support is essential for enhancing psychological wellbeing in adulthood. Mental health professionals, such as psychologists, therapists, or counselors, can provide guidance and support in navigating the challenges of adulthood. Some circumstances where seeking professional help is recommended include:

- Persistent Feelings of Sadness or Anxiety: If feelings of depression or anxiety persist for an extended period and interfere with daily functioning, it is crucial to seek professional help for assessment and treatment.

- Relationship Issues: When relationship difficulties persist and impact psychological wellbeing, couples therapy or individual counseling can provide tools and support for improving relationships.

- Work-related Stress: If work-related stress becomes overwhelming and affects mental health, seeking counseling or consulting with a career coach can help explore strategies for managing stress and finding job satisfaction.

- Major Life Transitions: Significant life transitions, such as divorce, loss of a loved one, or retirement, may necessitate the support of a mental health professional to navigate through the associated emotional challenges.

Professional support can provide the necessary tools, interventions, and coping strategies tailored to individual needs, ultimately enhancing psychological wellbeing in adulthood.

Conclusion

Enhancing psychological wellbeing in adulthood is a multifaceted process that requires a combination of self-help strategies and professional support. By building psychological resilience, managing stress, practicing mindfulness, and seeking professional help when needed, individuals can promote their mental health and overall wellbeing. Developing a proactive approach to psychological wellbeing empowers individuals to navigate the challenges of adulthood and cultivate a fulfilling and sustainable life. It is important to remember that every individual's journey toward psychological wellbeing is unique, and what works for one person may not work for another. Experimentation, self-reflection, and ongoing learning are key to finding effective strategies for enhancing psychological wellbeing in adulthood.

Coping with Life Transitions and Loss

Life is full of transitions and losses, and navigating through these experiences can be challenging and overwhelming. Coping with life transitions and loss requires resilience and a set of strategies to help individuals adapt and cope effectively. In this section, we will explore different coping mechanisms that can support individuals during life transitions and help them navigate the process of grieving and healing after experiencing loss.

Understanding Life Transitions

Life transitions are significant changes that individuals experience in various domains of life, such as education, career, relationships, parenthood, and aging. These transitions can be both planned, such as transitioning from school to the workforce, and unplanned, such as loss of a job or a sudden illness. Transition periods often involve a shift in roles, identities, routines, and expectations, which can be disruptive and cause stress.

To effectively cope with life transitions, individuals need to have a clear understanding of the change they are going through. This includes acknowledging the emotions and uncertainties that accompany the transition and recognizing the potential challenges that may arise. By understanding the transition process, individuals can better prepare themselves and develop coping strategies to navigate through the changes.

Grieving and Healing after Loss

Loss is an inevitable part of life, and individuals may experience various types of losses, including the death of a loved one, the end of a relationship, loss of a job or financial security, or the loss of physical or mental abilities. Coping with loss requires time and understanding, as it involves a grieving process that individuals go through to heal and come to terms with the emotional impact of the loss.

The grieving process is unique to each individual, but it typically involves different stages, including denial, anger, bargaining, depression, and acceptance. It is important to note that not everyone goes through all these stages, and the process may not follow a linear progression. However, understanding and acknowledging the emotions associated with grief can help individuals navigate through the healing process.

Coping with grief involves various strategies that support emotional healing and recovery. Some of these strategies include:

- **Seeking support:** Sharing feelings and experiences with trusted friends, family members, or support groups can provide comfort and validation during the grieving process. Support from others helps individuals feel understood and less isolated in their grief.

- **Self-care:** Taking care of physical and emotional well-being is crucial during the healing process. Engaging in activities that promote self-care, such as exercise, proper nutrition, and getting enough sleep, can help individuals cope with grief more effectively.

- **Expressing emotions:** Finding healthy ways to express emotions, such as through journaling, art, or music, can provide an outlet for grief. Expressing emotions allows individuals to process their feelings and release them in a constructive manner.

- **Maintaining routines:** Establishing and maintaining routines can provide a sense of stability and normalcy during a period of upheaval. Routines can help individuals regain a sense of control and structure in their lives, which can be particularly beneficial when coping with loss.

- **Seeking professional help:** In some cases, grief may become overwhelming or prolonged, and individuals may benefit from seeking professional help. Therapists, counselors, or grief support specialists can provide guidance and support through the healing process.

It is important to note that grief is a highly individual and personal experience. Different individuals may find different coping strategies helpful, and it is essential to respect and honor each person's unique journey through grief.

Examples and Real-World Applications

To illustrate the process of coping with life transitions and loss, let's consider a real-life example. Sarah is a recent college graduate who had been looking forward to starting her dream job in a prestigious company. However, due to unforeseen circumstances, the company went bankrupt, and Sarah's job offer was rescinded.

Facing this unexpected life transition, Sarah experiences a mix of emotions, including shock, disappointment, and uncertainty about her future. To cope with this transition, Sarah engages in various coping strategies:

- **Seeking support:** Sarah reaches out to her close friends and family, sharing her feelings and seeking comfort and advice. She also joins a professional networking group to connect with others who may have similar experiences or insights into potential job opportunities.

- **Self-care:** Sarah prioritizes her physical and emotional well-being by engaging in regular exercise, practicing mindfulness, and engaging in activities she enjoys, such as painting and hiking.

- **Exploring opportunities:** Sarah takes this transition as an opportunity to explore other career paths and expand her skills through online courses and volunteer work. She attends career fairs and networking events to connect with potential employers in her field of interest.

- **Maintaining routines:** Sarah establishes a daily routine that includes job searching, professional development activities, self-care practices, and social interactions. This routine provides a sense of structure and purpose during the transition period.

- **Seeking professional help:** As Sarah continues to face difficulties in coping with the job loss, she decides to seek guidance from a career counselor who specializes in helping individuals navigate career transitions. The counselor provides her with strategies, resources, and emotional support to assist her in her job search and career development.

Through these coping strategies, Sarah is able to navigate the life transition, maintain a positive outlook, and eventually secure a job that aligns with her interests and goals.

Additional Resources and Exercises

To further explore coping with life transitions and loss, here are some resources and exercises that can support individuals in their journey:

- **Books:** "Transitions: Making Sense of Life's Changes" by William Bridges and "The Grief Recovery Handbook" by John W. James and Russell Friedman offer valuable insights and practical strategies for coping with life transitions and grief.

- **Journaling exercise:** Encourage individuals to keep a grief journal where they can express their thoughts, feelings, and reflections on their loss and the transition process. This exercise can help facilitate self-reflection and promote emotional healing.

- **Support group participation:** Provide information about local support groups or online communities where individuals can connect with others who have experienced similar life transitions or losses. Participating in support groups allows individuals to share experiences, gain support, and learn coping strategies from others.

- **Self-reflection questions:** Encourage individuals to reflect on their own coping strategies and identify which ones have been most effective for them. Ask questions such as: What coping strategies have you found helpful when facing life transitions or losses? How can you incorporate these strategies into your daily life?

By engaging with these resources and exercises, individuals can deepen their understanding of coping with life transitions and loss, discover new strategies, and enhance their resilience in the face of adversity.

Conclusion

Coping with life transitions and loss is a challenging but necessary process for personal growth and development. By understanding the nature of life transitions, acknowledging the emotions associated with grief, and employing effective coping strategies, individuals can navigate through these experiences with resilience and find a path towards healing and growth. It is crucial to remember that each person's journey is unique, and support from loved ones, professionals, and communities can play a significant role in facilitating the healing process.

Promoting Work-Life Balance for Resilience

Work-life balance is a key component of promoting resilience and maintaining good mental health. In today's fast-paced and demanding world, many individuals struggle to find a balance between their professional obligations and personal lives. This section explores the importance of work-life balance, its impact on mental health, and strategies for promoting and achieving this balance.

Understanding Work-Life Balance

Work-life balance refers to the equilibrium between work-related activities and personal life domains, such as family, leisure, and self-care. Achieving work-life balance involves effectively managing time, energy, and attention to ensure that both work and personal life are adequately addressed.

While work is an essential aspect of life and can provide fulfillment, excessive work demands and long hours can lead to chronic stress, burnout, and other mental health issues. On the other hand, neglecting personal life can lead to a sense of emptiness, strained relationships, and decreased overall life satisfaction. Thus, maintaining a healthy work-life balance is crucial for the well-being of individuals.

The Impact of Work-Life Imbalance on Mental Health

When work-life balance is compromised, individuals are more susceptible to mental health problems. The excessive demands from work can lead to chronic stress, anxiety, and depression. High levels of stress can affect sleep patterns, increase irritability, and impair cognitive functioning.

Moreover, work-life imbalance can negatively impact personal relationships, leading to conflicts and reduced social support. This lack of social support can further contribute to feelings of loneliness and isolation, which can exacerbate mental health issues.

Strategies for Promoting Work-Life Balance

Promoting work-life balance requires a comprehensive approach that addresses both individual behaviors and organizational practices. Here are some strategies that can be employed to achieve a better work-life balance:

- **Setting boundaries:** Establish clear boundaries between work and personal life. This includes defining specific periods for work, leisure, and family time. Avoid checking work emails or taking calls outside of designated work hours.

- **Time management:** Develop effective time management skills to prioritize tasks and allocate time for different aspects of life. Use techniques such as to-do lists, calendars, and prioritization methods to ensure that work and personal obligations are balanced.

- **Flexible work arrangements:** Advocate for flexible work arrangements, such as remote work, compressed workweeks, or flexible hours. These arrangements empower individuals to have more control over their schedules and allow for better integration of work and personal life.

- **Promoting self-care:** Prioritize self-care activities, such as regular exercise, adequate sleep, and engaging in hobbies or leisure activities. Taking care of physical and mental well-being is essential for maintaining resilience and work-life balance.

- **Effective communication:** Communicate openly and assertively with supervisors, colleagues, and family members about work-life balance needs and expectations. Clear communication can help in negotiating realistic workloads and setting boundaries.

- **Supportive organizational culture:** Encourage employers to foster a supportive organizational culture that values work-life balance. This includes promoting policies such as parental leave, flexible work arrangements, and employee assistance programs. Organizations can also provide resources and training on stress management and work-life balance.

- **Disconnecting from technology:** Limit the use of technology outside of work hours to create boundaries between work and personal life. Designate technology-free periods or areas in the home to foster relaxation and rejuvenation.

Case Study: The Benefits of Work-Life Balance Programs

ABC Corporation, a multinational company, implemented a series of work-life balance programs to enhance employee well-being and productivity. These programs included flexible work arrangements, an on-site daycare center, and a wellness program.

After the implementation of these programs, the company observed several positive outcomes. Employee satisfaction increased, as individuals felt greater autonomy and control over their work schedules. Absenteeism rates decreased, and employee retention improved significantly. The wellness program also led to a reduction in stress-related illnesses and improved mental health outcomes.

This case study highlights the importance of organizations prioritizing work-life balance initiatives. By investing in such programs, employers can create a culture that supports employee well-being, productivity, and resilience.

Conclusion

Promoting work-life balance is vital for maintaining good mental health and building resilience. By implementing strategies such as setting boundaries, time management, flexible work arrangements, and promoting self-care, individuals can achieve a better balance between their work and personal lives. Supportive organizational cultures and policies are also crucial in fostering work-life balance. Ultimately, creating a sustainable future requires prioritizing work-life balance and recognizing its significant impact on overall well-being.

Cultivating Resilience in Midlife and Aging Adults

As individuals transition into midlife and older adulthood, they often face unique challenges that can impact their mental health and overall well-being. This section explores strategies and interventions that can help cultivate resilience in midlife and aging adults, enabling them to navigate these challenges and maintain their mental well-being.

Understanding the Challenges of Midlife and Aging

Midlife is a stage characterized by significant life changes, such as career shifts, empty nest syndrome, and the loss of loved ones. These transitions can lead to feelings of loss, grief, and a sense of purposelessness. Aging adults, on the other hand, may grapple with age-related physical and cognitive changes, chronic health conditions, and social isolation.

1. **Maintaining physical health:** Aging adults can cultivate resilience by prioritizing their physical health. Regular exercise, a nutritious diet, and adequate sleep contribute to a strong foundation for overall well-being. Encouraging the adoption of healthy lifestyle habits can help individuals maintain physical resilience and reduce the risk of chronic diseases.

2. **Supporting cognitive well-being:** Brain health plays a crucial role in resilience during aging. Engaging in mentally stimulating activities, such as puzzles, reading, or learning new skills, can support cognitive function and enhance resilience. Additionally, staying socially connected and maintaining strong social networks can provide cognitive stimulation and emotional support.

3. **Addressing emotional well-being:** Emotional resilience is vital for navigating the challenges of midlife and aging. This includes maintaining positive mental health, managing stress and anxiety, and seeking support when needed. Encouraging open conversations about mental health and promoting access to mental health resources can help individuals build emotional resilience.

Promoting Social Connections and Community Involvement

Social isolation is a common issue faced by midlife and older adults, which can negatively impact mental health and resilience. Building and maintaining social connections is crucial for fostering resilience during aging.

1. **Building supportive relationships:** Encouraging midlife and aging adults to invest in their relationships and actively seek out social connections can have a significant impact on their mental well-being. This can involve joining community groups, volunteering, participating in group activities, or seeking out support from family and friends.

2. **Creating intergenerational programs:** Building bridges between different generations can provide a sense of purpose and social connection. Intergenerational

programs, where younger and older individuals interact and learn from each other, can promote mutual understanding, combat ageism, and foster resilience.

3. **Engaging in community involvement:** Active participation in the community can enhance resilience by fostering a sense of belonging and purpose. Older adults can contribute their skills, knowledge, and experiences through mentoring programs, volunteering in local organizations, or engaging in advocacy work.

Promoting Mental Health Literacy and Seeking Help

Midlife and aging adults may hesitate to seek help for mental health concerns due to stigma or a lack of awareness. Promoting mental health literacy can empower individuals to recognize the signs of mental distress and take appropriate action.

1. **Educating about mental health:** Providing accurate information about common mental health conditions, their symptoms, and available treatments can help reduce the stigma and increase awareness. This can be done through community workshops, informational campaigns, or educational materials targeted towards midlife and aging adults.

2. **Accessible mental health services:** Ensuring that mental health services are accessible and tailored to the needs of midlife and older adults is crucial. This includes providing age-appropriate care, training mental health professionals in geriatric mental health, and increasing the availability of mental health resources in community settings.

3. **Supportive interventions:** Implementing evidence-based interventions can help individuals develop coping skills and enhance their resilience. Cognitive-behavioral therapy, mindfulness-based interventions, and support groups specifically designed for midlife and aging adults can be effective in addressing mental health challenges and promoting resilience.

Creating Meaningful Lifestyles and Engaging in Meaningful Activities

Finding purpose and meaning in life is essential for resilience in midlife and aging adults. Encouraging the pursuit of meaningful activities can enhance a sense of identity, achievement, and overall well-being.

1. **Retirement planning and engagement:** Retirement can be a significant life transition, and its impact on mental health and resilience should not be overlooked. Supporting midlife individuals in planning for retirement, exploring new interests, or engaging in part-time work can help maintain a sense of purpose and social connection.

2. **Lifelong learning and personal growth:** Encouraging midlife and aging adults to continue learning and pursuing personal growth can foster resilience. This can involve taking educational courses, engaging in hobbies or creative pursuits, or participating in workshops that promote personal development.

3. **Volunteer work and civic engagement:** Engaging in volunteer work or community-based activities can provide a sense of purpose and contribute to the well-being of others. This can include mentoring, participating in community service projects, or joining advocacy organizations focused on issues relevant to midlife and older adults.

In conclusion, cultivating resilience in midlife and aging adults requires a holistic approach that addresses physical, cognitive, emotional, and social well-being. By promoting social connections, fostering mental health literacy, and facilitating meaningful engagement, individuals can navigate the challenges of aging with strength and resilience. It is essential to recognize that resilience can be developed and nurtured throughout life, and supporting midlife and aging adults in cultivating resilience contributes to their overall sustainability and well-being.

Resilience and Aging

Aging and Mental Health

As individuals age, they are at an increased risk for experiencing mental health challenges. Aging is a complex process that can affect various aspects of mental well-being, including cognitive functioning, emotional regulation, and social interactions. In this section, we will explore the relationship between aging and mental health, and discuss strategies for enhancing resilience and promoting mental well-being among older adults.

The Impact of Aging on Mental Health

Aging is often accompanied by changes in physical health, functional abilities, and social roles, which can contribute to the development of mental health disorders. Common mental health challenges in older adults include depression, anxiety, dementia, and substance abuse. These conditions can significantly impact the quality of life and overall well-being of older individuals, as well as their families and caregivers.

One of the major factors influencing mental health in older adults is the presence of chronic medical conditions. Conditions such as cardiovascular disease, diabetes, arthritis, and stroke can increase the risk of developing mental health disorders. The burden of managing these conditions, combined with the physical limitations they impose, can contribute to feelings of frustration, helplessness, and depression.

Additionally, cognitive decline is a common concern in older adults. Mild cognitive impairment (MCI) and dementia, including Alzheimer's disease, can significantly impact memory, thinking, and decision-making abilities. These cognitive changes can lead to increased anxiety, depression, and social isolation among older individuals.

Social factors also play a crucial role in mental health during aging. Older adults may experience loss of loved ones, retirement, and decreased social interactions, which can lead to feelings of loneliness and isolation. The loss of social support networks and the disruption of meaningful activities can contribute to the development of mental health disorders.

Strategies for Enhancing Mental Health in Older Adults

1. Promoting Social Connections: Encouraging older adults to maintain social relationships and engage in community activities can help reduce isolation and loneliness. Community centers, senior organizations, and support groups provide opportunities for social interaction, meaningful engagement, and emotional support.

2. Holistic Healthcare: Integrating mental health services into primary care settings can improve access to mental health care for older adults. Collaborative care models that involve a team of healthcare professionals, including primary care physicians, psychologists, and social workers, can address the complex needs of older adults and ensure comprehensive support.

3. Cognitive Stimulation: Engaging in mentally stimulating activities, such as puzzles, reading, and learning new skills, can help maintain cognitive function and prevent cognitive decline. Participating in cognitive training programs and brain fitness exercises can be beneficial for older adults in preserving cognitive abilities.

4. Physical Activity: Regular exercise has been shown to have numerous benefits for mental health, including reducing symptoms of depression and anxiety. Encouraging older adults to engage in physical activities that they enjoy, such as walking, swimming, or dancing, can improve mood, cognitive function, and overall well-being.

5. Sleep Hygiene: Adequate sleep is essential for maintaining mental health. Older adults should establish a regular sleep routine, create a comfortable sleep environment, and practice relaxation techniques to promote restful sleep. Addressing sleep disorders, such as insomnia or sleep apnea, is crucial for optimizing mental health in older individuals.

6. Age-Friendly Environments: Creating age-friendly communities and environments that promote accessibility, safety, and social participation can support the mental well-being of older adults. Providing transportation services, accessible housing, and opportunities for community engagement can enhance the quality of life and reduce social isolation.

7. Caregiver Support: Recognizing the significant role of caregivers in the lives of older adults, it is important to provide support and resources to caregivers. Caregiver support groups, respite care services, and educational programs can help caregivers manage their own mental health and enhance their ability to provide care.

Case Study: Addressing Mental Health Challenges in an Aging Population

Consider the case of Mrs. Johnson, an 80-year-old woman living alone. Mrs. Johnson recently lost her husband, and she has been experiencing feelings of loneliness and sadness. She has also been struggling with managing chronic pain from arthritis, which has limited her mobility. As a result, Mrs. Johnson has become socially isolated, rarely leaving her home or engaging in activities she once enjoyed.

To address Mrs. Johnson's mental health challenges, a holistic approach is necessary. First, a collaborative care team consisting of her primary care physician, a mental health professional, and a social worker can assess her needs and develop a comprehensive care plan. This plan may include a combination of interventions such as medication management, cognitive-behavioral therapy for depression, and physical therapy for managing her pain.

The team can also connect Mrs. Johnson with local senior centers, support groups, and transportation services to help her re-engage in social activities. They can provide resources for home modifications to ensure her living environment is safe and accessible. Additionally, providing education and support to Mrs. Johnson's caregivers, such as her children or close friends, will help them better understand her needs and provide appropriate assistance.

By implementing this multidimensional approach, Mrs. Johnson's mental health can be improved, and her overall well-being can be enhanced. It is essential to address the physical, social, and psychological aspects of aging to promote mental health and resilience in older adults.

Conclusion

As the global population continues to age, it is imperative to prioritize mental health in older adults. Aging poses unique challenges for mental well-being, but by adopting a holistic approach that considers the physical, social, and psychological aspects of aging, we can enhance the mental health and quality of life of older individuals. By promoting social connections, ensuring access to comprehensive healthcare services, and addressing specific needs such as cognitive decline or sleep disorders, we can build resilience and support a sustainable mental health future for aging populations.

Chapter 4: Building Resilience for Overall Sustainability

4.9 Strategies for Enhancing Resilience in Older Adults

The aging process brings about various physical, cognitive, and psychosocial changes that can impact an individual's mental health and overall well-being. Older adults may face challenges such as chronic health conditions, loss of loved ones, social isolation, and declining cognitive function. However, resilience can play a crucial role in helping older adults navigate these challenges and maintain a positive outlook on life. In this section, we will discuss strategies for enhancing resilience in older adults.

Understanding Resilience in Older Adults

Resilience in older adults refers to their ability to adapt and bounce back from adversity, maintain a sense of purpose and meaning in life, and continue to thrive despite the challenges they face. It involves the ability to effectively cope with stress, maintain positive relationships, foster a sense of self-efficacy, and utilize available resources and support systems.

Promoting Physical Health

Physical health is closely linked to mental well-being and resilience in older adults. Encouraging regular exercise, healthy eating, and proper sleep can have a positive impact on their resilience. Physical activities such as walking, swimming, or yoga can improve mood, reduce stress, and increase overall physical fitness. A balanced diet rich in fruits, vegetables, whole grains, and lean proteins can provide the necessary nutrients for optimal brain function and emotional well-being. Sufficient sleep is also crucial for cognitive function, emotional regulation, and overall resilience.

Fostering Social Connections

Maintaining strong social connections is essential for promoting resilience in older adults. Loneliness and social isolation can have detrimental effects on mental health and overall well-being. Encouraging older adults to participate in social activities, join clubs or groups, and connect with their community can help reduce social isolation and foster a sense of belongingness. Additionally, maintaining close relationships with family and friends can provide emotional support during times of adversity.

Cultivating Emotional Well-being

Emotional well-being is an important aspect of resilience in older adults. Encouraging older adults to practice self-care, engage in positive self-talk, and express their emotions can contribute to their emotional well-being. Engaging in activities that bring joy and happiness, such as hobbies, creative pursuits, or volunteering, can also enhance emotional well-being and resilience. Providing emotional support and validation for the challenges they may face can help older adults build their emotional resilience.

Promoting Cognitive Stimulation

Engaging in cognitive activities can help older adults maintain cognitive function and enhance their resilience. Encouraging activities such as reading, puzzles, learning new skills, and engaging in stimulating conversations can promote brain health and cognitive resilience. Cognitive exercises can also help older adults build their problem-solving skills, adaptability, and mental flexibility, which are essential components of resilience.

Providing Supportive Care

Healthcare professionals and caregivers play a crucial role in promoting resilience in older adults. Providing supportive care involves ensuring access to quality healthcare, regular screenings for mental health conditions, and appropriate interventions when needed. It is important to create a safe and nurturing environment that recognizes and respects the individuality and autonomy of older adults. Additionally, providing the necessary information, resources, and support systems can help older adults navigate life's challenges and build their resilience.

Encouraging Life Review and Meaning-Making

Life review and meaning-making activities can help older adults reflect on their life experiences, derive a sense of meaning and purpose, and develop a positive outlook on life. Encouraging older adults to share their life stories, engage in reminiscence therapy, or participate in activities that promote self-reflection can support their resilience. Such activities can help older adults find a sense of meaning, develop a positive self-image, and understand the legacy they wish to leave behind.

Addressing Ageism and Challenging Stereotypes

Ageism and negative stereotypes about aging can have a detrimental impact on the resilience of older adults. It is essential to challenge ageist beliefs and promote positive attitudes towards aging. Educating society about the contributions and capabilities of older adults can help reduce ageism and create a more supportive and inclusive environment. Encouraging intergenerational interactions and promoting opportunities for older adults to engage in meaningful roles can foster a sense of purpose and enhance their resilience.

Integrating Technology

Technology can be a valuable tool for enhancing resilience in older adults. Teaching older adults how to utilize technology to connect with others, access information, and engage in cognitive activities can improve their overall resilience. Technology can facilitate social connection, provide mental stimulation, and enhance access to resources and support systems. However, it is important to ensure that older adults have access to user-friendly technology and receive appropriate training and support.

Conclusion

Enhancing resilience in older adults is crucial for promoting their mental health and overall well-being. By implementing strategies that focus on physical health, social connections, emotional well-being, cognitive stimulation, and supportive care, we can support older adults in navigating life's challenges and maintaining a positive outlook. Promoting resilience in older adults not only benefits them individually but also contributes to creating a more resilient and sustainable society.

CHAPTER 4: BUILDING RESILIENCE FOR OVERALL SUSTAINABILITY

The Role of Caregivers in Supporting Resilience

Caregivers play a crucial role in supporting resilience among individuals facing mental health challenges. Whether it is a family member, friend, or professional caregiver, their support and involvement can significantly impact the well-being and recovery of individuals. In this section, we will explore the various ways in which caregivers can contribute to building resilience and creating a supportive environment for individuals with mental health disorders.

Understanding the Needs of the Individual

The first step in supporting resilience is to understand the unique needs of the individual. Each person will have different strengths, weaknesses, and coping mechanisms. Caregivers should spend time getting to know the person they are caring for and communicate openly to gain insights into their experiences, preferences, and goals. This understanding allows caregivers to tailor their support and interventions accordingly.

Providing Emotional Support

Emotional support is a critical aspect of caregiving when it comes to resilience. Caregivers can offer a sympathetic ear, providing a safe space for individuals to express their feelings, fears, and frustrations. Validating their emotions and offering a non-judgmental presence can go a long way in enhancing resilience. It is essential for caregivers to actively listen, show empathy, and be present during difficult times.

Encouraging and Supporting Treatment

In many cases, individuals with mental health disorders require professional treatment. Caregivers can play a vital role in encouraging individuals to seek help and supporting them throughout the treatment process. By assisting with appointment scheduling, accompanying them to therapy sessions, and helping them remember medication schedules, caregivers provide practical support that removes barriers to treatment. This active involvement shows individuals that they are not alone in their journey to recovery and instills a sense of hope and resilience.

Promoting Self-Care

Caregivers must prioritize their own self-care to effectively support resilience in others. Taking care of their physical, mental, and emotional well-being enables caregivers to provide better support to individuals with mental health challenges. It is essential for caregivers to set boundaries, engage in activities they enjoy, seek their own support network, and practice effective stress management techniques. By modeling self-care, caregivers contribute to a culture of resilience and inspire those they care for to prioritize their own well-being.

Education and Advocacy

Caregivers can empower individuals with mental health challenges by providing them with information and resources. This includes educating them about their condition, treatment options, and available support services. Caregivers can actively advocate for the rights and needs of the individuals they care for, ensuring they have access to appropriate healthcare, social services, and community resources. By equipping individuals with knowledge and advocating on their behalf, caregivers foster resilience and empower individuals to make informed decisions about their care.

Creating a Supportive Environment

Caregivers can create a supportive environment that fosters resilience by promoting open communication, positive relationships, and a sense of belonging. This involves creating a safe and non-judgmental space where individuals can express themselves freely. Caregivers can encourage social connections, either through organized support groups or by facilitating informal social interactions. By fostering a sense of community and connection, caregivers contribute to the resilience of individuals with mental health challenges.

Maintaining Hope and Encouragement

Resilience is closely tied to hope and optimism. Caregivers can play a crucial role in maintaining hope by consistently providing encouragement and reinforcing positive progress. Celebrating even small achievements can significantly impact an individual's motivation and resilience. Caregivers should consistently remind individuals that resilience is a process and that setbacks are a natural part of the journey towards recovery. By fostering a hopeful mindset, caregivers empower individuals to continue striving for their goals.

In summary, caregivers have a significant impact on the resilience of individuals with mental health challenges. By understanding the unique needs of the individual, providing emotional support, encouraging and supporting treatment, promoting self-care, educating and advocating, creating a supportive environment, and maintaining hope and encouragement, caregivers can help individuals build resilience and navigate their journey towards mental well-being.

Palliative Care and Resilience in End-of-Life Care

In the final stages of life, individuals often face significant physical, emotional, and psychological challenges. Palliative care, a specialized area of healthcare, aims to improve the quality of life for patients with serious illnesses and to provide support to their families. Resilience plays a crucial role in helping patients and their loved ones navigate the complexities of end-of-life care, cope with grief, and find meaning and peace during this difficult time.

Understanding Palliative Care

Palliative care is an interdisciplinary approach that focuses on managing pain and other distressing symptoms, addressing psychosocial and spiritual needs, and optimizing the overall well-being of individuals with life-limiting illnesses. It considers the unique experiences and goals of each patient, aiming to enhance their quality of life, regardless of prognosis.

The principles of palliative care are rooted in holistic approaches to health, focusing on the physical, psychological, social, and spiritual aspects of care. By adopting a person-centered approach, healthcare professionals aim to provide comfort and support to patients and their families. Palliative care often involves a multidisciplinary team, including physicians, nurses, social workers, psychologists, chaplains, and other specialists, who work collaboratively to meet the diverse needs of patients.

Resilience in Palliative Care

Resilience in the context of palliative care refers to the emotional and psychological capacity of individuals to adapt, cope, and find meaning and purpose in the face of adversity. It involves embracing the reality of illness, managing symptoms and distress, fostering relationships, engaging in self-care, and seeking support from healthcare professionals and support networks.

For patients receiving palliative care, resilience can play a significant role in improving their well-being and quality of life. Resilient individuals often experience better pain management, reduced psychological distress, enhanced communication with healthcare professionals, and increased satisfaction with care. Additionally, resilience can positively impact the families and caregivers of patients, as they navigate the emotional complexities of end-of-life care.

Cultivating Resilience in Palliative Care

1. **Embracing open and honest communication:** Palliative care involves difficult conversations about prognosis, treatment options, and end-of-life decisions. Resilience can be fostered by encouraging patients and their families to engage in open and honest communication with healthcare professionals. This can help them gain a sense of control, make informed decisions, and find support.

2. **Promoting emotional well-being:** Resilience is closely tied to emotional well-being. Palliative care providers can support patients and families by offering emotional support, counseling, and therapeutic interventions. This may include individual or family therapy, support groups, mindfulness practices, and creative therapies such as art or music therapy.

3. **Enhancing coping strategies:** Resilience can be strengthened by developing effective coping strategies to manage the challenges associated with end-of-life care. Palliative care teams can assist patients and families in identifying and utilizing adaptive coping mechanisms, such as problem-solving skills, relaxation techniques, and maintaining meaningful routines.

4. **Supporting spiritual and existential needs:** Palliative care recognizes the importance of spirituality and existential concerns. Resilience can be nurtured by providing patients and families with opportunities to explore their beliefs, values, and find meaning in their experiences. Chaplains or spiritual care providers can offer guidance and support in this aspect of care.

5. **Promoting self-care and self-compassion:** Resilience flourishes when individuals prioritize self-care and self-compassion. Palliative care providers can encourage patients and families to engage in activities that bring them joy and comfort, practice self-care rituals, and be kind to themselves amidst the challenges they face.

6. **Involving the support network:** Resilience is often strengthened by the support of loved ones. Palliative care teams should engage and involve the patient's support network, providing guidance and education to help them navigate the complexities of end-of-life care. This may include caregiver support groups, bereavement support, and community resources.

Challenges and Considerations in Palliative Care Resilience

Palliative care resilience also faces challenges and considerations that need to be addressed:

1. **Cultural and religious diversity:** Resilience in palliative care must respect and embrace the diverse cultural and religious beliefs of patients and families.

Healthcare professionals should be mindful of cultural practices, rituals, and preferences when providing care and support.

2. **Grief and bereavement:** Resilience in palliative care extends beyond the patient's end-of-life journey and into the grieving process. Palliative care providers should be prepared to support families and caregivers during their bereavement, offering resources and counseling to foster resilience in the face of loss.

3. **Ethical considerations:** Resilience in palliative care necessitates ethical decision-making, such as respecting patient autonomy, ensuring informed consent, and navigating complex end-of-life choices. Healthcare professionals should be knowledgeable about ethical principles and guidelines to promote resilience within a framework of compassionate and patient-centered care.

4. **Interdisciplinary collaboration:** Building resilience in palliative care requires effective interdisciplinary collaboration. Communication and coordination among healthcare professionals, patients, families, and support networks are crucial for providing holistic care and ensuring the diverse needs of individuals are met.

Overall, palliative care is not solely about managing symptoms or providing end-of-life support; it is about promoting resilience and enhancing the overall well-being of patients and their families. By embracing resilience as an integral aspect of care, healthcare professionals can help individuals find strength, meaning, and peace in their journey, ultimately improving their quality of life during this challenging time.

Intersectionality and Resilience

Understanding Intersectionality in Mental Health

Intersectionality refers to the interconnected nature of social categories such as race, gender, class, and sexuality, and how they overlap and intersect to shape an individual's experiences and identities. In the context of mental health, intersectionality recognizes that various social identities and systems of oppression can significantly impact mental health experiences.

1. **The Influence of Intersectionality on Mental Health:** Intersectionality recognizes that mental health experiences are shaped not only by individual factors but also by broader social contexts. For example, a person's gender identity, racial background, or socioeconomic status can influence their access to resources, healthcare, and social support, which in turn impact their mental well-being.

Understanding intersectionality in mental health is crucial to develop inclusive and effective strategies for prevention, diagnosis, and treatment.

2. **Multiple Forms of Oppression and Mental Health:** Intersectionality highlights that individuals may face multiple forms of oppression simultaneously, leading to unique mental health challenges. For instance, LGBTQ+ individuals of color may experience discrimination based on their sexual orientation, race, and gender identity, which can negatively affect their mental well-being. It is important to consider these intersecting dimensions of identity to provide appropriate and culturally sensitive mental health care.

3. **Health Disparities and Intersectionality:** Intersectionality sheds light on health disparities that arise from the intersection of different social identities. For example, marginalized communities often face higher rates of mental health problems due to systemic discrimination, limited access to healthcare, and socioeconomic disadvantages. Recognizing these disparities is essential for developing targeted interventions, reducing barriers to care, and promoting equity in mental health services.

4. **Understanding Unique Experiences:** Intersectionality emphasizes the need to understand the unique experiences and perspectives of individuals with diverse social identities. Mental health practitioners must be aware of how intersecting social identities, cultural backgrounds, and experiences can shape an individual's mental health experiences and inform their approach to diagnosis, treatment, and support.

5. **Recognizing and Addressing Bias:** Intersectionality challenges mental health professionals to examine their own biases and assumptions. It is crucial to consider the ways in which bias and privilege can influence the diagnosis, treatment, and support provided to individuals from diverse backgrounds. Cultural competency and sensitivity training can help mental health practitioners provide inclusive and effective care.

6. **Inclusive Research and Policy Development:** Intersectionality calls for inclusive research that examines the impact of multiple identities on mental health. By considering the multiple dimensions of identity, research can provide a comprehensive understanding of the complex intersections that influence mental health outcomes. Policy development should also take into account the needs and experiences of individuals with intersecting identities to ensure equitable access to mental health care and support services.

In conclusion, understanding intersectionality in mental health acknowledges the complex ways in which social identities and systems of oppression intersect and impact mental well-being. Recognizing and addressing these intersections is crucial for promoting an inclusive, equitable, and effective approach to mental health care.

By embracing intersectionality, mental health professionals can better understand and support individuals with diverse social identities and experiences.

Other Factors Influencing Resilience

Resilience is a complex concept that is influenced by a wide range of factors. While personal strengths, resources, and social support networks play a significant role in cultivating resilience, there are also other important factors that contribute to individual and community levels of resilience. In this section, we will explore some of these additional factors and their impact on resilience.

Environmental Factors

The environment in which individuals live can greatly impact their resilience. This includes both physical and social environments. Physical environments that are prone to natural disasters, such as hurricanes, floods, or earthquakes, can pose significant challenges to individuals' resilience. Exposure to violence, crime, and poverty in the social environment can also negatively impact resilience.

On the other hand, access to green spaces, clean air, and safe neighborhoods can enhance resilience. Research has shown that exposure to nature can reduce stress, improve mental well-being, and enhance resilience. Creating and maintaining environments that promote safety, social cohesion, and access to resources is crucial for building resilient communities.

Cultural Factors

Cultural factors play a vital role in shaping resilience. Cultural values, customs, beliefs, and practices influence how individuals and communities cope with adversity. Cultural resilience refers to the adaptive capacity of a community or group to maintain their cultural identity and practices in the face of external challenges. Cultural resilience can be a powerful protective factor against mental health issues and can foster a sense of belonging and connectedness.

It is important to recognize and respect diverse cultural perspectives and practices in promoting resilience. Cultural sensitivity should be integrated into mental health policies, practices, and interventions to ensure that they are responsive to the needs of different cultural groups.

Economic Factors

Economic factors, such as income, employment, and socioeconomic status, have a significant impact on resilience. Financial stability and access to resources can provide individuals and communities with the means to cope with and recover from adversity. It enables people to access appropriate mental health care and support services.

On the other hand, financial stress, income inequality, and lack of economic opportunities can undermine resilience. Individuals and communities facing poverty and economic hardship may experience higher levels of psychological distress and have limited access to the resources necessary for resilience. Addressing economic disparities and promoting equitable access to economic opportunities is crucial for promoting resilience.

Educational Factors

Education is a fundamental factor that influences resilience. Access to quality education equips individuals with knowledge, skills, and resources necessary for coping with challenges. It fosters critical thinking, problem-solving abilities, and self-efficacy, which are essential components of resilience.

Educational opportunities also provide a sense of hope, purpose, and connectedness. It opens doors to personal and professional growth, enhances social networks, and expands opportunities for meaningful engagement. Investing in education, particularly in disadvantaged communities, is essential for promoting resilience at individual and community levels.

Political Factors

Political factors, including governance, policy, and social justice, significantly impact resilience. Effective governance ensures the provision of essential services, equitable distribution of resources, and protection of human rights. It creates an environment that fosters trust, social cohesion, and community engagement - all crucial elements for building resilience.

Policies that address social inequalities, promote social justice, and protect the rights of marginalized populations are essential for fostering resilience. Advocating for policy changes that support mental health and well-being, as well as addressing systemic injustices, is critical for building resilient societies.

In summary, resilience is influenced by a range of factors beyond personal strengths and social support networks. Environmental factors, cultural factors, economic factors, educational factors, and political factors all contribute to individual and community levels of resilience. Recognizing and addressing these factors is crucial for promoting resilience and building a sustainable mental health future.

Promoting Inclusive and Culturally Sensitive Resilience Programs

In order to promote resilience in diverse populations, it is crucial to develop inclusive and culturally sensitive resilience programs. These programs should recognize and respect the individual identities and backgrounds of individuals, while also providing the necessary support and resources to enhance their ability to bounce back from adversity.

Understanding Culture and Resilience

Culture plays a significant role in shaping an individual's experience, including their interpretation of adversity and their coping strategies. Therefore, it is important to consider cultural factors when designing resilience programs. It is essential to recognize that resilience may be different across cultures and to avoid imposing a uniform understanding of resilience on diverse populations.

To promote inclusive resilience programs, it is necessary to engage in cultural competence training. This training helps mental health professionals develop an understanding and appreciation of different cultural norms, beliefs, values, and practices. By incorporating cultural competence, resilience programs can ensure that they are respectful and sensitive to the needs of individuals from different cultural backgrounds.

Cultural Adaptation of Resilience Programs

To make resilience programs more inclusive, it is important to culturally adapt them to the specific needs and preferences of diverse populations. This involves modifying program content, delivery methods, and evaluation approaches to align with cultural values and beliefs. Cultural adaptation allows for greater relevance, acceptability, and effectiveness of resilience interventions.

Cultural adaptation can include various aspects, such as language, symbols, examples, and case studies that are culturally relevant to the target population. For instance, in a program designed for a Hispanic community, using examples and case studies that reflect their cultural experiences can enhance engagement and understanding. Additionally, incorporating culturally specific coping strategies and cultural rituals into the program can further enhance the effectiveness of resilience interventions.

Collaboration with Community Partners

In promoting inclusive and culturally sensitive resilience programs, it is essential to collaborate with community partners. Community organizations and leaders can provide valuable insights into the specific needs and preferences of the population they serve. They can also help in establishing trust and rapport with the community, leading to greater program acceptance and participation.

Engaging community partners can involve conducting focus groups, interviews, and surveys to gather input and feedback on program design and implementation. By involving community members in the planning process, resilience programs can ensure that they are addressing the specific cultural needs and challenges faced by the community.

Addressing Structural and Systemic Barriers

Inclusive resilience programs must also address structural and systemic barriers that may hinder access to mental health services and resources. These barriers can include language barriers, lack of culturally competent providers, limited financial resources, and discrimination experienced by marginalized groups. To overcome these barriers, resilience programs should advocate for policies and initiatives that support the mental health needs of diverse populations.

This may involve partnering with policymakers, advocacy groups, and stakeholders to address disparities and promote equity in mental health care. Resilience programs can also collaborate with community organizations to provide resources and support that are tailored to the unique needs of different cultural groups.

Measuring the Effectiveness of Inclusive Resilience Programs

To ensure the effectiveness of inclusive resilience programs, it is important to develop culturally appropriate evaluation measures. Standard evaluation tools may not accurately capture the impact of resilience programs on diverse populations. Culturally appropriate evaluation measures should consider cultural values, beliefs, and manifestations of resilience specific to different cultural groups.

Additionally, qualitative research methods, such as in-depth interviews and focus groups, can provide rich insights into the experiences and perceptions of program participants. This qualitative data, combined with quantitative measures, can offer a comprehensive understanding of the impact of resilience programs in diverse cultural contexts.

Case Study: Culturally Sensitive Resilience Program for Refugee Communities

To illustrate the implementation of inclusive and culturally sensitive resilience programs, consider a case study of a program designed for refugee communities. This program takes into account the unique challenges faced by individuals who have experienced forced migration and provides culturally appropriate support.

The program begins with cultural competence training for mental health professionals involved in delivering the program. This training helps them understand the socio-cultural context and traumatic experiences of refugee populations. It also equips them with knowledge of cultural norms, values, and coping mechanisms specific to the communities they serve.

The program incorporates group interventions that provide a safe space for participants to share their experiences and build social connections. These interventions utilize storytelling, art therapy, and communal rituals, which are valued in the participants' cultural backgrounds. By incorporating culturally familiar practices, the program creates a sense of belonging and facilitates the healing process.

Furthermore, the program collaborates with community organizations and refugee advocacy groups to address systemic barriers and provide comprehensive support. This collaboration helps to ensure that participants have access to resources such as language interpretation services, legal assistance, and employment support.

The effectiveness of the program is evaluated through a mixed-methods approach. Quantitative measures assess changes in mental health symptoms and levels of resilience, while qualitative methods capture participants' perspectives on the program's impact and cultural appropriateness.

By implementing this culturally sensitive resilience program, refugee communities are better equipped to overcome trauma and continued adversity, fostering their well-being and long-term resilience.

Conclusion

Promoting inclusive and culturally sensitive resilience programs is crucial for addressing the mental health needs of diverse populations. By recognizing and respecting cultural differences, adapting program content, collaborating with community partners, addressing structural barriers, and developing culturally appropriate evaluation measures, resilience programs can effectively support individuals from different cultural backgrounds. These programs can play a vital role in enhancing the overall well-being and resilience of diverse communities.

Resilience and LGBTQ+ Communities

In the context of mental health, resilience refers to an individual's ability to adapt and bounce back from challenging or traumatic experiences. Resilience is not a fixed trait but can be developed and strengthened over time through various strategies and support systems. When it comes to LGBTQ+ (Lesbian, Gay, Bisexual, Transgender, Queer/Questioning, and others) communities, resilience plays a crucial role in navigating the unique challenges and discrimination they may face.

Members of the LGBTQ+ community often experience higher rates of mental health issues such as depression, anxiety, and suicidal ideation compared to their heterosexual and cisgender counterparts. They may face societal stigma, discrimination, rejection, and violence, which can adversely impact their mental wellbeing. However, LGBTQ+ individuals have demonstrated remarkable resilience in the face of these challenges, finding strength and support within their communities.

The LGBTQ+ Minority Stress Model

Understanding the unique challenges faced by LGBTQ+ individuals is essential to comprehending the factors that contribute to their resilience. The LGBTQ+ Minority Stress Model offers insights into the specific stressors that can impact this population and how they may affect mental health outcomes.

According to this model, LGBTQ+ individuals face both external and internal minority stressors. External stressors include experiences of prejudice, discrimination, victimization, and social stigma. Internal stressors refer to the internalized homophobia, shame, and self-stigma that can result from societal attitudes and beliefs.

These stressors have a cumulative effect on mental health and can lead to adverse outcomes. However, individuals who develop resilience are better able to cope with and overcome these stressors, leading to improved mental health and overall wellbeing.

Building Resilience in LGBTQ+ Communities

Building resilience within LGBTQ+ communities involves addressing both individual and systemic factors. Here are some strategies to promote resilience:

1. Creating Safe Spaces: Creating safe and inclusive spaces, such as LGBTQ+ community centers or support groups, can help foster a sense of belonging and provide social support. These spaces allow individuals to openly express their identities without fear of judgment or rejection.

2. LGBTQ+-Inclusive Mental Health Services: Mental health professionals should receive training on LGBTQ+ cultural competency to better understand the unique needs and experiences of this community. LGBTQ+-inclusive counseling and therapy can help individuals navigate their mental health challenges and develop effective coping strategies.

3. Peer Support Networks: Establishing peer support networks within LGBTQ+ communities can provide opportunities for individuals to connect with others who share similar experiences. Peer support can offer validation, empathy, and practical advice in times of distress, promoting resilience.

4. Advocacy and Activism: Engaging in advocacy work and activism can empower individuals to challenge discriminatory practices and policies that negatively affect LGBTQ+ mental health. By advocating for their rights and well-being, individuals can develop a sense of agency and resilience.

5. Mental Health Education: Increasing LGBTQ+ cultural competency and mental health literacy among the general population can help reduce stigma and improve support for LGBTQ+ individuals. Education initiatives can promote understanding, acceptance, and support, leading to increased resilience within the community.

Case Study: The Trevor Project

The Trevor Project is an example of an organization that promotes resilience within LGBTQ+ communities. Founded in 1998, it focuses on suicide prevention and crisis intervention for LGBTQ+ youth. The organization provides a range of support services, including a 24/7 helpline, online chat, and text-based support.

By providing accessible and LGBTQ+-affirming resources, the Trevor Project offers vital support to those who may face rejection or isolation within their communities. The organization's commitment to fostering resilience and empowering LGBTQ+ individuals enhances their overall mental health and wellbeing.

Conclusion

Resilience is a vital factor in promoting the mental health and wellbeing of LGBTQ+ individuals. By acknowledging and addressing the unique challenges faced by this community, we can support the development of resilience and create a more inclusive and supportive society. Through safe spaces, inclusive mental health services, peer support networks, advocacy efforts, and education, we can foster resilience and empower LGBTQ+ individuals on their mental health journeys.

Resilient Communities and Societies

Community-Based Interventions for Resilience

In recent years, there has been a growing recognition of the importance of community-based interventions in promoting resilience and well-being. These interventions aim to empower individuals and communities to develop the skills, resources, and support networks needed to navigate and overcome challenges. By mobilizing community assets and fostering social cohesion, these interventions play a crucial role in enhancing resilience at both individual and collective levels.

Understanding Resilience in Community Context

Resilience in a community context refers to the ability of a community to adapt, recover, and grow stronger in the face of adversity. It encompasses the collective capacity to withstand and bounce back from stressors such as natural disasters, economic downturns, social conflicts, and health crises. Community resilience involves not only the individuals within the community but also the social and physical environments that shape their experiences.

A key principle of community-based interventions for resilience is recognizing that communities are not homogenous entities. They consist of diverse groups with varying levels of vulnerability and resources. Therefore, a comprehensive approach to community resilience must consider the needs and strengths of different population groups and address systemic inequalities.

Components of Community-Based Interventions

Community-based interventions for resilience comprise various components, including:

1. *Community Engagement and Participation*: These interventions prioritize involving community members in decision-making processes, fostering a sense of ownership and empowerment. Community engagement promotes active participation, collaboration, and collective problem-solving.

2. *Social Support Networks*: Building and strengthening social connections within the community is essential for resilience. Interventions focus on nurturing supportive relationships, fostering a sense of belonging, and promoting mutual aid. This can involve creating social spaces, organizing community events, or establishing support groups.

3. *Asset-Based Approaches*: Community assets, including individual skills, knowledge, cultural practices, and local resources, form the foundation of resilience. Interventions focus on identifying and mobilizing these assets to address community needs and challenges effectively.

4. *Capacity Building*: Enhancing individual and community capacities is a central component of community-based interventions. This may involve providing training programs, workshops, or educational initiatives aimed at developing skills, promoting leadership, and fostering self-efficacy within the community.

5. *Creating Resilient Physical Infrastructure*: Community resilience is closely linked to the physical environment. Interventions focus on creating or improving infrastructure that can withstand and recover from shocks, such as designing disaster-resistant buildings or implementing sustainable urban planning strategies.

Examples of Community-Based Interventions

1. *Community Emergency Response Teams (CERT)*: CERT programs train community members in disaster preparedness, response, and recovery. These teams play a critical role in supporting first responders and providing immediate assistance to their neighbors during emergencies.

2. *Community Gardens*: Community gardens promote social interaction, enhance food security, and contribute to the physical and mental well-being of individuals and communities. They provide opportunities for education, skill-building, and strengthening social connections.

3. *Youth Development Programs*: These programs focus on empowering young people by building their skills, fostering their resilience, and helping them become active contributors to their community. They offer mentoring, leadership training, and opportunities for civic engagement.

4. *Community-Based Mental Health Programs*: These programs aim to improve mental health outcomes by providing accessible and culturally sensitive mental health services within the community. They often involve peer support, counseling, and community education initiatives to reduce stigma and enhance help-seeking behaviors.

Challenges and Considerations

While community-based interventions hold great promise, there are important challenges and considerations to be addressed:

1. *Inclusivity and Equity*: It is crucial to ensure that community-based interventions are inclusive and address the needs of marginalized and vulnerable populations. Efforts should be made to reduce disparities, foster social equity, and empower all community members.

2. *Sustainability*: Sustaining community-based interventions over the long term can be challenging. Adequate funding, stakeholder engagement, and strong community leadership are necessary to ensure the continued success and impact of these initiatives.

3. *Evaluation and Research*: Rigorous evaluation and research are essential to determine the effectiveness and outcomes of community-based interventions. This evidence can inform future interventions and contribute to the wider field of community resilience.

4. *Collaboration and Partnerships*: Building strong partnerships among community organizations, local government, and other stakeholders is critical for the success of community-based interventions. Collaboration facilitates resource sharing, leverages expertise, and enhances collective impact.

In conclusion, community-based interventions play a vital role in promoting resilience and well-being. By leveraging community assets, fostering social support networks, and empowering individuals and communities, these interventions contribute to the overall sustainability of mental health. However, careful consideration of inclusivity, sustainability, and collaboration is necessary to maximize the impact of these interventions and address the challenges faced by communities.

Resilience and Disaster Preparedness

In the face of natural disasters, communities must be prepared to respond effectively and recover swiftly. Resilience plays a critical role in disaster preparedness, helping individuals, families, and communities withstand and bounce back from the impact of catastrophes. In this section, we will explore the concept of resilience in the context of disaster preparedness and examine strategies to build resilience at various levels.

Understanding Resilience in Disaster Preparedness

Resilience is the ability to adapt and recover in the face of adversity. In the context of disaster preparedness, resilience refers to the capacity of individuals, communities, and systems to withstand and recover from the physical, emotional, and economic challenges posed by disasters. It involves preparing for potential hazards, mitigating risks, and fostering a culture of preparedness.

Disaster resilience encompasses a multidimensional approach that aims to reduce vulnerabilities, enhance adaptive capacity, and enable effective response and recovery. It encompasses not only physical infrastructure but also the social, economic, and environmental factors that contribute to overall community well-being.

Building Resilience at the Individual Level

Individuals play a critical role in disaster preparedness and response. Here are some key strategies to build resilience at the individual level:

1. Education and Awareness: Stay informed about potential hazards in your area and how to respond to them. Educate yourself and your family on emergency preparedness, evacuation procedures, and first aid techniques.

2. Emergency Kits and Supplies: Prepare emergency kits that include essential items such as food, water, medications, and basic tools. Ensure that you have backup power sources, such as batteries or generators, as well as a communication plan.

3. Mental and Emotional Wellbeing: Prioritize your mental and emotional wellbeing before, during, and after a disaster. Develop coping strategies to manage stress and anxiety, seek social support, and practice self-care.

4. Risk Reduction and Mitigation: Take proactive measures to reduce risks, such as securing heavy furniture, reinforcing structures, or installing smoke detectors and fire extinguishers. Familiarize yourself with fire safety, flood-proofing, and earthquake safety techniques.

5. Communication and Networking: Establish communication networks with neighbors, friends, and family members to stay connected and provide mutual support during emergencies. Join community organizations or local emergency response groups to contribute to collective resilience efforts.

Building Resilience at the Community Level

Communities that are resilient can minimize the impact of disasters and recover more effectively. Here are strategies to promote community resilience in disaster preparedness:

1. Risk Assessment and Planning: Conduct comprehensive risk assessments to understand the potential hazards and vulnerabilities in the community. Develop and implement disaster response and recovery plans that involve all stakeholders, including government agencies, non-profit organizations, and community members.

2. Infrastructure and Building Codes: Ensure that infrastructure is designed and built to withstand potential hazards, such as earthquakes, floods, or hurricanes. Enforce strict building codes and regulations to enhance structural resilience.

3. Early Warning Systems and Communication: Establish effective early warning systems that can quickly alert the community about imminent threats. Create clear communication channels to disseminate information, instructions, and warnings to residents.

4. Public Health and Medical Support: Strengthen public health systems to provide necessary medical support during disasters. Ensure access to healthcare facilities, medications, and mental health services. Develop emergency response plans for vulnerable populations, including the elderly, children, and individuals with disabilities.

5. Social Cohesion and Community Engagement: Foster social cohesion by promoting community engagement and participation. Encourage the formation of community-based organizations, neighborhood watch groups, and volunteer networks that support disaster preparedness and response.

Building Resilience at the National and Global Level

Resilience in disaster preparedness extends beyond the individual and community level. National and global efforts are essential to building resilience. Here are strategies for resilience-building at broader scales:

1. Policy and Governance: Develop comprehensive policies and legislation that promote disaster risk reduction and resilience. Allocate sufficient resources for emergency response, recovery, and infrastructure development.

2. International Cooperation: Foster international collaboration and knowledge-sharing to address global challenges posed by disasters. Promote resilient practices and support capacity-building programs in vulnerable regions.

3. Research and Innovation: Invest in research and innovation to enhance understanding of disaster risks and develop cutting-edge technologies for early warning systems, shelter design, and disaster recovery. Support interdisciplinary research on resilience and sustainable development.

4. Risk Financing and Insurance: Establish risk financing mechanisms, such as insurance programs, to enable swift recovery and reduce the burden on affected

individuals and communities. Encourage public-private partnerships to strengthen financial resilience.

By building resilience at the individual, community, national, and global levels, we can enhance our ability to withstand and recover from disasters. Remember, resilience is not a one-time effort but an ongoing process that requires continuous adaptation and improvement. Let us work together to create a more resilient and sustainable future for all.

Creating Sustainable Environments for Resilience

Creating sustainable environments is crucial for promoting resilience in individuals and communities. Resilience refers to the ability to bounce back from adversity and maintain positive mental health and well-being. In this section, we will explore the importance of sustainable environments in fostering resilience, examine the key elements of such environments, and provide practical strategies for creating and sustaining them.

Understanding Sustainable Environments

Sustainable environments are those that support the well-being of individuals and communities over the long term. They are designed to promote physical, mental, and social well-being while minimizing negative impacts on the environment. When it comes to resilience, sustainable environments play a vital role in building adaptive capacities and providing resources and support systems that help individuals and communities effectively cope with and recover from challenges and crises.

Key Elements of Sustainable Environments

To create sustainable environments that foster resilience, several key elements need to be considered:

1. **Physical Infrastructure:** The physical infrastructure of a community or an organization plays a significant role in determining its resilience. Infrastructure that is designed to withstand natural disasters, has robust emergency response systems in place, and ensures access to essential services like healthcare and clean water improves the ability to withstand and recover from adverse events.

2. **Social Support Networks:** Building strong social support networks is essential for resilience. A supportive community that fosters social connections, promotes inclusivity, and shares resources and information helps individuals cope with stressors and provides a safety net during challenging times.

3. **Access to Resources:** Availability and equitable access to essential resources such as food, water, healthcare, education, and employment opportunities are critical for building resilience. Ensuring equal distribution of resources and addressing socioeconomic disparities are key considerations in creating sustainable environments.

4. **Environmental Sustainability:** Protecting and preserving the natural environment is vital for long-term resilience. Implementing sustainable practices such as reducing carbon emissions, promoting renewable energy sources, preserving biodiversity, and adopting environmentally friendly policies contribute to the overall well-being of individuals and communities.

5. **Collaborative Governance:** Establishing effective governance systems that involve collaboration and participation from all stakeholders is crucial for creating sustainable environments. Inclusive decision-making processes that take into account diverse perspectives and prioritize the well-being of the community promote resilience and ensure the long-term sustainability of the environment.

Strategies for Creating and Sustaining Sustainable Environments

Implementing strategies to create and sustain sustainable environments requires a comprehensive approach that involves multiple stakeholders and sectors. Here are some practical strategies for achieving this goal:

1. **Education and Awareness:** Promote education and awareness campaigns to increase understanding and knowledge about sustainable practices and their benefits. This can be done through school programs, community workshops, and public awareness campaigns to empower individuals to make informed choices and take action.

2. **Policy and Planning:** Develop and implement policies and urban planning strategies that prioritize sustainability and resilience. This can include zoning regulations, green building standards, and requirements for green spaces and infrastructure resilience. Encouraging the use of renewable energy sources and implementing sustainable transportation options can also contribute to creating sustainable environments.

3. **Collaboration and Partnerships:** Foster collaboration and partnerships among government agencies, non-profit organizations, businesses, and community groups to address sustainability challenges. These collaborations can lead to innovative solutions, shared resources, and collective efforts towards building resilient and sustainable environments.

4. **Community Engagement:** Engage individuals and communities in sustainability initiatives by involving them in decision-making processes,

encouraging volunteerism, and providing opportunities for active participation. This promotes ownership, pride, and a sense of responsibility towards creating and sustaining sustainable environments.

5. **Sustainable Infrastructure Development:** Invest in the development of sustainable infrastructure that promotes resilience. This includes implementing green building practices, incorporating renewable energy sources, and designing physical spaces to withstand climate-related events and natural disasters.

6. **Monitoring and Evaluation:** Regularly monitor and evaluate the progress of sustainability initiatives to ensure their effectiveness and make necessary adjustments. Tracking sustainability indicators, conducting impact assessments, and soliciting feedback from community members contribute to continuous improvement and the long-term sustainability of environments.

Example: Sustainable Urban Planning

An example of sustainable environment creation is through urban planning. Sustainable urban planning aims to create cities and communities that are environmentally friendly, socially inclusive, and economically viable. It seeks to balance the needs of the present generation without compromising the ability of future generations to meet their needs.

In this approach, urban planners consider factors such as transportation systems, green spaces, energy efficiency, waste management, and social infrastructure. They work collaboratively with architects, environmentalists, policymakers, and community members to develop sustainable and resilient urban areas.

For instance, a sustainable urban plan might prioritize the development of public transportation systems to reduce emissions and congestion, promote the construction of energy-efficient buildings, incorporate green spaces such as parks and gardens, and ensure affordable housing options for all residents.

By implementing sustainable urban planning strategies, communities can reduce their ecological footprint, enhance quality of life, improve access to essential services, and build resilience to climate change impacts and other challenges.

Conclusion

Creating sustainable environments is crucial for fostering resilience in individuals and communities. By addressing physical, social, and environmental aspects of sustainability, we can build adaptive capacities and provide the necessary resources and support systems to effectively cope with and recover from adversity. Through education, collaboration, and strategic planning, we can create sustainable environments that promote resilience and contribute to overall well-being.

Resilience and Climate Change Adaptation

Climate change is one of the greatest challenges of our time, with far-reaching impacts on ecosystems, economies, and human health and well-being. As the world's climate rapidly changes, it poses significant threats to mental health and requires us to build resilience at individual, community, and societal levels. In this section, we will explore the relationship between resilience and climate change adaptation, highlighting strategies to promote mental well-being in the face of this global crisis.

Understanding the Impact of Climate Change on Mental Health

Climate change impacts, such as extreme weather events, rising temperatures, sea-level rise, and changing precipitation patterns, have profound implications for mental health. These environmental changes can lead to increased stress, anxiety, depression, and other mental health disorders. Additionally, climate change-induced displacement and forced migration further exacerbate psychological distress and trauma.

The direct and indirect impacts of climate change on mental health are complex and multidimensional. Individuals may experience psychological reactions, such as eco-anxiety, grief, and loss, as they witness the destruction of ecosystems and the loss of biodiversity. Moreover, vulnerable populations, including low-income communities, Indigenous peoples, and coastal communities, face disproportionate mental health challenges due to climate-related stressors and unequal access to resources.

Building Resilience in the Face of Climate Change

Resilience plays a crucial role in mitigating the negative mental health impacts of climate change and promoting adaptive behaviors. By enhancing resilience, individuals and communities can better cope with the stressors and uncertainties associated with climate change and develop strategies to adapt and thrive in changing environments. Here are some key approaches to building resilience in the face of climate change:

1. **Enhancing Individual Resilience** Individuals can enhance their resilience by developing proactive coping strategies and adaptive skills. This includes building

emotional resilience, cultivating optimism, practicing mindfulness techniques, and fostering problem-solving abilities. By developing a positive mindset and increasing their self-efficacy, individuals can better navigate the challenges and uncertainties associated with climate change.

2. **Strengthening Social Support Networks**   Strong social support networks are critical in promoting resilience in the face of climate change. These networks provide emotional support, practical assistance, and a sense of belonging. Building and strengthening social connections within communities can facilitate mutual aid and collective action in response to climate-related challenges. Peer support groups, community organizations, and online platforms can play a vital role in fostering social support and resilience.

3. **Investing in Climate Change Education**   Education and awareness are fundamental in building resilience and promoting adaptive behaviors. Climate change education should be integrated into schools, universities, and community programs to foster understanding and empower individuals to take collective action. Teaching climate change science, environmental ethics, sustainable practices, and interpersonal skills can equip individuals with the knowledge and skills needed to navigate climate-related challenges.

4. **Implementing Climate-Informed Mental Health Services**   Mental health services must be informed by climate change realities and tailored to the unique needs of climate-affected communities. Clinicians and mental health professionals should receive training on climate change impacts and develop trauma-informed approaches to care. This includes recognizing and addressing eco-anxiety, climate-related grief, and the psychological toll of environmental disasters. Additionally, incorporating nature-based therapies and ecotherapy can harness the healing power of nature in promoting mental well-being.

5. **Community-Based Resilience Approaches**   Community-based resilience approaches empower local communities to adapt and thrive in the face of climate change. This involves engaging community members in decision-making processes, fostering social cohesion, and building adaptive capacity. Implementing climate-smart infrastructure, such as improved drainage systems or renewable energy projects, can enhance community resilience while providing co-benefits for mental health.

6. **Advocating for Climate Change Policy and Action** Promoting resilient communities requires addressing the root causes of climate change through policy and advocacy efforts. By advocating for sustainable development, greenhouse gas reduction, and climate justice, individuals and communities can contribute to systemic change. Engaging in climate activism, participating in policy discussions, and supporting environmental organizations can amplify the voice of those affected by climate change and drive the necessary action at local, national, and international levels.

Case Study: The Pacific Islands and Climate Change Resilience

The Pacific Islands, including Fiji, Samoa, and Tuvalu, are highly vulnerable to the impacts of climate change, with rising sea levels, increased frequency of extreme weather events, and coastal erosion posing significant challenges. These small island nations are at the forefront of climate change adaptation, and their experiences provide valuable lessons in building resilience.

In the Pacific Islands, community-based approaches to climate change resilience are rooted in traditional knowledge, cultural practices, and indigenous wisdom. The concept of "talanoa," a Pacific Islander practice of dialogue and storytelling, fosters community engagement and collaboration in response to climate challenges. By integrating indigenous knowledge with scientific expertise, Pacific Island communities have successfully implemented adaptation strategies such as mangrove restoration, sustainable fishing practices, and climate-smart agriculture.

Furthermore, Pacific Island nations have been leading global initiatives to address climate change, advocating for stronger mitigation targets and financial assistance for vulnerable regions. The Pacific Islands Development Forum and the Pacific Islands Forum are platforms that enable collective action, knowledge sharing, and policy advocacy.

The Pacific Island experience highlights the power of community resilience, cultural preservation, and advocacy in climate change response. By recognizing and valuing different forms of knowledge, Pacific Island communities have demonstrated creative and holistic approaches to climate change adaptation, maintaining their cultural identity while building resilience for their people.

Conclusion

Climate change presents unprecedented challenges to mental health, requiring holistic and resilient responses. By understanding the impact of climate change on mental well-being and implementing strategies to build resilience, individuals, communities, and societies can navigate the complexities of climate change while promoting sustainable development and well-being. By integrating climate change adaptation into mental health policy, research, and practice, we can envision a sustainable future where mental health is protected in the face of environmental uncertainty. Let us join hands and work towards a world that supports the resilience and well-being of both people and the planet.

Exercises

1. Reflect on your own resilience in the face of environmental challenges. Identify one coping strategy or skill that you can develop to enhance your resilience to climate change impacts.

2. Research a community-based climate change resilience project in your local area or another region. Describe the strategies implemented and assess their effectiveness in promoting both environmental sustainability and mental well-being.

3. Engage in a climate change advocacy campaign by joining a local environmental organization or participating in a community event. Reflect on the impact of collective action on your own well-being and the overall resilience of your community.

Further Reading

1. Clayton, S., Manning, C. M., & Hodge, C. (2014). Beyond Storms and Droughts: The Psychological Impacts of Climate Change. American Psychological Association.

2. Reser, J. P., & Swim, J. K. (2011). Adapting to and Coping with the Threat and Impacts of Climate Change. American Psychologist, 66(4), 277-289.

3. Petherick, A. (2019). Climate Change Resilience. Oxford Research Encyclopedia of Public Health.

4. Berry, H. L., Waite, T. D., Dear, K. B., Capon, A. G., & Murray, V. (2011). The Case for Systems Thinking about Climate Change and Mental Health. Nature Climate Change, 1, 462-464.

Chapter 5: Conclusion: Towards a Sustainable Mental Health Future

Chapter 5: Conclusion: Towards a Sustainable Mental Health Future

Chapter 5: Conclusion: Towards a Sustainable Mental Health Future

In this final chapter, we reflect on the journey we have embarked upon in exploring mental health and wellbeing in contemporary history. We have delved into the definitions and scope of mental health, examined the historical context of mental health care, explored various psychological challenges, discussed the importance of promoting holistic health, and highlighted the significance of building resilience. Now, we turn our attention towards envisioning a sustainable mental health future, where individuals and communities thrive.

1. Embracing Diversity, Inclusion, and Social Justice: As we move forward, it is imperative that we commit ourselves to embracing diversity, inclusion, and social justice in mental health care. We recognize that mental health challenges affect individuals across different cultures, ethnicities, genders, and socioeconomic backgrounds. A sustainable mental health future requires us to address the unique needs and experiences of all individuals, ensuring equitable access to quality care. We must challenge stigma, discrimination, and systemic barriers, while promoting culturally sensitive and trauma-informed approaches.

2. Balancing Individual and Collective Responsibility: While mental health starts at the individual level, it is also a collective responsibility. Families, communities, educational institutions, workplaces, and governments each play a

crucial role in fostering mental health and wellbeing. A sustainable mental health future emphasizes collaborative approaches, where all stakeholders work together to create supportive environments. It requires us to prioritize prevention, early intervention, and mental health literacy to empower individuals to take charge of their own mental wellbeing.

3. Envisioning a Holistic and Sustainable Approach to Mental Health: We have recognized throughout this textbook the importance of holistic approaches to mental health. To achieve sustainability, we must continue to integrate the biopsychosocial model and recognize the interconnectedness of physical, mental, and social aspects of health. This involves promoting the use of complementary and alternative therapies, nurturing the mind-body connection, and addressing the impact of nutrition, exercise, and mind-body practices. Additionally, we must harness the potential of art, music, animal-assisted therapy, and spirituality in supporting mental health and encouraging overall wellbeing.

4. Inspiring Hope and Resilience: Resilience lies at the core of a sustainable mental health future. As we navigate the complexities of life, building resilience becomes crucial in promoting recovery, adaptability, and growth. We must equip individuals with the personal strengths and resources necessary to navigate challenges, overcome adversity, and bounce back from setbacks. By fostering social support networks, ensuring access to mental health care, and promoting positive coping strategies, we can lay the foundations for a resilient society.

In conclusion, a sustainable mental health future demands our collective commitment to embracing diversity, promoting holistic approaches, and inspiring resilience. It requires us to challenge stigma, advocate for effective policies and systems, and prioritize the wellbeing of individuals and communities. As we move forward, let us remember the valuable lessons learned from history, seize the opportunities for transformative change, and work towards a world where mental health and wellbeing are prioritized as essential components of overall sustainability.

The Evolution of Mental Health Care

Lessons from History

In the study of mental health and wellbeing, history plays a crucial role in helping us understand the evolution of our understanding and approaches to mental health care. By examining the lessons from the past, we can gain valuable insights into the successes and failures of different models and interventions. These lessons can guide us in building a more effective and sustainable mental health future. In this section, we will explore some key lessons from history that have shaped the field of mental health.

Lesson 1: The Importance of Human Rights

One of the most important lessons from history is the recognition of the fundamental human rights of individuals with mental health challenges. Throughout history, people with mental illness have often been subjected to discrimination, stigmatization, and human rights abuses. The mistreatment of individuals with mental health conditions in asylums and other institutions serves as a stark reminder of the need to respect the dignity and rights of all individuals regardless of their mental health status.

The movement towards deinstitutionalization in the mid-20th century emerged as a response to these abuses and emphasized the need for community-based care and support. This lesson highlights the importance of creating inclusive, non-coercive, and empowering mental health systems that promote the autonomy and agency of individuals with mental health challenges.

Lesson 2: The Power of Social Support

Another crucial lesson from history is the power of social support in promoting mental health and resilience. In the past, individuals with mental health conditions were often isolated and excluded from their communities. The establishment of community mental health centers and the emphasis on peer support and group therapy represented a significant shift in recognizing the importance of social connections in mental health care.

Research has consistently shown that social support can protect against stress, reduce the risk of mental health issues, and enhance overall wellbeing. This lesson reaffirms the need to foster supportive communities, promote social connections, and provide spaces for individuals to share their experiences and support one another.

Lesson 3: The Role of Trauma

The recognition of the impact of trauma on mental health has been another important lesson from history. Historically, trauma was often dismissed or overlooked as a contributing factor to mental health challenges. However, our understanding of trauma has evolved significantly, and trauma-informed care has gained prominence.

By acknowledging the prevalence and impact of trauma, mental health systems can provide more compassionate and effective care. This lesson emphasizes the need for trauma-informed approaches that prioritize safety, trustworthiness, choice, collaboration, and empowerment in mental health care settings.

Lesson 4: The Need for Holistic Approaches

Throughout history, there has been a growing recognition of the need for holistic approaches to mental health. The shift from the medical model towards a biopsychosocial perspective highlighted the importance of considering biological, psychological, and social factors in understanding and addressing mental health challenges.

This lesson emphasizes the need to move beyond a narrow focus on symptoms and diagnoses and consider the multifaceted nature of mental health. Holistic approaches that incorporate nutrition, exercise, mind-body practices, art therapy, animal-assisted therapy, and spirituality have shown promise in promoting overall wellbeing and resilience.

Lesson 5: The Power of Advocacy

Advocacy has played a crucial role in driving the transformation of mental health care throughout history. The voices and experiences of individuals with mental health challenges, their families, and mental health professionals have been instrumental in shaping policy, challenging stigma, and promoting awareness.

This lesson highlights the power of grassroots movements, public campaigns, and policy advocacy in driving positive change in mental health. It encourages individuals, communities, and organizations to join forces and advocate for greater investments in mental health, improved access to care, and the implementation of evidence-based practices.

Conclusion

The lessons from history provide us with valuable insights into the challenges and opportunities in the field of mental health. As we strive towards a sustainable mental health future, it is important to remember the importance of human rights, social support, trauma-informed care, holistic approaches, and advocacy. By incorporating these lessons into our practice, research, policies, and systems, we can build a more inclusive, compassionate, and effective mental health care system that promotes the wellbeing and resilience of individuals and communities.

THE EVOLUTION OF MENTAL HEALTH CARE   481

Challenges and Opportunities in the Future

As we look towards the future of mental health care, there are both challenges and opportunities that lie ahead. In this section, we will explore some of the key issues that mental health professionals and policymakers will need to address, as well as the potential for transformative change in the field.

Challenge 1: Mental Health Stigma

One of the major challenges in the future of mental health is the persistent stigma surrounding mental illness. Despite the progress made in recent years, many individuals still face discrimination, prejudice, and social exclusion due to their mental health conditions. This stigma can prevent individuals from seeking help, receiving adequate treatment, and fully participating in society.

Addressing mental health stigma requires a multi-faceted approach. It involves raising awareness, challenging stereotypes, and promoting empathy and understanding. Educating the public about mental health and sharing stories of recovery can help to reduce stigma. Moreover, integrating mental health education into school curricula and training programs for healthcare providers can contribute to destigmatization efforts.

Challenge 2: Access to Mental Health Care

Another significant challenge is the limited access to mental health care services. Many individuals, especially those in low-income communities and marginalized groups, face barriers such as high costs, shortage of mental health professionals, and inadequate insurance coverage. This lack of accessibility leads to delayed or inadequate treatment, perpetuating the cycle of mental health disparities.

To address this challenge, it is crucial to improve the availability and affordability of mental health services. This can be achieved through the expansion of mental health care facilities, the integration of mental health services into primary care settings, and the use of telemedicine to provide remote access to care. Additionally, policy interventions that prioritize mental health funding and reimbursement for mental health services can help ensure that everyone can access the care they need.

Opportunity 1: Technology and Digital Mental Health

Advancements in technology have the potential to revolutionize the field of mental health care. Digital mental health interventions, such as smartphone applications, virtual reality therapy, and online support communities, offer new avenues for prevention, early intervention, and ongoing support. These technologies have the advantage of being scalable, accessible, and cost-effective.

Digital mental health also presents opportunities for data collection and analysis. By harnessing the power of big data and artificial intelligence, we can gain insights into patterns, risk factors, and treatment outcomes. This information can inform personalized interventions and improve the overall quality of care. However, it is important to address ethical considerations, such as privacy and data security, to ensure the responsible use of these technologies.

Opportunity 2: Holistic and Integrated Approaches

Moving forward, the integration of mental health care with other healthcare disciplines presents an opportunity to enhance overall well-being. Adopting a holistic approach that recognizes the interconnectedness of mental, physical, and social health can lead to more effective treatment outcomes.

Integrative medicine, which combines conventional and complementary therapies, can play a significant role in promoting holistic health. By incorporating approaches such as nutrition, exercise, mindfulness, and art therapy, we can address mental health challenges from multiple angles. Moreover, fostering collaboration among different healthcare providers, including mental health professionals, primary care physicians, and community workers, can lead to comprehensive and coordinated care.

Challenge 3: Global Mental Health Disparities

Disparities in mental health care exist not only within countries but also between countries. Low- and middle-income countries often face limited resources, infrastructure, and trained professionals, resulting in significant gaps in mental health services. Additionally, cultural and contextual factors influence the perception and understanding of mental health, warranting culturally sensitive approaches.

Addressing global mental health disparities requires a commitment to equity and social justice. This involves collaborating with international organizations, governments, and local communities to prioritize mental health on the global health agenda. Investing in mental health infrastructure, training programs, and research in low-resource settings can help bridge the gap and ensure that everyone, regardless of their socioeconomic status or geographic location, has access to quality mental health care.

Conclusion

The future of mental health care is both challenging and full of opportunities. By tackling stigma, improving access to care, leveraging technology, adopting holistic approaches, and addressing global disparities, we can build a more sustainable and inclusive mental health future. It requires a collective effort, involving individuals, communities, policymakers, and healthcare providers, to transform the way we understand and support mental health. As we reflect on our journey, let us embrace diversity, inclusion, and social justice, envisioning a future where mental health and well-being are at the forefront of our collective consciousness.

Incorporating Lessons Learned for Future Practice

As we reflect on the evolution of mental health care and the challenges and opportunities that lie ahead, it is essential to consider how we can incorporate the lessons learned from the past into future practice. By embracing these lessons, we can build a more sustainable and effective mental health system. In this section, we will explore key areas where these lessons can be applied.

1. Integrate Research and Practice

One important lesson is the need to bridge the gap between research and practice in mental health care. It is crucial to incorporate the latest evidence-based treatments into clinical settings and ensure that practitioners are knowledgeable about cutting-edge research. This can be achieved through ongoing professional development and training programs that prioritize research literacy and the dissemination of best practices.

Additionally, the integration of research and practice can be facilitated by establishing collaborative partnerships between researchers and clinicians. By working together, they can develop innovative interventions, conduct clinical trials, and translate research findings into real-world applications. Such collaboration fosters a culture of continuous learning and improvement in mental health care.

2. Embrace a Holistic Approach

Another crucial lesson is the importance of adopting a holistic approach to mental health care. Acknowledging the interconnectedness of physical, emotional, and social well-being enables us to provide comprehensive and person-centered care. Integrated care models that incorporate medical, psychological, and social support services can enhance treatment outcomes and promote overall well-being.

In a holistic approach, mental health care extends beyond the clinic walls and encompasses the broader social determinants of health. It recognizes the influence of factors such as socioeconomic status, education, housing, and access to nutritious food on mental well-being. By addressing these determinants and promoting social justice, we can create a more equitable and sustainable mental health system.

3. Prioritize Prevention and Early Intervention

Prevention and early intervention are vital components of effective mental health care. By identifying risk factors and implementing preventive measures, we can reduce the incidence and severity of mental health disorders. This entails educating the public about mental health, promoting resilience-building strategies, and destigmatizing help-seeking behaviors.

Furthermore, early intervention is crucial in improving treatment outcomes and reducing the long-term impact of mental health disorders. By promptly identifying and addressing symptoms, we can prevent the progression of illnesses and mitigate their negative consequences. This requires strengthening mental health literacy, expanding access to early intervention services, and integrating mental health screening into routine healthcare settings.

4. Promote Collaboration and Interdisciplinary Care

Collaboration and interdisciplinary care are essential for providing holistic and comprehensive mental health services. By involving professionals from various disciplines, such as psychiatrists, psychologists, social workers, nurses, and occupational therapists, we can address the diverse needs of individuals experiencing mental health challenges.

Interdisciplinary care teams can collaborate to develop personalized treatment plans, coordinate services, and provide ongoing support to individuals and their families. This collaborative approach ensures that care is well-coordinated and avoids fragmentation, resulting in improved treatment adherence and better outcomes.

5. Address Mental Health Disparities

Another important lesson is the need to address mental health disparities that exist within and between populations. It is essential to recognize and eliminate barriers to mental health care, including unequal access, discriminatory practices, and cultural stigma. This requires culturally competent care that respects diverse backgrounds and integrates cultural beliefs and practices into treatment approaches.

Additionally, reducing mental health disparities necessitates targeted interventions for underserved communities, including racial and ethnic minorities, LGBTQ+ individuals, and individuals with disabilities. By prioritizing equity in mental health care, we can ensure that everyone has access to high-quality services and experiences equitable outcomes.

Conclusion

Incorporating the lessons learned from the past is crucial for building a sustainable mental health future. By integrating research and practice, embracing a holistic approach, prioritizing prevention and early intervention, promoting collaboration and interdisciplinary care, and addressing mental health disparities, we can work towards a more effective and equitable mental health system. These lessons serve as a foundation for improving the well-being of individuals, communities, and societies as a whole.

Advancing Mental Health Research and Training

Building a Strong Evidence Base

In order to effectively address mental health challenges and promote sustainable mental health care, it is crucial to have a strong evidence base. A robust evidence base provides the foundation for making informed decisions, developing effective interventions, and improving mental health outcomes. This section will explore the importance of building a strong evidence base in mental health, the key components of evidence-based practice, and strategies for generating and disseminating high-quality evidence.

The Importance of Evidence-Based Practice

Evidence-based practice (EBP) is a framework that integrates the best available evidence, clinical expertise, and patient values and preferences to guide decision-making and improve outcomes. In the context of mental health care, EBP involves translating research findings into everyday practice to enhance the quality, effectiveness, and efficiency of care.

Building a strong evidence base is essential for several reasons. Firstly, it helps to identify effective treatments and interventions that can improve mental health outcomes. By conducting rigorous research studies and evaluating the effectiveness of different approaches, mental health professionals can identify strategies that have the greatest impact on the well-being of individuals and communities.

Secondly, a strong evidence base helps to reduce variability in practice. By providing clear guidelines and recommendations based on empirical evidence, EBP promotes standardized care and reduces the potential for bias and inconsistency in treatment decisions. This not only improves the quality of care but also ensures that individuals receive the most appropriate interventions based on their specific needs.

Furthermore, a strong evidence base is essential for informing policy and resource allocation decisions. Governments, healthcare organizations, and other stakeholders rely on evidence to prioritize and allocate resources effectively. By identifying interventions that are both clinically effective and cost-effective, decision-makers can make informed choices that optimize the use of limited resources and improve population health outcomes.

Components of Evidence-Based Practice

Evidence-based practice consists of several key components that work together to inform decision-making and promote high-quality care. These components include:

- **Research evidence:** The cornerstone of EBP is empirical research. This includes randomized controlled trials (RCTs), systematic reviews, meta-analyses, and other high-quality studies that generate reliable and valid evidence. Research evidence provides the basis for understanding the effectiveness and safety of different interventions and helps to identify the best approaches for addressing mental health challenges.

- **Clinical expertise:** In addition to research evidence, EBP involves integrating the knowledge, skills, and expertise of mental health professionals. Clinicians' experience, expertise, and judgment play a crucial role in applying research findings to individual cases, considering patient preferences, and making informed decisions about interventions. Clinical expertise ensures that evidence-based recommendations are tailored to the unique needs and circumstances of each individual.

- **Patient values and preferences:** EBP recognizes the importance of considering patient values, preferences, and goals in decision-making. Mental health care should be person-centered, taking into account the individual's beliefs, values, culture, and personal circumstances. By involving patients in the decision-making process and aligning interventions with their preferences, EBP improves treatment adherence and enhances overall outcomes.

- **Quality improvement:** EBP is an iterative process that involves continuous quality improvement. This includes monitoring outcomes, assessing the impact of interventions, and making adjustments to improve care delivery. By systematically evaluating the effectiveness of interventions, monitoring patient outcomes, and implementing evidence-based changes, organizations can ensure that their services are continuously improving and delivering the best possible care.

Strategies for Generating High-Quality Evidence

To build a strong evidence base in mental health, it is essential to generate high-quality evidence through rigorous research methods. Here are some strategies for generating high-quality evidence:

1. **Randomized controlled trials (RCTs):** RCTs are considered the gold standard for determining the efficacy of interventions. By randomly assigning participants to different treatment groups, researchers can minimize bias and establish causality. Conducting well-designed RCTs with appropriate sample sizes and control groups is crucial for generating robust evidence.

2. **Longitudinal studies:** Longitudinal studies follow participants over an extended period, allowing researchers to examine the long-term effects of interventions or track the progression of mental health conditions. Longitudinal studies provide valuable insights into the natural history of mental health disorders and the impact of interventions over time.

3. **Observational studies:** Observational studies, such as cohort studies and case-control studies, can provide important evidence in situations where RCTs are not feasible or ethical. These studies can help identify risk factors, explore associations between variables, and generate hypotheses for further investigation.

4. **Qualitative research:** Qualitative research methods, such as interviews, focus groups, and ethnographic studies, provide rich insights into the lived experiences of individuals with mental health challenges. Qualitative research can help researchers understand the social, cultural, and contextual

factors that influence mental health and inform the development of culturally sensitive interventions.

5. **Implementation research:** Implementation research focuses on the real-world application of interventions and explores factors that facilitate or hinder their adoption and implementation. By studying the implementation process, researchers can identify strategies for effectively translating evidence into practice and addressing barriers to implementation.

6. **Participatory research:** Participatory research actively involves individuals with lived experience in the research process. By partnering with individuals, communities, and organizations, researchers can ensure that research questions are relevant, interventions are acceptable and feasible, and findings are used to drive positive change.

Dissemination of Evidence

Disseminating research findings is a crucial step in building a strong evidence base. High-quality evidence must reach the appropriate audiences, including policymakers, healthcare providers, researchers, and individuals with lived experience. Here are some strategies for effective dissemination:

- **Publication in peer-reviewed journals:** Researchers should aim to publish their findings in reputable peer-reviewed journals. This ensures that the research undergoes rigorous review by experts in the field and meets established scientific standards.

- **Presentations at conferences and workshops:** Researchers can share their findings and engage with the mental health community by presenting at conferences and workshops. These platforms provide opportunities for discussion, collaboration, and knowledge exchange.

- **Policy briefs and reports:** Summarizing research findings in concise and accessible formats, such as policy briefs and reports, can help policymakers and stakeholders understand the implications of the research and make informed decisions.

- **Media engagement:** Collaborating with the media can help raise awareness about important research findings and promote public understanding of mental health issues. Researchers should work with journalists to ensure accurate and responsible reporting that avoids stigmatizing language or misinterpretation of the findings.

- **Knowledge translation:** Knowledge translation refers to the process of moving evidence into practice. Researchers can collaborate with knowledge brokers, such as healthcare organizations or advocacy groups, to ensure that research findings are translated into actionable recommendations and integrated into clinical guidelines and practice.

In conclusion, building a strong evidence base in mental health is essential for improving outcomes, reducing variability in practice, and guiding resource allocation decisions. Evidence-based practice integrates research evidence, clinical expertise, and patient values to guide decision-making. Strategies for generating high-quality evidence include conducting RCTs, longitudinal studies, and qualitative research, as well as implementing participatory and implementation research approaches. Disseminating research findings through peer-reviewed publications, conferences, policy briefs, and media engagement helps ensure that evidence is translated into practice and informs policy decisions. By prioritizing the development and dissemination of high-quality evidence, mental health care can become more effective, efficient, and equitable.

5.3.2 The Importance of Interdisciplinary Collaboration

Introduction

In order to effectively address the complex and multifaceted challenges in the field of mental health, it is crucial to foster interdisciplinary collaboration among various disciplines. Interdisciplinary collaboration brings together professionals from different fields, such as psychology, psychiatry, social work, neuroscience, and public health, to work collaboratively towards a common goal. This section explores the importance of interdisciplinary collaboration in advancing mental health research, education, and practice.

Enhancing Research and Knowledge Creation

Interdisciplinary collaboration plays a vital role in advancing mental health research and knowledge creation. By bringing together experts from different disciplines, researchers can pool their expertise and perspectives to develop a more holistic understanding of mental health issues. This interdisciplinary approach helps in generating innovative research questions, designing comprehensive studies, and analyzing data from multiple angles.

For example, a collaboration between psychologists and neuroscientists can combine behavioral data with neuroimaging techniques to gain a better understanding of the neural mechanisms underlying mental health disorders. This integration of different methodologies and perspectives can lead to groundbreaking discoveries and advancements in the field.

Additionally, interdisciplinary collaboration facilitates the translation of research findings into interventions and policies. Collaborative research teams can identify the practical implications of their findings and work together to develop evidence-based interventions that are applicable across disciplines and settings.

Enriching Education and Training

Interdisciplinary collaboration also enriches education and training in the field of mental health. By exposing students to diverse perspectives and approaches, interdisciplinary education prepares future professionals to work collaboratively and effectively in multidisciplinary teams.

For instance, interdisciplinary courses that bring together students from psychology, social work, and occupational therapy can provide a comprehensive understanding of the complexities of mental health and the importance of a holistic approach to care. These courses allow students to learn from each other's experiences and develop strong interdisciplinary communication and collaboration skills.

Furthermore, interdisciplinary training programs enable students to develop a broader skill set that encompasses knowledge and techniques from different disciplines. This enhanced skill set allows them to provide comprehensive and integrated care to individuals with mental health challenges.

Promoting Holistic and Person-Centered Care

Interdisciplinary collaboration promotes a holistic and person-centered approach to mental health care. By integrating the knowledge and expertise of professionals from various disciplines, the care provided becomes more comprehensive, addressing the physical, psychological, social, and environmental aspects of an individual's well-being.

For example, a collaborative mental health team consisting of a psychiatrist, psychologist, social worker, and occupational therapist can develop a personalized care plan that incorporates pharmacological interventions, psychotherapy, social support, and occupational therapy. This interdisciplinary approach ensures that all

5.3.2 THE IMPORTANCE OF INTERDISCIPLINARY COLLABORATION

aspects of an individual's mental health are addressed, leading to better treatment outcomes.

Interdisciplinary collaboration also helps in identifying and addressing the unique needs of specific populations. For instance, a collaboration between mental health professionals and cultural experts can provide culturally sensitive and tailored care to individuals from diverse backgrounds. This approach acknowledges the influence of culture on mental health and ensures that interventions are appropriate and effective across different cultural contexts.

Overcoming Challenges and Limitations

While interdisciplinary collaboration offers numerous benefits, it also presents challenges and limitations that need to be addressed. One of the primary challenges is the differences in language, methodologies, and approaches across disciplines. Effective interdisciplinary collaboration requires bridging these gaps through effective communication and mutual understanding.

Additionally, power dynamics within interdisciplinary teams can impact collaboration. It is essential to create an inclusive and supportive environment where all team members are valued and their expertise respected. This requires fostering a culture of openness, trust, and mutual respect, where all team members have equal opportunities to contribute and learn from each other.

Moreover, interdisciplinary collaboration requires time, resources, and infrastructure support. This can be challenging in contexts where interdisciplinary collaboration is not prioritized or where funding is primarily discipline-focused. It is crucial to advocate for the importance of interdisciplinary collaboration and allocate resources to support collaborative initiatives.

Conclusion

Interdisciplinary collaboration is essential for advancing mental health research, education, and practice. By bringing together professionals from various disciplines, interdisciplinary collaboration enriches knowledge creation, enhances education and training, promotes holistic care, and overcomes the challenges associated with complex mental health issues. It is through embracing interdisciplinary collaboration that we can collectively work towards a sustainable and comprehensive approach to mental health care.

CHAPTER 5: CONCLUSION: TOWARDS A SUSTAINABLE MENTAL HEALTH FUTURE

Integrating Mental Health into Professional Training

In order to address the growing mental health needs of our society, it is crucial that mental health be integrated into professional training across various disciplines. Professionals in fields such as medicine, psychology, social work, counseling, and education all play a vital role in supporting the mental health and wellbeing of individuals and communities. Integrating mental health into professional training ensures that these professionals are equipped with the knowledge, skills, and competencies necessary to effectively address mental health challenges.

Understanding the Importance of Mental Health in Professional Training

The first step in integrating mental health into professional training is for educators and trainers to recognize the importance of mental health in their respective fields. It is essential to understand that mental health is not just the concern of mental health professionals, but is relevant and applicable across disciplines. For example, medical professionals need to be trained to recognize the signs and symptoms of mental health disorders in their patients, while educators need to understand how mental health can impact students' learning and overall well-being.

By integrating mental health into professional training, professionals in various fields can work collaboratively and holistically to support individuals in all aspects of their lives. This approach recognizes that mental health is interconnected with physical health, social relationships, and environmental factors, and requires a multidimensional understanding.

Core Competencies for Mental Health Integration

To effectively integrate mental health into professional training, there are several core competencies that professionals should develop:

1. **Mental Health Literacy:** Professionals need to have a basic understanding of mental health concepts, including common mental health disorders, risk factors, and protective factors. This knowledge enables professionals to identify signs of mental health issues in their respective domains and provide appropriate support and referrals.

2. **Assessment and Diagnosis:** Professionals should be trained in conducting mental health assessments and making accurate diagnoses when necessary. This involves understanding diagnostic criteria, conducting comprehensive assessments, and using evidence-based assessment tools.

3. **Treatment and Intervention:** Professionals should be equipped with knowledge and skills related to evidence-based treatment modalities and intervention strategies for mental health disorders. This may include therapies such as cognitive-behavioral therapy, psychopharmacology, and other interventions specific to their field.

4. **Screening and Prevention:** Professionals should be trained in the identification and implementation of mental health screening tools and prevention strategies. This includes understanding risk and protective factors, implementing early intervention programs, and promoting mental health promotion and prevention initiatives.

5. **Cultural Competence:** Professionals need to develop cultural competence to effectively work with individuals from diverse backgrounds. This involves understanding cultural norms, values, and beliefs related to mental health, and adapting interventions and treatment plans accordingly.

6. **Ethics and Professional Boundaries:** Professionals should be educated on ethical guidelines and professional boundaries specific to mental health. This includes understanding confidentiality, informed consent, and duty of care.

7. **Interprofessional Collaboration:** Professionals should develop the skills to work collaboratively with other professionals and disciplines to provide comprehensive care. This involves effective communication, interdisciplinary teamwork, and shared decision-making.

Interactive and Experiential Learning

Integration of mental health into professional training should incorporate interactive and experiential learning methods to enhance understanding and application of knowledge. For example, role-playing exercises can allow professionals to practice communication and intervention skills in simulated scenarios. Case studies and real-world examples can further illustrate the complexities and challenges of mental health issues in different contexts. Guest speakers from mental health professions can also provide valuable insights and share their experiences.

Professional training programs should also provide opportunities for self-reflection and self-care. Professionals need to develop self-awareness and learn strategies to manage their own mental health in order to effectively support others.

CHAPTER 5: CONCLUSION: TOWARDS A SUSTAINABLE MENTAL HEALTH FUTURE

Challenges and Considerations

Integrating mental health into professional training is not without its challenges. One of the main challenges is the limited time and resources available within existing curricula. However, incorporating mental health content can be done through careful curriculum planning and collaboration across disciplines.

Another challenge is the stigma surrounding mental health, which may impact professionals' attitudes and comfort in addressing mental health issues. Educators and trainers need to create a safe and supportive learning environment that encourages open discussions and destigmatizes mental health.

Additionally, ongoing training and professional development are crucial for professionals to stay up-to-date with the latest research, interventions, and best practices in the field of mental health. Access to continuing education opportunities should be provided to ensure professionals can continuously enhance their knowledge and skills.

Resources and Further Reading

To support the integration of mental health into professional training, there are a variety of resources available. These include textbooks, journal articles, online courses, and professional organizations that provide guidelines and standards of practice.

Some recommended resources for further reading on integrating mental health into professional training include:

1. World Health Organization (WHO) Mental Health Gap Action Programme (mhGAP): Provides resources and training materials for non-specialists to improve mental health care delivery.
2. American Psychological Association (APA) guidelines for the undergraduate psychology major: Includes recommendations for mental health education in psychology undergraduate curricula.
3. National Alliance on Mental Illness (NAMI) Provider Education Programs: Offers training programs for professionals to better understand mental health conditions and provide support to individuals and families.
4. Substance Abuse and Mental Health Services Administration (SAMHSA) online courses and resources: Provides free online courses and resources on mental health assessment, treatment, and recovery.

It is important for professionals to continually engage in self-directed learning and stay connected to the evolving field of mental health in order to provide the best possible care to their clients or patients.

5.3.2 THE IMPORTANCE OF INTERDISCIPLINARY COLLABORATIONS

In conclusion, integrating mental health into professional training is essential for addressing the mental health needs of individuals and communities. By equipping professionals in various disciplines with the necessary knowledge, skills, and competencies, we can promote a holistic and sustainable approach to mental health care. Through interactive and experiential learning, professionals can develop the core competencies needed to effectively assess, diagnose, treat, and prevent mental health disorders. However, it is important to acknowledge and address the challenges and considerations associated with this integration process. By providing resources and promoting ongoing professional development, we can ensure that professionals are prepared to meet the mental health needs of the individuals they serve.

Promoting Research Translation and Dissemination

In order to ensure the advancement and impact of mental health research, it is crucial to promote the translation and dissemination of research findings. This involves bridging the gap between scientific discoveries and their practical application in clinical settings and communities. Effective research translation and dissemination strategies play a key role in improving mental health outcomes, informing evidence-based practices, and shaping mental health policies. In this section, we will explore various approaches to promote research translation and dissemination in the field of mental health.

Importance of Research Translation and Dissemination

Research translation refers to the process of transforming research findings into practical applications and interventions that can be used in real-world settings. Dissemination, on the other hand, focuses on the communication and distribution of research findings to relevant stakeholders, including policymakers, clinicians, researchers, and the public. Research translation and dissemination are crucial for several reasons:

1. **Informing Evidence-Based Practices:** By translating and disseminating research findings, we can provide clinicians and mental health practitioners with evidence-based practices that have been shown to be effective. This ensures that individuals receive the most appropriate and up-to-date treatments and interventions.

2. **Improving Mental Health Outcomes:** Research translation and dissemination contribute to improving mental health outcomes by enabling

the implementation of effective interventions and treatments. This ensures that individuals facing mental health challenges receive the best care and support available.

3. **Shaping Mental Health Policies:** Research findings can provide valuable insights into the development of mental health policies and interventions at the local, national, and global levels. By disseminating research to policymakers, we can influence the formulation of evidence-based policies that promote mental health and wellbeing.

4. **Building a Strong Evidence Base:** Research translation and dissemination contribute to building a robust evidence base in the field of mental health. This allows for further research and development of innovative interventions, ultimately improving our understanding of mental health and wellbeing.

Strategies for Research Translation and Dissemination

To effectively translate and disseminate research in the field of mental health, it is important to employ a range of strategies that target different stakeholders and utilize various communication channels. Here are some key strategies for research translation and dissemination:

1. **Engaging Stakeholders:** Engaging relevant stakeholders, such as clinicians, policymakers, researchers, and community members, is crucial for successful research translation and dissemination. By involving stakeholders in the research process from the beginning, researchers can ensure that the findings are relevant, practical, and easily applicable in real-world settings.

2. **Communicating in Plain Language:** Research findings can often be complex and filled with jargon, making it challenging for non-experts to understand and apply the information. Using plain language and clear communication strategies is essential for effective research translation and dissemination. This includes summarizing research findings, using visual aids and infographics, and providing practical implications and recommendations.

3. **Utilizing Multiple Communication Channels:** To reach a wide audience, it is important to utilize multiple communication channels for research dissemination. This can include traditional methods such as academic publications, conferences, and workshops, as well as newer platforms such as online blogs, social media, and podcasts. By using a combination of

5.3.2 THE IMPORTANCE OF INTERDISCIPLINARY COLLABORATION

channels, researchers can effectively engage with diverse stakeholders and increase the visibility and impact of their research.

4. **Collaborating with Knowledge Users:** Engaging with knowledge users, such as policymakers, clinicians, and community organizations, is critical for the successful translation of research into practice. By actively involving knowledge users in the research process, researchers can ensure that their findings are relevant and applicable to real-world contexts. This collaboration can also facilitate the co-production of knowledge and the development of innovative interventions.

5. **Tailoring Messages for Different Audiences:** Different audiences have varying levels of knowledge and understanding of mental health issues. It is important to tailor research messages to suit the needs and preferences of different audiences. This includes adapting the language, format, and content of research findings to make them accessible and engaging for specific groups, such as policymakers, clinicians, or community members.

6. **Promoting Open Access and Data Sharing:** Open access publishing and data sharing are important practices that promote research transparency and accessibility. By making research findings freely available to the public and sharing research data, researchers can maximize the impact and reproducibility of their work. This allows for wider dissemination, collaboration, and the potential for further innovation and discovery.

Challenges and Considerations

While research translation and dissemination are essential, they are not without challenges and considerations. Some of the key challenges include:

1. **Language and Communication Barriers:** Communicating research findings effectively to diverse audiences can be challenging due to language barriers, literacy levels, and cultural differences. Researchers need to consider these factors and employ strategies that overcome these barriers, such as using plain language, visual aids, and culturally appropriate messaging.

2. **Knowledge Gaps and Research-Practice Gap:** There can often be a gap between research findings and their integration into practice. This research-practice gap can be due to various factors, including limited awareness and understanding of research findings among practitioners, lack of resources for implementation, and resistance to change. Researchers need

to address these gaps by actively engaging with knowledge users, providing support for implementation, and fostering collaborations between researchers and practitioners.

3. **Ethical Considerations:** When translating and disseminating research, ethical considerations need to be taken into account. This includes ensuring the privacy and confidentiality of research participants, obtaining informed consent, and appropriately attributing the work of others. Researchers should adhere to ethical guidelines and seek institutional approval when disseminating research findings.

4. **Misinterpretation and Misuse of Findings:** Research findings can sometimes be misinterpreted or misused, leading to inappropriate or ineffective interventions. Researchers should be mindful of how their findings are presented and provide clear explanations and limitations to prevent misinterpretation. Collaboration with knowledge users and engaging in ongoing dialogue can help bridge gaps in understanding and address any potential misuse of research findings.

In summary, the promotion of research translation and dissemination is critical for enhancing mental health outcomes, informing evidence-based practices, and shaping mental health policies. Researchers play a pivotal role in ensuring that their findings reach the intended audiences in a meaningful and accessible manner. By employing strategies such as engaging stakeholders, communicating in plain language, utilizing multiple communication channels, and collaborating with knowledge users, researchers can maximize the impact of their research and contribute to a more sustainable future for mental health.

Strengthening Mental Health Policies and Systems

The Role of Government and Legislators

Government and legislators play a crucial role in shaping and influencing mental health policies and systems. As representatives of the people, they have the responsibility to create an enabling environment that promotes mental health and ensures access to quality mental health services for all individuals. In this section, we will explore the specific roles and responsibilities of government and legislators in promoting and supporting mental health.

Policy Development

One of the primary roles of government and legislators is the development and implementation of mental health policies. These policies serve as a roadmap for addressing mental health issues within a country or a particular jurisdiction. They provide strategic direction, outline goals and objectives, and serve as a guide for allocating resources. Government and legislators should work together with mental health experts, professionals, and stakeholders to develop evidence-based policies that address the needs of the population.

Policy development in mental health should prioritize the integration of mental health into overall health policies and frameworks. This integration recognizes the interconnectedness of mental health with physical health and emphasizes the importance of a holistic approach towards healthcare. It also involves developing policies that address the social determinants of mental health, such as poverty, education, housing, and social support systems.

In addition to policy development, government and legislators are responsible for ensuring the implementation and monitoring of mental health policies. This includes establishing mechanisms to track progress, evaluate outcomes, and make necessary adjustments based on evidence and best practices.

Legislation and Regulation

Government and legislators are instrumental in enacting laws and regulations that protect the rights of individuals with mental health conditions and ensure the provision of quality mental health services. These laws serve as a legal framework for addressing mental health issues and promoting the well-being of individuals with mental illness.

Legislation and regulation in mental health may encompass a wide range of areas, including:

- **Human rights and anti-discrimination laws:** Government and legislators should enact laws that protect the rights of individuals with mental health conditions, including their right to privacy, dignity, and non-discrimination. These laws should also address issues such as stigma and ensure equal access to employment, education, and housing.

- **Mental health care standards and regulations:** Government and legislators should establish standards and regulations for mental health care providers and facilities to ensure the delivery of safe, effective, and quality care. This includes licensing and accreditation processes, guidelines for treatment approaches, and supervision and oversight mechanisms.

- **Involuntary commitment and treatment laws:** Government and legislators should establish laws that govern the involuntary commitment and treatment of individuals with severe mental illness who pose a risk to themselves or others. These laws should strike a balance between protecting individuals' rights and ensuring public safety.

- **Access to mental health medications and services:** Government and legislators should work towards removing barriers to access mental health medications and services by enacting laws that promote affordability and availability. This may include regulations on drug pricing, insurance coverage for mental health services, and the integration of mental health services into primary care settings.

It is important for government and legislators to regularly review and update mental health legislation to reflect advances in research, changes in societal attitudes, and emerging challenges. They should also ensure that legislation aligns with international human rights standards and conventions, such as the United Nations Convention on the Rights of Persons with Disabilities.

Resource Allocation and Funding

Government and legislators have the authority and responsibility to allocate resources and funding for mental health programs and services. They must prioritize mental health within overall health budgets and ensure that sufficient resources are allocated to meet the needs of the population.

Resource allocation should be guided by evidence-based practices and the specific mental health needs of the population. It should also consider the social determinants of mental health and address disparities in access to care. Government and legislators should work with relevant stakeholders, including mental health experts and service providers, to determine resource allocation priorities and strategies.

In addition to direct funding, government and legislators can also seek funding from external sources, such as international organizations, to support mental health initiatives. They should actively explore partnerships and collaborations to leverage resources and expand the reach of mental health programs and services.

Advocacy and Awareness

Government and legislators have a unique platform to advocate for mental health awareness and promote positive attitudes towards mental illness. They can use their influence and positions to educate the public, challenge stigma, and promote understanding of mental health issues.

By engaging in public awareness campaigns, government and legislators can help reduce the barriers to seeking help and increase the recognition and acceptance of mental health as an integral part of overall well-being. They can also work with community leaders, faith-based organizations, and schools to disseminate accurate and culturally sensitive information about mental health.

Furthermore, government and legislators can advocate for the inclusion of mental health education in school curricula, workplace wellness programs, and community initiatives. By integrating mental health into various aspects of society, they can help create a culture that values and prioritizes mental well-being.

Conclusion

Government and legislators have a crucial role to play in building a sustainable mental health future. Through policy development, legislation and regulation, resource allocation and funding, and advocacy and awareness, they can create an enabling environment that promotes mental health, ensures access to quality care, and reduces stigma.

However, it is essential for governments and legislators to work in collaboration with mental health experts, professionals, and stakeholders to develop and implement effective policies and programs. They must listen to the needs and experiences of individuals with mental health conditions and prioritize their rights and well-being.

By taking an active role in mental health, government and legislators can contribute to the overall sustainability of their societies, leading to improved outcomes for individuals, families, and communities. They have the power to make a positive impact and drive transformative change in mental health care.

Financing and Resource Allocation for Mental Health

Ensuring adequate financing and resource allocation for mental health is crucial in order to provide optimal care and support for individuals experiencing psychological challenges. In this section, we will explore the various aspects related to financing mental health services, including funding sources, budget allocation, and the importance of equitable resource distribution.

Current Challenges in Financing Mental Health

The financing of mental health services is often plagued by several challenges, which can hinder the availability and accessibility of quality care. Some of the key challenges include:

1. **Underfunding:** Mental health services are often overlooked when it comes to budgetary allocations. This underfunding can lead to a lack of resources, inadequate staffing, and a limited range of services. As a result, many individuals do not receive the necessary support they require.

2. **Fragmented funding streams:** Mental health services are often funded through a combination of public and private sources, leading to a fragmented funding landscape. This can result in disparities in service availability and variations in resource allocation across different regions or populations.

3. **Inequitable resource distribution:** Resources for mental health care are not always distributed equitably, with marginalized populations often receiving less support. This can perpetuate existing health disparities and exacerbate social inequalities.

4. **Lack of integration:** Mental health is often treated as a separate entity from general healthcare, resulting in a lack of integration within health systems. This can lead to gaps in care coordination, limited collaboration between mental health and other healthcare providers, and inefficiencies in resource utilization.

Funding Sources for Mental Health

There are different sources of funding for mental health services, which can vary across countries and healthcare systems. Some common funding sources include:

1. **Government funding:** Governments play a critical role in financing mental health services, both at the national and local levels. Public funding can come from general tax revenues or dedicated mental health budgets. This funding is essential for ensuring the provision of basic mental health care services to the population.

2. **Private health insurance:** Many individuals have private health insurance coverage, which can include mental health benefits. Private insurance providers contribute to financing mental health services by reimbursing healthcare providers for services rendered to their insured members. However, the availability and extent of mental health coverage can vary depending on the insurance plan.

3. **Out-of-pocket payments:** Individuals may also pay for mental health services out of their own pockets, particularly in countries with limited public funding or inadequate insurance coverage. This can place a financial burden on individuals and may lead to disparities in access to care.

4. **Philanthropic organizations and non-profit agencies:** Non-governmental organizations (NGOs), community foundations, and charitable organizations often contribute to financing mental health services through grants, donations, and fundraising efforts. These funding sources can help bridge gaps in funding and support innovative initiatives.

Budget Allocation and Resource Planning

Effective budget allocation and resource planning are essential to ensure that mental health services receive adequate funding and resources. Some key considerations in this process include:

1. **Needs assessment:** Conducting a comprehensive assessment of mental health needs is crucial to inform resource planning. This involves analyzing the population's mental health profile, identifying service gaps, and understanding the specific needs of different population groups.

2. **Evidence-based decision making:** Budget allocation should be based on evidence-based practices and interventions that have been proven effective. This ensures that resources are allocated to services and programs that have a significant impact on mental health outcomes.

3. **Integration and coordination:** Mental health should be integrated into overall health system planning and resource allocation. This includes ensuring collaboration between mental health and primary care providers, as well as coordination with other sectors such as education, social services, and criminal justice.

4. **Promoting cost-effectiveness:** Resource planning should prioritize cost-effective interventions that maximize the value of investment. This involves analyzing the costs and benefits of different interventions and considering long-term outcomes and sustainability.

5. **Advocacy and stakeholder engagement:** Engaging stakeholders, including mental health professionals, service users, advocacy groups, and policymakers, is vital to ensure that resource allocation reflects the diverse needs and priorities of the population. Advocacy efforts can help raise awareness and garner support for increased funding for mental health.

Strategies for Equitable Resource Allocation

Achieving equitable resource allocation is crucial to address the disparities in access to mental health care. To promote equitable distribution of resources, the following strategies can be employed:

1. **Needs-based resource allocation:** Allocate resources based on the identified mental health needs of different populations. This includes considering factors such as the prevalence of mental health disorders, socio-economic disparities, and geographical distribution of services.

2. **Targeted interventions:** Allocate resources to specific populations or communities that are known to face higher mental health risks or have unique mental health needs. This can include marginalized groups, children and adolescents, older adults, and individuals experiencing homelessness.

3. **Integration of mental health into primary care:** Ensure that mental health services are integrated into primary care settings, where individuals often seek healthcare. This can help improve access to mental health services, particularly in underserved areas.

4. **Promoting community-based services:** Allocate resources to community-based mental health services, such as mobile clinics, outreach programs, and peer support networks. These services can reach individuals who may have difficulties accessing traditional healthcare settings.

5. **Capacity building:** Invest in training and development programs to build the capacity of mental health professionals, particularly in areas with limited resources. This can help address the shortage of mental health professionals and improve the quality of care.

6. **Monitoring and evaluation:** Establish robust monitoring and evaluation systems to assess the impact of resource allocation strategies. This involves regularly collecting data on mental health outcomes, service utilization, and resource allocation to inform decision-making and facilitate continuous improvement.

Case Study: Mental Health Financing in Country X

Let's consider the case of Country X, where mental health services are currently underfunded and face significant resource constraints. The government has recognized the need to improve mental health care and promote equitable resource allocation. To address this challenge, the following steps are being taken:

1. **Increasing government funding:** The government has allocated a dedicated budget for mental health, alongside the general healthcare budget. This increase in funding aims to address the existing resource gaps and ensure the provision of quality mental health services.

2. **Expanding health insurance coverage:** Efforts are being made to expand private health insurance coverage to include comprehensive mental health benefits.

This will help reduce out-of-pocket expenses for individuals seeking mental health care.

3. **Developing targeted programs:** Special programs are being developed to address the specific mental health needs of vulnerable populations, such as refugees, low-income individuals, and those living in remote areas. These programs include community-based services, mobile clinics, and telehealth initiatives.

4. **Capacity building and workforce development:** Training programs are being implemented to enhance the skills and competencies of mental health professionals. This includes training in evidence-based interventions, cultural competence, and trauma-informed care.

5. **Comprehensive monitoring and evaluation system:** A robust monitoring and evaluation system is being established to assess the impact of resource allocation strategies. This includes tracking mental health outcomes, service utilization rates, and resource distribution across different regions.

By implementing these strategies, Country X aims to improve access to mental health services, address disparities, and promote equitable resource allocation.

Conclusion

Financing and resource allocation play a crucial role in determining the availability and accessibility of mental health services. Adequate funding, along with equitable distribution and effective resource planning, can help bridge the gaps in mental healthcare provision. It is essential for governments, policymakers, and stakeholders to invest in mental health, promote integration within the healthcare system, and engage in evidence-based decision-making to ensure the sustainability of mental health services for the future. By prioritizing mental health financing, we can support individuals in their journey towards holistic wellbeing and overall sustainability.

Strengthening Mental Health Services

In order to promote holistic mental health and provide effective care to individuals, it is essential to strengthen mental health services. This involves improving the accessibility, quality, and availability of mental health care to meet the diverse needs of individuals and communities. Strengthening mental health services requires a coordinated effort from various stakeholders, including governments, healthcare providers, professionals, and community organizations.

Addressing the Treatment Gap

One of the key challenges in mental health care is the treatment gap, which refers to the disparity between the number of individuals with mental health disorders and the availability of services to meet their needs. To address the treatment gap, several strategies can be implemented:

- **Increasing funding:** Allocating sufficient resources to mental health services is crucial for expanding capacity and improving accessibility. Governments should prioritize mental health funding and invest in the development of mental health infrastructure, workforce training, and research.

- **Strengthening community-based services:** Enhancing community-based mental health services can help reach individuals who may face barriers to accessing traditional healthcare settings. This includes establishing mental health clinics, mobile units, and telehealth services to provide care in underserved areas.

- **Integrating mental health into primary care:** Integrating mental health services into primary care settings can help increase early detection, improve access to treatment, and reduce stigma associated with seeking mental health care. This can be achieved through training primary care providers in mental health screening, assessment, and basic interventions.

- **Expanding the mental health workforce:** Investing in the recruitment, training, and retention of mental health professionals is essential to meet the growing demand for services. This includes psychiatrists, psychologists, social workers, and counselors. Additionally, supporting the development of peer support workers and community health workers can help bridge the treatment gap in resource-constrained settings.

Improving Quality of Care

Improving the quality of mental health services is vital to ensure that individuals receive effective, evidence-based care. The following strategies can help enhance the quality of mental health services:

- **Implementing evidence-based practices:** Mental health services should be based on the best available evidence. This involves promoting the use of evidence-based assessment tools, treatment guidelines, and interventions. Regular training and supervision should be provided to ensure healthcare providers are up-to-date with the latest research and best practices.

- **Monitoring and evaluation:** Monitoring and evaluating the quality of mental health services is crucial to identify areas for improvement. This can be accomplished through routine data collection, performance indicators, and patient feedback. Regular evaluation can help identify gaps in service delivery, measure outcomes, and inform quality improvement initiatives.

- **Ensuring cultural competence:** Mental health services must be culturally sensitive and responsive to the diverse needs of individuals and communities. Healthcare providers should receive training in cultural competence to understand and address the unique factors that influence mental health within different cultural contexts. This includes considering language barriers, cultural beliefs, and practices that may impact help-seeking behavior and treatment adherence.

- **Promoting interdisciplinary collaboration:** Mental health services often require a multidisciplinary approach, involving collaboration between psychiatrists, psychologists, social workers, nurses, and other professionals. Creating opportunities for interdisciplinary training and collaboration can enhance the comprehensive care provided to individuals with mental health disorders.

Ensuring Accessibility and Equity

Ensuring accessibility and equity in mental health services is essential to promote social justice and reduce disparities. The following strategies can help improve accessibility and enhance equity in mental health care:

- **Reducing stigma and discrimination:** Stigma associated with mental illness can be a significant barrier to help-seeking behavior. Anti-stigma campaigns, education, and public awareness initiatives can help reduce the prejudice and discrimination faced by individuals with mental health disorders. Promoting positive portrayals of mental health in the media and fostering inclusive communities can also contribute to reducing stigma.

- **Addressing socioeconomic barriers:** Financial constraints can be a significant barrier to accessing mental health services. Governments should strive to provide financial assistance programs, insurance coverage, and subsidies for mental health care. Additionally, addressing social determinants of mental health, such as poverty, unemployment, and housing instability, can help improve overall mental wellbeing.

- **Tailoring services to diverse populations:** Mental health services should be tailored to meet the specific needs of diverse populations, including racial and ethnic minorities, LGBTQ+ individuals, refugees, and individuals with disabilities. This involves providing culturally competent care, language services, and ensuring the availability of specialized programs that address the unique challenges faced by these populations.

- **Promoting community engagement:** Engaging communities in mental health promotion and service delivery can help ensure that services are relevant, accessible, and accepted. Community-based organizations, faith-based institutions, and non-governmental organizations can play a crucial role in raising awareness, providing support, and promoting mental health literacy.

Integrating Mental Health into Public Health Approaches

To strengthen mental health services, it is essential to integrate mental health into broader public health approaches. This involves recognizing the interconnections between mental health and other health domains, such as physical health, social determinants of health, and environmental factors. The following strategies can facilitate the integration of mental health into public health:

- **Health promotion and prevention:** Promoting mental health and preventing mental illness should be key components of public health strategies. This can be achieved through targeted interventions, such as mental health awareness campaigns, stress reduction programs, and resilience-building initiatives. Public health policies should prioritize mental health promotion across the lifespan, from early childhood to old age.

- **Data collection and surveillance:** Collecting comprehensive data on the prevalence, risk factors, and burden of mental health disorders is crucial for informing policy development and resource allocation. This includes integrating mental health indicators into routine health surveillance systems, conducting population-based surveys, and utilizing data to monitor trends and guide intervention efforts.

- **Policy development and advocacy:** Advocacy for mental health at all levels, including local, national, and international, is important for shaping policies that support the strengthening of mental health services. Mental health should be prioritized in policy agendas, and evidence-based recommendations should be used to guide policy development. Collaboration between mental health professionals, policymakers, and advocacy organizations can help drive meaningful change.

- **Research and innovation:** Advancing mental health research is essential to identify new interventions, improve existing services, and address emerging challenges. Public health approaches should support the development of innovative solutions, technology applications, and the dissemination of research findings. Collaboration between researchers, practitioners, and policymakers can help bridge the gap between research and practice.

Strengthening mental health services requires a comprehensive and multifaceted approach that addresses the treatment gap, improves quality of care, ensures accessibility and equity, and integrates mental health into public health approaches. By implementing these strategies, we can work towards a future where mental health services are sustainable, effective, and responsive to the needs of individuals and communities.

Ensuring Equity in Mental Health Care

Ensuring equity in mental health care is essential in providing fair and equal access to services for all individuals, regardless of their background or circumstances. Achieving equity requires addressing the barriers and disparities that exist in mental health care delivery, including unequal distribution of resources, lack of cultural competency, and systemic biases. In this section, we will explore strategies and approaches to promote equity in mental health care.

Understanding Mental Health Disparities

Mental health disparities refer to the unequal burden of mental illness and unequal access to mental health care experienced by certain populations. These disparities can be influenced by factors such as race, ethnicity, socioeconomic status, gender identity, sexual orientation, disability, and geographic location. It is crucial to examine these disparities and their underlying causes to develop targeted interventions and policies.

Research has shown that marginalized and underserved communities are more likely to experience mental health challenges due to various social determinants of health, such as poverty, discrimination, and limited access to quality education and healthcare. Discrimination and stigma can also prevent individuals from seeking help and receiving adequate mental health care.

Reducing Barriers to Access

To ensure equity in mental health care, it is important to reduce barriers to access for underserved populations. This can be achieved through various strategies:

- **Increasing availability of mental health services:** There is a need to expand mental health services in underserved areas, including rural and remote communities. This can be done by improving access to mental health professionals, establishing telemedicine programs, and integrating mental health services into primary care settings.

- **Addressing affordability:** The high cost of mental health care can be a significant barrier for many individuals, especially those with limited financial resources. Implementation of affordable and accessible mental health services, including sliding fee scales, insurance coverage, and financial assistance programs, is crucial to ensure equitable access to care.

- **Improving cultural competency:** Mental health care providers need to be culturally competent and sensitive to the diverse backgrounds and experiences of their patients. This includes understanding and addressing cultural beliefs, values, and practices that may influence help-seeking behaviors and treatment preferences. Training programs and continuing education can help enhance cultural competence among mental health professionals.

- **Reducing stigma and discrimination:** Stigma and discrimination associated with mental illness can prevent individuals from seeking help. Efforts should be made to challenge stereotypes, promote mental health literacy, and create a supportive and inclusive environment that encourages help-seeking behaviors.

- **Engaging communities and promoting outreach:** Community-based initiatives and outreach programs play a vital role in reaching underserved populations. Collaborating with community organizations, religious institutions, schools, and other stakeholders can help raise awareness about mental health, provide support, and connect individuals to appropriate services.

Integrating Equity in Mental Health Policies

To ensure equity in mental health care, it is essential to integrate equity considerations into mental health policies and systems. Some key approaches include:

- **Policy development and implementation:** Governments and policymakers should prioritize mental health equity in policy development and implementation. This includes allocating resources appropriately, monitoring and evaluating the impact of policies on underserved populations, and making adjustments as needed.

- **Data collection and research:** Collecting disaggregated data on mental health outcomes and access to services is critical to identify and address disparities. Research should focus on understanding the unique needs and experiences of underserved populations and informing evidence-based interventions.

- **Culturally appropriate services:** Mental health services should be tailored to meet the specific needs of different communities. This requires the involvement of community leaders, advocating for culturally appropriate interventions, and ensuring representation in policymaking processes.

- **Equity-oriented workforce development:** The mental health workforce should reflect the diversity of the population it serves. Efforts should be made to recruit, train, and retain mental health professionals from underrepresented backgrounds. Training programs should incorporate cultural humility and emphasize the importance of addressing health disparities.

- **Collaboration and coordination:** Collaboration between government agencies, healthcare organizations, community-based organizations, and advocacy groups is crucial for addressing mental health disparities. Coordinated efforts can maximize resources, share best practices, and improve service delivery.

Case Study: Improving Mental Health Care for Underserved Communities

Let's consider a case study of a community mental health center in a low-income neighborhood that has experienced significant mental health disparities. The center takes a comprehensive approach to ensure equity in mental health care:

- **Community engagement:** The center actively engages with community members to understand their needs and challenges. This includes conducting community needs assessments, holding town hall meetings, and establishing advisory boards with diverse representation.

- **Integrated care model:** The center adopts an integrated care model that combines mental health services with primary healthcare. By addressing physical and mental health needs in one setting, individuals have access to comprehensive and holistic care.

- **Culturally competent services:** The center recruits and trains a diverse workforce that reflects the demographics of the community. Staff members receive ongoing cultural competency training to effectively serve individuals from different backgrounds. Interpretation and translation services are also available to overcome language barriers.

- **Financial assistance programs:** The center offers a sliding fee scale based on income to ensure that individuals can afford services. Staff members provide guidance and assistance in navigating insurance options and applying for financial aid programs.

- **Outreach and education:** The center conducts outreach activities to raise awareness about mental health and combat stigma. They collaborate with local schools, religious institutions, and community organizations to provide education and support. They also provide information and resources in multiple languages to reach diverse populations.

- **Data monitoring and evaluation:** The center collects data on patient demographics, treatment outcomes, and satisfaction to monitor the impact of their services. Regular evaluations help identify areas for improvement and guide decision-making processes.

This case study highlights the importance of a multidimensional approach to ensure equity in mental health care. By addressing barriers, tailoring services to community needs, and involving various stakeholders, the center promotes equitable access to quality care.

Conclusion

Ensuring equity in mental health care requires a comprehensive and multifaceted approach that addresses the barriers and disparities faced by underserved populations. By reducing barriers to access, promoting cultural competency, integrating equity considerations in policies, and engaging communities, we can work towards a more equitable mental health care system. By striving for equity, we can improve the overall well-being and outcomes of individuals and communities.

Promoting Mental Health Advocacy and Awareness

The Power of Stigma Reduction

Stigma surrounding mental health has been a significant barrier to seeking help, accessing treatment, and achieving overall well-being. It has perpetuated discrimination, exclusion, and social isolation for individuals experiencing mental health challenges. Stigma can be defined as a set of negative beliefs, attitudes, and stereotypes that lead to the marginalization and devaluation of those with mental health conditions.

In recent years, there has been a growing recognition of the detrimental effects of stigma on mental health and a concerted effort to combat it. Stigma reduction plays a crucial role in creating a supportive and inclusive environment for individuals with mental health conditions. Let's explore the power of stigma reduction and the different strategies employed to challenge and change societal attitudes and perceptions.

Understanding the Impact of Stigma

The consequences of stigma are far-reaching and can have profound effects on individuals' lives. Stigmatized attitudes can:

- Prevent individuals from seeking help: Stigma often leads to self-stigmatization, causing individuals to internalize negative beliefs about themselves and feel ashamed of their mental health condition. This self-imposed stigma can prevent people from seeking the support they need, resulting in delayed or inadequate treatment.

- Limit opportunities for social inclusion: Stigmatization can lead to discrimination in housing, education, employment, and other areas of life. This exclusion can perpetuate a cycle of poverty, isolation, and poor mental health outcomes.

- Hinder recovery and well-being: The fear of being judged or rejected can make it difficult for individuals to open up about their experiences, leading to feelings of loneliness and isolation. This lack of support can impede the recovery process and exacerbate mental health conditions.

Recognizing the impact of stigma is the first step towards creating a stigma-free society and ensuring the well-being of those affected by mental health challenges.

Strategies for Stigma Reduction

Stigma reduction efforts aim to challenge existing stereotypes, change negative attitudes, and promote a more inclusive society. Here are some strategies that have been effective in combating stigma:

1. **Education and Awareness:** Increasing public knowledge and understanding of mental health conditions is essential in reducing stigma. Educational campaigns and initiatives can help dispel myths, provide accurate information, and promote empathy and compassion. These efforts should target various audiences, including schools, workplaces, and communities.

2. **Contact-Based Interventions:** Personal contact with individuals with lived experiences of mental health challenges has been shown to be an effective way to reduce stigma. Encouraging dialogue and interaction between those with mental health conditions and the general public can help challenge stereotypes and foster empathy.

3. **Media Representation:** Media plays a powerful role in shaping public perceptions. Promoting accurate and positive portrayals of mental health conditions in films, television shows, and advertisements can help counter stigmatizing narratives. Responsible reporting by media outlets can also contribute to reducing stigma and promoting understanding.

4. **Language Matters:** The use of stigmatizing language can reinforce negative attitudes towards mental health. Encouraging the use of person-centered language that focuses on the individual rather than their condition is crucial. This includes avoiding derogatory terms and using terminology that promotes dignity, respect, and inclusivity.

5. **Support and Peer Networks:** Encouraging the formation of support groups and peer networks can create safe spaces for individuals living with mental health conditions. These networks provide opportunities for sharing experiences, finding support, and challenging stigma collectively.

6. **Legislation and Policy Changes:** Advocacy for mental health policy reform is crucial in addressing systemic issues that contribute to stigma. Legal protections

against discrimination, ensuring equal access to healthcare, and promoting mental health parity can help create a more equitable society.

Measuring the Impact

Assessing the effectiveness of stigma reduction efforts is essential in refining strategies and ensuring positive outcomes. Several measures can be employed to evaluate the impact of stigma reduction interventions:

1. **Surveys and Questionnaires:** By using standardized scales, researchers can measure changes in attitudes, beliefs, and behaviors related to mental health stigma. Pre- and post-intervention surveys can provide valuable data on the effectiveness of specific interventions.

2. **Qualitative Research:** In-depth interviews, focus groups, and narrative analysis can provide insights into individuals' experiences, shedding light on the mechanisms through which stigma operates and how it can be challenged.

3. **Observational Studies:** Direct observations in settings such as schools, workplaces, or communities can help assess changes in behavior and interactions related to mental health stigma.

4. **Longitudinal Studies:** By following individuals over time, researchers can examine changes in stigma-related attitudes and behaviors, as well as the long-term effects of stigma reduction interventions.

Evaluation of the impact of stigma reduction efforts provides valuable information on the effectiveness of different interventions and enables the development of evidence-based practices.

Conclusion

Stigma reduction is a crucial element in creating a society that supports the mental health and well-being of all individuals. By challenging stereotypes, promoting understanding, and fostering empathy, we can create an environment where individuals feel comfortable seeking help and where recovery and overall sustainability are prioritized.

By employing educational campaigns, contact-based interventions, responsible media representation, and supportive policies, we can work towards dismantling the barriers imposed by stigma. The power of stigma reduction lies in its potential to create a more inclusive society where mental health is understood, accepted, and supported by all.

As we continue our journey towards a sustainable mental health future, let us remember the power we hold as individuals and communities to challenge stigma and promote positive change. Each step we take towards reducing stigma is a step towards a more compassionate and resilient society.

Effective Communication Strategies

Effective communication is a vital component of promoting mental health and wellbeing. It involves the exchange of information, ideas, and emotions between individuals or groups, fostering understanding and connection. In the context of mental health, effective communication plays a crucial role in reducing stigma, enhancing help-seeking behaviors, and promoting awareness and support. This section explores key strategies for effective communication in the field of mental health.

1. Creating a Safe and Nonjudgmental Environment

One of the fundamental principles of effective communication in mental health is creating a safe and nonjudgmental environment. This involves establishing trust, compassion, and respect when engaging with individuals experiencing mental health challenges. Practitioners should avoid labeling, blaming, or stigmatizing language that could further distress the person seeking help. Using person-first language, such as saying "a person with schizophrenia" instead of "a schizophrenic," can help reduce stigma and promote a person-centered approach.

2. Active Listening and Empathy

Active listening is a critical skill for effective communication in mental health. It involves fully paying attention to the speaker, being present in the moment, and actively processing the information being shared. Active listening shows empathy, validates the person's feelings and experiences, and creates a sense of being understood.

Practitioners can enhance active listening by using non-verbal cues, such as nodding, maintaining eye contact, and mirroring body language, to convey attentiveness. Reflective listening techniques, such as paraphrasing or summarizing the speaker's words, can also promote understanding and empathy. Additionally, focusing on the speaker's emotions and asking open-ended questions can encourage further exploration of their thoughts and feelings.

3. Clear and Simple Language

Using clear and simple language is essential when communicating about mental health. Complex medical or technical terms can be confusing and alienating for individuals seeking help. It is important to avoid jargon and use plain language that is easily understood by the target audience.

Practitioners should strive to explain concepts in a way that is relatable and accessible. Metaphors or analogies can be employed to simplify complex ideas and make them more relatable. Using visual aids, such as diagrams or illustrations, can also enhance understanding and facilitate effective communication.

4. Education and Psychoeducation

Education is a powerful tool in promoting mental health and combating stigma. Providing accurate and evidence-based information about mental health can help dispel misconceptions and foster understanding. Psychoeducation, which involves educating individuals and their families about specific mental health conditions and treatment options, is an effective communication strategy.

Practitioners can use various mediums to deliver education and psychoeducation, including workshops, support groups, online resources, and informational handouts. Tailoring the content to the specific needs and cultural background of the target audience is crucial for effective communication and engagement.

5. Collaboration and Shared Decision-Making

Promoting collaboration and shared decision-making is vital for effective communication in mental health. It involves actively involving individuals in the treatment planning process and respecting their autonomy and preferences. This approach shifts the power dynamic from a traditional provider-patient relationship to a partnership based on mutual trust and respect.

Practitioners should engage in active discussions with individuals, ensuring they understand their treatment options, risks, benefits, and alternatives. Informed consent should be obtained for any interventions, and individuals should be encouraged to express their opinions, concerns, and goals. Collaboration and shared decision-making enhance treatment adherence, satisfaction, and overall mental health outcomes.

6. Cultural Competence and Sensitivity

In a diverse and multicultural society, cultural competence and sensitivity are essential components of effective communication in mental health. Understanding and respecting cultural differences can help bridge communication gaps and avoid misunderstandings.

Practitioners should educate themselves about various cultures, beliefs, values, and traditions to provide culturally appropriate care. It is important to be aware of potential biases and stereotypes and to approach each individual with an open mind. Tailoring communication styles and interventions to align with cultural preferences can enhance engagement and promote better mental health outcomes.

7. Utilizing Technology and Digital Tools

In the digital age, technology offers new avenues for effective communication in mental health. Telemedicine and virtual platforms, such as video conferencing or online support groups, can improve access to mental health services, particularly for individuals in remote or underserved areas. These tools allow for real-time communication and can be more convenient for individuals with mobility or transportation challenges.

Practitioners should be mindful of the ethical considerations and privacy issues associated with technology-mediated communication. Ensuring secure and confidential platforms, obtaining informed consent, and maintaining professional boundaries are essential for maintaining the integrity of the therapeutic relationship.

8. Storytelling and Personal Narratives

Storytelling and personal narratives have the power to connect individuals, reduce stigma, and inspire hope. Sharing personal experiences with mental health challenges can help others feel less alone and create a sense of community.

Practitioners can encourage individuals with lived experiences to share their stories, either through public forums, support groups, or written testimonials. Personal narratives can be incorporated into educational materials, campaigns, or awareness events to foster empathy, challenge stereotypes, and promote understanding.

Conclusion

Effective communication is a cornerstone of promoting mental health and wellbeing. By creating a safe and nonjudgmental environment, practicing active listening and empathy, using clear and simple language, providing education and psychoeducation, fostering collaboration and shared decision-making, demonstrating cultural competence and sensitivity, utilizing technology and digital tools, and embracing storytelling and personal narratives, practitioners can enhance their communication skills and make a positive impact on individuals and communities. It is through effective communication strategies that we can break down barriers, reduce stigma, and foster a more inclusive and supportive society for mental health.

Engaging Communities in Mental Health Promotion

In order to address the complex challenges of mental health promotion, it is essential to engage communities at various levels. Communities play a crucial role in supporting individuals and shaping their mental health outcomes. By fostering community involvement, we can create a conducive environment that promotes mental well-being and resilience. In this section, we will explore different strategies to effectively engage communities in mental health promotion efforts.

Understanding the Role of Communities

Communities are dynamic units that include individuals, families, local organizations, and institutions. They provide a social support system and influence the overall well-being of individuals. In the context of mental health promotion, communities can offer a supportive network, promote awareness, provide resources, and advocate for change.

To effectively engage communities in mental health promotion, it is important to understand their unique characteristics, needs, and cultural contexts. Community engagement should be inclusive and respect diversity in terms of age, gender, ethnicity, socioeconomic status, and other relevant factors. By recognizing the strengths and challenges within a community, we can tailor interventions and initiatives that align with their specific circumstances.

Building Collaborative Partnerships

Engaging communities in mental health promotion requires building collaborative partnerships among various stakeholders. This includes mental health professionals, community leaders, policymakers, educators, and individuals with lived experiences. By working together, we can leverage collective expertise, share resources, and co-create solutions that are more comprehensive, sustainable, and culturally appropriate.

Collaborative partnerships can be established through community-based organizations, local government agencies, schools, and faith-based institutions. These partnerships can facilitate the implementation of mental health programs, raise awareness, and advocate for policy changes. By fostering dialogue and active participation, communities can take ownership of their mental health promotion efforts, leading to more effective and impactful outcomes.

Raising Awareness and Reducing Stigma

One crucial aspect of engaging communities in mental health promotion is raising awareness and reducing the stigma associated with mental health issues. Stigma often acts as a barrier to seeking help and support, leading to delayed intervention and poorer mental health outcomes. By challenging misconceptions and promoting understanding, communities can create a more supportive and inclusive environment.

Educational campaigns, workshops, and community events can be organized to provide accurate information about mental health, common mental disorders, and available resources. These initiatives should be tailored to the specific needs and cultural context of the community. By involving community members in planning and implementation, it ensures relevancy and enhances the impact of these awareness activities.

Creating Supportive Environments

Engaging communities in mental health promotion requires creating supportive environments that foster mental well-being. This involves addressing social determinants of mental health such as employment, housing, education, and access to healthcare. Communities can work towards creating policies and programs that promote social equity, reduce inequalities, and ensure the availability of affordable and accessible mental health services.

Moreover, communities can actively promote social connections and positive relationships. This can be done through organizing community-based activities, support groups, and promoting the sense of belonging and connectedness among community members. By creating safe spaces for open discussions and supportive interactions, communities can contribute to the overall mental well-being of individuals.

Empowering Community Members

To effectively engage communities in mental health promotion, it is important to empower community members to take an active role in promoting their own mental health and the well-being of others. This can be achieved through capacity-building initiatives, training programs, and peer support networks.

Community members can be trained to identify early signs of mental health problems, provide initial support, and refer individuals to appropriate resources. Peer support networks can be established to provide a platform for individuals with lived experiences to share their stories, provide support and mentorship, and inspire hope in others.

Evaluation and Continuous Improvement

Engaging communities in mental health promotion should be an ongoing process that involves evaluation and continuous improvement. It is important to assess the impact of community engagement initiatives, gather feedback from community members, and make necessary adjustments to ensure effectiveness.

Evaluation can be done through surveys, focus groups, and qualitative interviews to measure changes in knowledge, attitudes, and behaviors related to mental health. This feedback can inform future interventions and guide the allocation of resources towards areas of greatest need.

Conclusion

Engaging communities in mental health promotion is crucial for building a sustainable and holistic approach to mental well-being. By recognizing the unique strengths and challenges within communities, fostering collaborative partnerships, raising awareness, creating supportive environments, empowering community members, and continuously evaluating our efforts, we can effectively promote mental health at the community level. This collective approach not only improves individual well-being but also contributes to overall societal resilience and sustainability. Let us embrace the power of community engagement and work towards a future where mental health is a shared priority.

Peer Support and Advocacy Programs

Peer support and advocacy programs play a crucial role in promoting mental health and well-being. These initiatives provide individuals with valuable support, understanding, and encouragement from peers who have shared similar experiences. Moreover, peer support and advocacy programs empower individuals to become active participants in their own mental health journey and advocate for positive change in their communities. In this section, we will explore the principles and benefits of peer support, as well as the importance of advocacy in mental health.

Principles of Peer Support

Peer support is grounded in the principles of empathy, shared experiences, and mutual understanding. It recognizes that individuals experiencing mental health challenges can provide invaluable support to one another. Here are some key principles of peer support:

- **Mutuality:** Peer support fosters a relationship of equals, where individuals support one another without a hierarchy or power imbalance.

- **Empowerment:** Peer support aims to empower individuals by providing a safe space where they can voice their concerns, gain confidence, and make informed decisions about their mental health.

- **Respect:** Peer support establishes an environment of respect, where individuals' experiences, perspectives, and choices are honored and valued.

- **Confidentiality:** Peer support relies on trust and confidentiality, ensuring that personal information shared within the support network remains confidential.

- **Non-judgment:** Peer support encourages a non-judgmental atmosphere, free from stigma and discrimination, where individuals feel accepted and understood.

By embracing these principles, peer support programs create a safe and supportive environment for individuals to share their challenges, seek guidance, and build resilience.

Benefits of Peer Support

Peer support programs have numerous benefits for individuals experiencing mental health challenges. These benefits include:

- **Validation and Understanding:** Peer support provides a space where individuals can share their experiences and be understood by others who have gone through similar situations. This validation helps reduce feelings of isolation and promotes a sense of belonging.

- **Shared Knowledge and Coping Strategies:** Peer support offers an opportunity to gain practical knowledge and learn effective coping strategies from individuals who have overcome similar challenges. This shared wisdom can be empowering and help individuals develop new skills for managing their mental health.

- **Increased Self-Esteem:** Peer support boosts self-esteem by allowing individuals to contribute their knowledge and support to others. It also facilitates personal growth and self-acceptance by providing a platform for self-reflection and recognition of individual strengths and resilience.

- **Recovery-oriented Approach:** Peer support is guided by a recovery-oriented approach, which focuses on a person's strengths, abilities, and potential for growth. This approach promotes not just symptom management, but overall wellness and achieving meaningful life goals.

- **Reduced Stigma:** Peer support plays a vital role in challenging societal stigma surrounding mental health. By sharing their stories of recovery and resilience, individuals in peer support programs help combat negative stereotypes and promote a more compassionate and understanding society.

Overall, peer support programs create a supportive community where individuals feel validated, empowered, and equipped with the necessary tools to navigate their mental health challenges.

Importance of Advocacy in Mental Health

Advocacy in mental health is a powerful tool for promoting positive change, addressing systemic issues, and raising awareness about mental health concerns. Advocacy efforts can be carried out at various levels, including individual, community, and societal. Here are some key aspects of advocacy in mental health:

CHAPTER 5: CONCLUSION: TOWARDS A SUSTAINABLE MENTAL HEALTH FUTURE

- **Raising Awareness:** Advocacy involves educating the public about mental health issues, challenging misconceptions, and fostering a greater understanding of the importance of mental well-being. By raising awareness, advocacy helps reduce stigma and promotes a more inclusive society.

- **Reducing Barriers to Care:** Advocacy aims to remove barriers that hinder individuals from accessing mental health care, such as affordability, availability, and cultural barriers. It advocates for improved access to quality services and supports for all individuals, regardless of their background or circumstances.

- **Influencing Policy:** Advocacy plays a crucial role in shaping mental health policies and ensuring that the needs of individuals with mental health challenges are addressed. It involves engaging with policymakers, advocating for policy reforms, and participating in decision-making processes.

- **Promoting Systemic Change:** Advocacy seeks to address systemic issues within the mental health care system and promote changes that enhance the overall well-being of individuals. This includes advocating for community-based care, holistic approaches, and the integration of mental health into broader public health initiatives.

- **Amplifying Voices:** Advocacy empowers individuals and communities to share their stories and experiences, giving them a platform to advocate for their rights and demand better mental health services and supports. It amplifies the voices of those who are often marginalized and overlooked.

Advocacy in mental health is indispensable for creating a more equitable and inclusive society, where individuals can access the resources and support they need to thrive.

Examples of Peer Support and Advocacy Programs

There are various types of peer support programs and advocacy initiatives that have been successful in promoting mental health. Here are a few examples:

- **Peer Support Groups:** These groups bring together individuals with similar mental health challenges to share experiences, provide emotional support, and learn coping strategies. Peer support groups can take place in-person or online.

- **Mental Health Helplines:** Helplines staffed by trained peers offer support, information, and referral services to individuals experiencing mental health challenges. These helplines operate 24/7 and provide a confidential and non-judgmental space for individuals to seek help.

- **Youth Peer Advocacy:** Youth-led advocacy programs empower young people to be advocates for their own mental health and well-being. These programs provide training, support networks, and opportunities for youth to engage in advocacy efforts within their schools and communities.

- **Peer-supported Crisis Services:** Some crisis intervention services incorporate peer support workers, who provide immediate assistance and emotional support to individuals in crisis. Peer support workers can relate to the experiences of individuals in crisis and offer a unique perspective and connection.

These examples demonstrate the diverse range of peer support and advocacy programs available and highlight the significant impact they can have on individuals, communities, and society as a whole.

Challenges and Considerations

While peer support and advocacy programs have many benefits, it is important to consider and address some challenges and considerations:

- **Training and Support:** Peer supporters and advocates require appropriate training and ongoing support to ensure they have the necessary skills and resources to provide effective support and advocacy services.

- **Ethics and Boundaries:** Peer supporters and advocates need to understand and maintain appropriate ethical guidelines and boundaries to protect themselves and the individuals they support.

- **Intersectionality and Inclusivity:** Peer support and advocacy programs must be mindful of diverse experiences and identities to ensure inclusivity and avoid perpetuating systemic biases or exclusionary practices.

- **Sustainability and Funding:** Peer support and advocacy programs rely on sustainable funding to ensure long-term viability and impact. Securing ongoing funding can be a challenge and requires partnerships with relevant stakeholders.

By addressing these challenges and considerations, peer support and advocacy programs can be strengthened and have a lasting positive impact on mental health promotion and support.

Summary

In this section, we explored the principles and benefits of peer support and advocacy programs in promoting mental health and well-being. Peer support programs, guided by principles of empathy, mutuality, and respect, provide individuals with a supportive and understanding space to share experiences, gain knowledge, and promote recovery-oriented approaches. Advocacy in mental health plays a vital role in raising awareness, reducing barriers to care, influencing policies, and promoting systemic change to enhance mental well-being for all. While peer support and advocacy programs have numerous benefits, they also face challenges that need to be addressed to ensure their effectiveness and sustainability. By embracing peer support programs and becoming advocates for mental health, individuals can contribute to building a more inclusive, equitable, and sustainable mental health future.

A Call to Action: Building a Sustainable Mental Health Future

Collaborative Approaches to Mental Health Care

Collaborative approaches to mental health care are essential in addressing the complex and multidimensional nature of mental health issues. These approaches involve the integration of different stakeholders, disciplines, and perspectives to provide comprehensive and person-centered care. By working together, healthcare professionals, researchers, policy-makers, and individuals with lived experience can create a more effective and sustainable mental health care system.

The Importance of Collaboration in Mental Health Care

Collaboration in mental health care is crucial due to the interconnected nature of mental health and the various factors that contribute to well-being. Mental health challenges are influenced by biological, psychological, social, and environmental factors, and addressing each of these components requires a multi-faceted approach. Collaboration encourages individuals and organizations to share knowledge, expertise, and resources, leading to better outcomes for individuals experiencing mental health difficulties.

Moreover, collaborative approaches empower individuals to actively participate in their own care. By involving individuals with lived experience, their families, and support networks in the decision-making process, mental health care becomes more person-centered and responsive to individual needs. Collaborative care models recognize that mental health challenges affect the broader social context and require collective action for effective solutions.

Interdisciplinary Collaboration in Mental Health Care

Interdisciplinary collaboration is a cornerstone of effective mental health care. Bringing together professionals from various disciplines such as psychiatry, psychology, nursing, social work, occupational therapy, and peer support, allows for a comprehensive understanding of mental health issues. Each discipline brings its unique expertise, skills, and perspectives to the table, fostering holistic and well-rounded care.

For example, a collaborative care team may consist of a psychiatrist who diagnoses and provides pharmacological treatment, a psychologist who offers therapy, a social worker who connects individuals with community resources, and a peer support worker who offers guidance based on their own lived experience. This team-based approach ensures that individuals receive comprehensive care that addresses their diverse needs.

Integration of Mental Health and Primary Care

Collaborative approaches often involve integrating mental health care into primary care settings, recognizing the strong relationship between physical and mental health. Primary care providers are often the first point of contact for individuals seeking healthcare, and they play a crucial role in early identification and intervention for mental health concerns. By integrating mental health services into primary care, individuals have easier access to mental health support and receive more coordinated and holistic care.

Collaborative care models, such as the Collaborative Care Model and the Primary Care Behavioral Health Model, encourage communication and collaboration between primary care providers, mental health specialists, and other healthcare professionals. These models support shared decision-making, collaborative treatment planning, and regular follow-up, ensuring that individuals receive both physical and mental health care that is responsive to their needs.

Community-Based Collaboration

Collaboration in mental health care extends beyond healthcare settings to involve various community stakeholders. Community-based collaboration recognizes that the social determinants of mental health, such as housing, education, employment, and social support networks, significantly impact overall well-being. Engaging community organizations, schools, employers, and advocacy groups can help create supportive environments that promote mental health and reduce stigma.

For example, mental health awareness campaigns, community forums on mental health, and peer-led support groups can be powerful collaborative initiatives that engage the wider community. By fostering dialogue, education, and support, community-based collaboration reduces barriers to access, raises awareness about mental health, and promotes early intervention.

Collaborative Research and Policy Development

Collaboration is also vital in the research and policy development arenas. Researchers from various disciplines can work together to conduct high-quality studies that generate evidence-based practices and interventions. Collaborative research efforts can help identify gaps in knowledge and areas for improvement in mental health care. By working together, researchers can pool resources, share expertise, and conduct studies that have a more significant impact on mental health policy and practice.

Policy development in mental health care requires collaboration among policymakers, healthcare providers, researchers, advocacy groups, and individuals with lived experience. By involving diverse stakeholders in policy discussions and decision-making, policies can be more responsive to the needs of individuals with mental health challenges. Collaborative policy development also ensures that policies are evidence-based, grounded in human rights principles, and address systemic barriers to accessing quality mental health care.

Challenges and Opportunities in Collaborative Approaches

While collaborative approaches to mental health care offer numerous benefits, they also present challenges that need to be addressed. Some of these challenges include:

- Communication and information sharing between different stakeholders.
- Addressing power dynamics and promoting equal participation in decision-making.

- Integrating different professional cultures and perspectives.

- Managing resources effectively and ensuring equitable distribution of services.

- Overcoming stigma and discrimination that may affect collaboration.

To overcome these challenges, it is essential to invest in training and education that promotes collaborative skills, effective communication, and interdisciplinary understanding. Additionally, creating supportive policies and funding mechanisms that incentivize collaboration can help foster sustainable collaborative approaches to mental health care.

In summary, collaborative approaches to mental health care are essential in addressing the complex and interconnected nature of mental health challenges. By leveraging the expertise and resources of multiple stakeholders, collaborative care models can provide more comprehensive, person-centered, and sustainable support. Collaboration in mental health care extends beyond healthcare settings to involve community organizations, policymakers, researchers, and individuals with lived experience. Overcoming challenges and promoting effective collaboration can lead to a more inclusive, accessible, and responsive mental health care system.

Addressing Global Mental Health Disparities

One of the key challenges in the field of mental health is the existence of global disparities in accessing and receiving appropriate care. These disparities can be attributed to various factors such as socio-economic conditions, cultural beliefs, geographical barriers, and limited resources. Addressing these disparities is crucial in order to ensure equitable and effective mental health care for all individuals, regardless of their background or circumstances.

Understanding Global Mental Health Disparities

Global mental health disparities refer to the unequal distribution of mental health resources, services, and outcomes across different populations and regions worldwide. These disparities can manifest in several ways:

- **Access Disparities:** Many individuals in lower-income countries or marginalized communities face significant barriers in accessing mental health services. This could be due to financial constraints, lack of transportation, or the absence of mental health facilities in their vicinity.

- **Treatment Disparities:** Even when mental health services are available, disparities may still exist in terms of the quality and appropriateness of treatment. This could be due to a lack of trained professionals, limited availability of evidence-based interventions, or biases in the delivery of care.

- **Outcome Disparities:** Disparities in mental health outcomes refer to variations in the effectiveness of treatment and the level of recovery experienced by individuals. Factors such as access to social support, socio-economic conditions, and stigma can influence these outcomes.

Causes of Global Mental Health Disparities

Global mental health disparities arise from a complex interplay of social, economic, political, and cultural factors. Some key causes include:

- **Poverty and Inequality:** Poverty and socio-economic disadvantage are closely linked to mental health disparities. Individuals living in poverty often face multiple stressors that increase their risk of developing mental health problems, and they may lack the resources needed to access appropriate care.

- **Limited Resources and Infrastructure:** Many low- and middle-income countries have limited resources allocated to mental health services. This includes a shortage of trained mental health professionals, lack of mental health facilities, and limited availability of psychotropic medications.

- **Stigma and Discrimination:** Stigma surrounding mental health is a significant barrier to care worldwide. In some cultures, mental illness is heavily stigmatized, leading to discrimination, social isolation, and reluctance to seek help.

- **Geographical and Cultural Barriers:** People living in remote or underserved areas may face challenges in accessing mental health services due to geographical barriers, such as long distances or lack of transportation. Furthermore, cultural beliefs and practices may affect help-seeking behaviors and perceptions of mental health.

Strategies to Address Global Mental Health Disparities

Addressing global mental health disparities requires a comprehensive and multi-faceted approach. Here are some strategies that can be employed:

- **Strengthening Mental Health Systems:** Building robust mental health systems is essential to improve access to care. This involves training and increasing the number of mental health professionals, improving the availability of mental health facilities, and integrating mental health into primary healthcare services.

- **Reducing Stigma and Increasing Awareness:** Efforts should be made to reduce stigma associated with mental illness through public education campaigns, media engagement, and community-based anti-stigma programs. By increasing awareness and understanding, more individuals may feel encouraged to seek help and support.

- **Empowering Communities:** Engaging communities in mental health care can help address disparities. This can involve training community health workers to provide basic mental health support, promoting peer support networks, and involving local leaders in mental health initiatives.

- **Adapting Interventions to Cultural Contexts:** Recognizing the influence of culture on mental health is crucial in addressing disparities. Mental health interventions should be adapted to local cultural contexts, taking into account beliefs, traditions, and practices relevant to specific communities.

- **Advocacy and Policy Reform:** Advocacy efforts can play a vital role in raising awareness about mental health disparities and influencing policy change. It is important to advocate for increased funding, policy reforms, and the integration of mental health into broader health and development agendas.

Promoting Collaboration and Partnerships

Addressing global mental health disparities requires collaboration and partnerships among various stakeholders, including governments, non-governmental organizations, healthcare providers, researchers, and communities. Some avenues for collaboration include:

- **International Cooperation:** Collaboration between countries, international organizations, and global health agencies can help mobilize resources, share best practices, and foster knowledge exchange to address mental health disparities globally.

CHAPTER 5: CONCLUSION: TOWARDS A SUSTAINABLE MENTAL HEALTH FUTURE

- **Research and Innovation:** Investing in research to understand the underlying causes of mental health disparities and evaluate the effectiveness of interventions is vital. Collaborative research partnerships can help generate evidence-based solutions and innovative approaches to mental health care.

- **Community Engagement:** Engaging communities and involving them in the design, implementation, and evaluation of mental health programs can lead to more contextually and culturally appropriate interventions. Community-driven initiatives have the potential to empower individuals and reduce disparities at the grassroots level.

- **Advocacy Networks:** Networking with advocacy groups, professional associations, and civil society organizations can help amplify voices and advocate for mental health policy reforms. By working together, these networks can influence change and prioritize mental health on national and global agendas.

Case Study: The Friendship Bench Project

One example of a program addressing global mental health disparities is the Friendship Bench Project in Zimbabwe. This community-based intervention trains lay health workers, known as "Grandmothers," to offer mental health support and counseling to individuals experiencing common mental health problems. By utilizing existing community structures and promoting peer support, the project has successfully improved access to mental health care in resource-constrained settings.

Conclusion

Addressing global mental health disparities is a critical step towards achieving equitable and sustainable mental health care worldwide. By recognizing the causes and consequences of these disparities, implementing evidence-based strategies, and promoting collaboration among stakeholders, it is possible to create a future where everyone has equal access to the mental health support they deserve.

The Potential for Transformative Change

In the field of mental health, there exists a great potential for transformative change. This potential lies in the ability to revolutionize our understanding, perception, and approach to mental health care. By embracing innovative practices, challenging conventional norms, and advocating for systemic change, we can create a sustainable future that prioritizes mental well-being for all.

Shifting the Narrative

Transformative change begins with shifting the narrative surrounding mental health. Historically, mental health has been stigmatized and misunderstood, leading to exclusion and discrimination. To foster change, we must challenge these negative beliefs and provide education and awareness campaigns to promote a more compassionate and inclusive society.

One approach to transformative change is reframing mental health as a fundamental aspect of overall well-being. By emphasizing the importance of mental health in our personal and collective lives, we can change societal perceptions and prioritize mental well-being as a core value.

Integrated and Person-Centered Care

A transformative approach to mental health care involves embracing integrated and person-centered care. Integrated care encourages collaboration between mental health professionals, primary care providers, and other disciplines to address the multiple dimensions of mental health. By breaking down silos and promoting interdisciplinary collaboration, we can provide comprehensive and holistic care to individuals.

Additionally, person-centered care recognizes the unique experiences, needs, and preferences of each individual. It involves empowering individuals to actively participate in their treatment planning, fostering a sense of agency, and respecting their autonomy. This approach ensures that mental health care is tailored to the specific circumstances and identities of each person, promoting personalized and effective interventions.

Community-Based Interventions

Transformative change also involves shifting the focus from solely individual-level interventions to community-based approaches. Communities play a critical role in promoting mental health and well-being, as they provide social support networks, resources, and opportunities for connection.

Community-based interventions can take various forms, such as establishing support groups, implementing mental health promotion programs in schools and workplaces, and creating safe spaces for open dialogue about mental health. By engaging communities, we can reduce stigma, increase resilience, and create environments that foster mental well-being.

Embracing Technology and Innovation

The potential for transformative change in mental health care lies in embracing technology and innovation. Technological advancements offer new opportunities to enhance services, increase accessibility, and improve outcomes.

Telehealth and digital platforms, for example, enable individuals to access mental health care remotely, breaking down barriers of distance and transportation. Online therapy, mobile applications for self-care, and virtual support groups provide flexible and convenient options for individuals seeking support. Furthermore, artificial intelligence has the potential to improve diagnostic accuracy, develop personalized treatment plans, and enhance mental health research.

Innovation also extends to novel therapeutic modalities and approaches. Strategies such as virtual reality therapy, biofeedback, and neurofeedback hold promise in transforming traditional treatment methods. By embracing these technologies and innovative practices, we can revolutionize the mental health landscape.

Advocacy and Policy Reform

Transformative change in mental health care requires advocacy and policy reform at both local and global levels. Advocacy efforts help to raise awareness, challenge systemic barriers, and prioritize mental health on political and social agendas.

Policy changes should aim to strengthen mental health systems, increase funding for prevention and treatment, and promote integration across different sectors. It is essential to advocate for policies that address the social determinants of mental health and reduce disparities, ensuring equitable access to care for all.

Collaboration and Partnerships

Finally, transformative change necessitates collaboration and partnerships among various stakeholders. Mental health care involves multiple sectors, including healthcare, education, employment, and social services. Collaborative efforts can foster a comprehensive approach to mental health, taking into account the interconnectedness of various factors impacting mental well-being.

Partnerships with organizations, community leaders, policymakers, and individuals with lived experience of mental health challenges are crucial in driving change. By working together, we can harness collective knowledge, resources, and expertise to create a sustainable mental health future.

In conclusion, the potential for transformative change in mental health care is vast. By shifting the narrative, embracing integrated and person-centered care, implementing community-based interventions, leveraging technology and innovation, advocating for policy reform, and fostering collaboration and partnerships, we can create a future where mental well-being is prioritized, stigma is minimized, and equitable access to high-quality care is a reality. It is through these transformative changes that we can build a sustainable mental health future for generations to come.

Advocacy for Mental Health Policy Reform

The field of mental health has seen significant progress over the years, but there is still much work to be done to create a sustainable future for mental health. One crucial aspect of this is advocacy for mental health policy reform. Advocacy plays a vital role in shaping policies that can address the needs of individuals with mental health challenges and promote overall well-being. In this section, we will explore the importance of advocacy, discuss key strategies and approaches, and provide examples of successful advocacy efforts.

Understanding the Importance of Advocacy

Advocacy involves speaking up for individuals with mental health challenges and working towards improving mental health policies at various levels, including local, national, and international. It is a means of influencing decision-makers, policymakers, and the general public to prioritize mental health and allocate resources for effective mental health care.

Efficient mental health policies are crucial for ensuring that individuals with mental health challenges have access to appropriate and timely care. They can help address systemic issues, reduce stigma, promote equality, and create supportive environments. Advocacy for mental health policy reform is essential for the following reasons:

- **Increased Awareness and Understanding:** Advocacy efforts can help educate the public and policymakers about mental health, raising awareness about the importance of addressing mental health challenges. This increased understanding can lead to better support systems and improved access to care.

- **Reduced Stigma and Discrimination:** Advocacy plays a critical role in challenging stigma and discrimination associated with mental health. By promoting understanding and acceptance, advocacy can create a more inclusive and supportive society.

- **Improved Access to Services:** Effective mental health policies can ensure equitable access to quality mental health services, regardless of one's background or socioeconomic status. Advocacy can influence the allocation of resources to provide better mental health care options and support systems.

- **Prevention and Early Intervention:** Advocacy for mental health policy reform can focus on prevention and early intervention strategies. By implementing policies that prioritize prevention programs and early identification of mental health challenges, advocacy can help mitigate more severe mental health issues in the long run.

- **Addressing Systemic Barriers:** Mental health policies can help identify and address systemic barriers that prevent individuals from accessing appropriate care. Advocacy efforts can push for policy changes that promote equity and fairness in mental health care delivery.

Key Strategies for Advocacy

Advocacy for mental health policy reform requires a strategic approach to effectively influence decision-makers and achieve meaningful change. Here are some key strategies to consider:

1. **Building Coalitions:** Collaborating with like-minded organizations, individuals, and stakeholders can amplify the impact of advocacy efforts. By forming coalitions, advocates can pool resources, share knowledge, and work collectively towards common goals.

2. **Developing Evidence-Based Arguments:** It is crucial to gather and present evidence supporting the need for policy reform. This can include research findings, statistical data, and real-life stories that demonstrate the impact of mental health challenges and the potential benefits of policy changes.

3. **Engaging Stakeholders:** Involving key stakeholders, such as mental health professionals, policymakers, community leaders, and individuals with lived experience, can enhance the credibility and effectiveness of advocacy efforts.

Engaging stakeholders in dialogue and decision-making processes can lead to more informed and comprehensive policies.

4. **Storytelling and Personal Narratives:** Sharing personal experiences and stories of individuals facing mental health challenges can be a powerful advocacy tool. Personal narratives can humanize the issue, create empathy, and drive home the need for policy reform.

5. **Using Media and Technology:** Leveraging media platforms, including social media, can help raise awareness, mobilize support, and reach a broader audience. Advocates can use technology to share information, organize campaigns, and facilitate communication and collaboration among stakeholders.

6. **Creating Policy Briefs and Recommendations:** Developing concise policy briefs and recommendations can provide decision-makers with clear and actionable steps for policy reform. These documents should outline essential issues, evidence-based solutions, and the potential benefits of proposed changes.

7. **Engaging in Policy Monitoring and Evaluation:** Advocacy efforts should not stop at policy implementation. Monitoring and evaluating the impact of policies are crucial for assessing their effectiveness and identifying areas for improvement. Advocates can actively participate in policy evaluation processes and provide feedback to ensure ongoing progress and accountability.

Examples of Successful Advocacy Efforts

Advocacy for mental health policy reform has yielded positive outcomes in various contexts. Let's explore a few successful examples:

1. **Mental Health Parity Laws:** Advocacy efforts in the United States led to the passing of the Mental Health Parity and Addiction Equity Act in 2008. This law requires health insurers to provide equal coverage and treatment options for mental health conditions and substance use disorders, ensuring equitable access to care.

2. **Global Mental Health Agenda:** The mental health community has made significant progress in advocating for mental health as a global priority. The inclusion of mental health in the United Nations' Sustainable Development

Goals (SDGs) highlights the growing recognition of its importance worldwide.

3. **Community-Based Mental Health Programs:** Advocacy has played a crucial role in promoting community-based mental health programs as an alternative to institutionalization. These programs focus on providing accessible and holistic care within the community, reducing stigma, and empowering individuals to lead fulfilling lives.

4. **Policy Changes for Workplace Mental Health:** Advocacy efforts have led to policy changes that prioritize workplace mental health. For example, some countries have implemented legislation requiring employers to provide mental health support and accommodations, fostering mentally healthy work environments.

Challenges and Considerations

While advocacy can bring about positive change, there are challenges and considerations to navigate:

- **Stigma and Discrimination:** The stigma surrounding mental health can hinder advocacy efforts. Advocates must address these societal barriers and work towards creating more empathetic and supportive communities.

- **Resource Allocation:** Resource constraints within the mental health sector can pose challenges to policy reform. Advocates need to make a strong case for resource allocation and prioritize effective, evidence-based interventions.

- **Sustainability and Long-Term Commitment:** Achieving sustainable policy reform requires long-term commitment and ongoing efforts. Advocacy should focus not only on initial policy changes but also on their implementation, evaluation, and continuous improvement.

- **Global and Cultural Context:** Advocacy efforts need to be sensitive to cultural nuances and take into account diverse global contexts. Local factors, cultural beliefs, and contextual realities should shape advocacy strategies to ensure relevance and effectiveness.

Conclusion

Advocacy for mental health policy reform is indispensable for creating a sustainable future for mental health. By raising awareness, challenging stigma, and promoting evidence-based policies, advocates can drive meaningful change and improve outcomes for individuals with mental health challenges. Through strategic approaches, engagement with stakeholders, and the use of various advocacy tools, mental health advocates have the power to shape policies that prioritize mental health, reduce disparities, and foster resilience in individuals and communities. Let us embrace the call to action and work towards a future where mental health is a fundamental priority.

Reflecting on our Journey: Mental Health and Wellbeing in Contemporary History

Embracing Diversity, Inclusion, and Social Justice

In the pursuit of a sustainable mental health future, it is imperative to embrace diversity, inclusion, and social justice. These principles are essential for creating a society that supports the well-being of all individuals, regardless of their background, identity, or circumstances. By recognizing and addressing the unique challenges faced by diverse populations, we can work towards eliminating disparities in mental health care and promoting equal access to support and resources.

Understanding Diversity and Inclusion

Diversity encompasses a wide range of factors that contribute to individuals' unique experiences and identities, including race, ethnicity, gender, sexual orientation, socioeconomic status, and disability, among others. Inclusion, on the other hand, refers to creating an environment where individuals from diverse backgrounds feel valued, respected, and empowered to participate fully.

Promoting diversity and inclusion in mental health care involves recognizing the intersectionality of different identities and understanding how these intersecting factors can shape an individual's mental health experiences. For example, individuals from racial and ethnic minority groups often face social and economic inequalities that can impact their mental well-being. It is essential to acknowledge these disparities and take active steps to address them.

Challenges in Mental Health Disparities

Mental health disparities are prevalent globally, affecting marginalized communities disproportionately. Socioeconomic factors, discrimination, lack of access to healthcare, and cultural barriers can contribute to these disparities. The impact of discrimination and stigma can lead to increased rates of mental health conditions and reduced access to resources and support.

For instance, communities of color often face systemic barriers to mental health care, such as limited access to culturally competent services or experiences of racial discrimination that increase stress levels. It is crucial to address these challenges through targeted interventions and policies that promote equity and social justice.

Strategies for Promoting Diversity, Inclusion, and Social Justice

To create a more inclusive and equitable mental health system, several strategies can be implemented:

1. Culturally Sensitive Care: Mental health professionals should receive training on cultural competency to ensure they can effectively engage with individuals from diverse backgrounds. This includes understanding the cultural nuances of different communities and adapting treatment approaches accordingly.

2. Collaborative Partnerships: Building alliances with community organizations, religious institutions, and advocacy groups can help facilitate access to mental health services for underserved populations. These partnerships can bridge cultural and language barriers and foster trust within the community.

3. Addressing Discrimination and Stigma: Efforts to reduce discrimination and stigma associated with mental health are crucial. Public awareness campaigns, education programs, and legislative initiatives can help challenge negative stereotypes and promote a more inclusive and tolerant society.

4. Equitable Resource Allocation: Ensuring equitable distribution of mental health resources, including funding and services, is essential. By prioritizing underserved communities and addressing disparities in access, we can work towards closing the mental health gap.

5. Inclusive Research and Data Collection: Research should be expansive and inclusive, involving diverse populations in studies to understand the unique mental health challenges they face. Collecting comprehensive data on mental health disparities can inform evidence-based interventions and policies.

6. Policy Reforms: Advocacy for changes in mental health policies and legislation is necessary to address systemic inequities. These reforms should focus on reducing barriers to care, increasing access to quality services, and promoting social justice.

7. Educational Initiatives: Integrating diversity, inclusion, and social justice principles into mental health education can foster cultural sensitivity among

mental health professionals. By training a diverse workforce that understands the needs of underserved populations, we can improve the quality of care provided.

Case Study: LGBTQ+ Mental Health

One specific population that faces unique mental health challenges is the LGBTQ+ community. Discrimination, social stigma, and the lack of legal protections can significantly impact the mental well-being of LGBTQ+ individuals. Embracing diversity, inclusion, and social justice is critical in addressing these challenges and promoting their mental health.

To support LGBTQ+ mental health, mental health care providers can undergo specialized training to become LGBTQ+ affirming. This training equips them with the knowledge and skills to create a safe and respectful environment for LGBTQ+ clients. It also helps them understand the specific mental health concerns faced by this population, such as higher rates of depression, anxiety, and suicide.

Collaboration with LGBTQ+ community organizations and support groups is essential for creating a supportive network that provides resources, advocacy, and a sense of belonging. Mental health professionals can work with these organizations to address the unique challenges faced by LGBTQ+ individuals and develop culturally sensitive interventions and services.

Additionally, policies that protect LGBTQ+ rights, such as anti-discrimination laws and marriage equality, are crucial steps towards creating a more inclusive society. By acknowledging and affirming the identities and experiences of LGBTQ+ individuals, we can promote their mental well-being and work towards a more sustainable mental health future.

Conclusion

Embracing diversity, inclusion, and social justice is fundamental to building a sustainable mental health future. By understanding and addressing the unique challenges faced by diverse populations, we can create a more equitable and supportive mental health system. Through targeted interventions, policy reforms, and collaborative efforts, we can work towards eliminating mental health disparities and promoting the well-being of all individuals, regardless of their background or circumstances. Let us strive for a future that embraces diversity, promotes inclusion, and advocates for social justice in mental health care.

Balancing Individual and Collective Responsibility

In the pursuit of building a sustainable mental health future, it is crucial to strike a balance between individual and collective responsibility. Mental health is a deeply personal and individual experience, but it is also a social issue that requires collective action. This section explores the importance of finding this balance and provides insights into how individuals and communities can contribute to the overall wellbeing of society.

Embracing the Individual Aspect

Acknowledging the individual aspect of mental health is essential because every person's experience is unique. Each individual has their own set of strengths, challenges, and coping mechanisms that shape their mental health journey. It is crucial to recognize that individuals play a fundamental role in their own mental health and wellbeing.

Enabling individuals to take responsibility for their mental health involves fostering self-awareness, self-care practices, and providing access to resources that support personal growth. Encouraging individuals to develop a sense of agency and autonomy empowers them to make informed decisions and take positive actions to enhance their mental health. This could include engaging in activities they find fulfilling and meaningful, seeking professional help when needed, practicing self-reflection, and actively engaging in self-care routines.

Understanding Collective Responsibility

However, mental health is not solely an individual responsibility. To promote sustainable mental health, it is important to recognize the collective responsibility of communities, institutions, and society as a whole. We must create an environment that supports mental health and fosters overall wellbeing for everyone.

Collective responsibility involves several key elements. Firstly, it requires the recognition that we are all interconnected, and the actions of one individual can impact the mental health of others. This understanding encourages empathy, compassion, and the willingness to support those in need. It also necessitates creating inclusive spaces where diverse perspectives are valued, and stigma and discrimination are actively challenged.

Secondly, collective responsibility involves creating a supportive network of resources and services. This includes adequately funding and providing accessible mental health care, implementing policies that address social determinants of mental health, and promoting mental health literacy within communities. Collaborative efforts between healthcare professionals, policymakers, educators, and community leaders are essential to developing an integrated and comprehensive system of support.

Thirdly, collective responsibility requires fostering a culture of openness and dialogue around mental health. This includes promoting awareness, reducing stigma, and encouraging conversations about mental health in various settings such as schools, workplaces, and community spaces. Developing a society where individuals feel safe and comfortable seeking help, sharing their experiences, and supporting one another is crucial for the overall mental health of a community.

Strengthening the Balance

Balancing individual and collective responsibility necessitates recognizing that both are equally important and interconnected. Emphasizing individual responsibility without addressing the systemic factors that contribute to mental health challenges can lead to blame and overlook the broader societal context. Conversely, focusing solely on collective responsibility without empowering individuals to take ownership of their mental health can foster dependency and undermine personal agency.

To strike this balance, it is critical to create an environment that supports both personal growth and collective action. This involves providing education and resources that empower individuals to take responsibility for their mental health while also fostering a sense of community and shared responsibility. It requires a shift from an individualistic mindset to a collective mindset where mental health is viewed as a shared value and responsibility.

By finding this balance, we can build a sustainable mental health future that recognizes the importance of both individual actions and collective efforts. It enables personal growth, resilience, and empowerment, while also promoting a supportive, inclusive, and mentally healthy society.

Case Study: Mental Health Initiatives in Schools

An example of balancing individual and collective responsibility can be seen in the implementation of mental health initiatives in schools. Schools play a critical role in promoting the mental health and wellbeing of students. By integrating mental health education into the curriculum, schools can empower individuals to take responsibility for their mental health while also creating a supportive and inclusive environment.

CHAPTER 5: CONCLUSION: TOWARDS A SUSTAINABLE MENTAL HEALTH FUTURE

In this case, individual responsibility is fostered through lessons on self-care, stress management, and emotional regulation. Students are encouraged to develop healthy coping strategies, seek help when needed, and practice self-reflection. By equipping individuals with the necessary skills and knowledge, schools enable students to navigate their mental health challenges and contribute to their personal growth.

At the same time, schools also embrace collective responsibility by creating a supportive network for students. This includes implementing counseling services, peer support programs, and mental health awareness campaigns. By fostering a culture of empathy and understanding, schools create an environment where students feel safe seeking help and supporting one another. Additionally, involving parents, teachers, and the wider community in mental health initiatives ensures a collaborative approach that acknowledges the collective responsibility of all stakeholders.

By balancing individual responsibility with collective efforts, schools can create a holistic and sustainable mental health framework that benefits both individuals and the community as a whole.

Summary

Balancing individual and collective responsibility is crucial for building a sustainable mental health future. Recognizing the unique experiences and agency of individuals empowers them to take ownership of their mental health. Simultaneously, fostering a sense of collective responsibility in communities and society at large creates an inclusive and supportive environment for all.

Striking this balance involves developing educational resources, providing accessible services, reducing stigma, and fostering a culture of empathy and understanding. By creating a society where individuals are supported in their personal growth and wellbeing, and communities actively work together to address systemic factors, we can build a sustainable mental health future that benefits everyone.

Envisioning a Holistic and Sustainable Approach to Mental Health

In envisioning a holistic and sustainable approach to mental health, we must consider the interconnectedness of various factors that contribute to overall well-being. This approach recognizes that mental health is influenced by multiple determinants, including biological, psychological, social, and environmental factors. By addressing these interconnected factors, we can develop strategies and interventions that promote mental health in a comprehensive and sustainable way.

Understanding the Biopsychosocial Model

The biopsychosocial model provides a framework for understanding the complex interactions between biological, psychological, and social factors in mental health. This model emphasizes the integration of these domains and highlights the importance of considering all aspects of an individual's life when addressing mental health issues. By adopting this model, healthcare providers can take a more comprehensive and holistic approach to mental health care.

Integrative Medicine in Mental Health Care

Integrative medicine combines conventional medical practices with evidence-based complementary and alternative therapies. This approach recognizes the potential benefits of incorporating interventions such as acupuncture, herbal remedies, and mindfulness-based therapies alongside traditional treatment modalities. Integrative medicine promotes a patient-centered approach, where individuals actively participate in their own care and have access to a broader range of treatment options.

Promoting Mental Health Literacy

Mental health literacy refers to the knowledge and understanding of mental health issues. By promoting mental health literacy among individuals, communities, and healthcare providers, we can reduce stigma, increase awareness, and facilitate early intervention. This includes educating individuals about common mental health disorders, their signs and symptoms, and available treatment options.

Prevention and Early Intervention

A proactive approach to mental health involves prevention and early intervention strategies. Prevention efforts aim to address risk factors and promote protective factors through community-level interventions. This may include implementing mental health promotion programs in schools, workplaces, and communities, as well as initiatives to reduce social and economic inequalities. Early intervention focuses on identifying and addressing mental health issues at the earliest signs, before they become more severe. Providing accessible and timely intervention can improve outcomes and prevent the progression of mental health disorders.

Collaborative Care and Integrated Services

Collaborative care models involve a multidisciplinary team working together to provide comprehensive and coordinated care. This approach ensures that individuals receive the support they need from a range of professionals, including psychiatrists, psychologists, social workers, and other healthcare providers. Integrated services aim to bridge the gap between mental health care and other healthcare settings, such as primary care, to ensure a holistic and seamless approach to care.

Promoting Mental Health in Policy and Legislation

Mental health should be a priority in policy and legislation at local, national, and international levels. This includes advocating for increased funding for mental health services, developing policies that support early intervention and prevention, and implementing strategies to reduce stigma and discrimination. Legislation can also play a crucial role in protecting the rights and well-being of individuals with mental health issues, ensuring access to quality care and support.

Enhancing Research and Innovation

Advancing mental health care requires ongoing research and innovation. This includes identifying effective interventions, exploring new treatment modalities, and improving the understanding of the underlying mechanisms of mental health disorders. Research should also focus on addressing health disparities and understanding the impact of social determinants on mental health outcomes. By fostering a culture of research and innovation, we can continuously improve and refine our approaches to mental health care.

Promoting Sustainable Mental Health Systems

To achieve sustainable mental health outcomes, we need to establish robust and resilient mental health systems. This includes ensuring an adequate workforce, developing infrastructure for mental health services, and promoting evidence-based practices. Sustainable mental health systems also involve addressing social determinants of mental health, such as poverty, inequality, and discrimination. By addressing these broader social factors, we can create a supportive environment that promotes mental well-being for all.

In conclusion, envisioning a holistic and sustainable approach to mental health requires recognizing the interconnectedness of various factors and addressing them in a comprehensive and integrated manner. By adopting the biopsychosocial model, promoting mental health literacy, implementing preventive and early intervention strategies, fostering collaborative and integrated care, advocating for mental health in policy and legislation, enhancing research and innovation, and promoting sustainable mental health systems, we can work towards a future where mental health is prioritized, stigma is reduced, and individuals receive the support they need to thrive.

Inspiring Hope and Resilience

In our journey towards a sustainable mental health future, it is essential to focus on inspiring hope and resilience in individuals and communities. Hope is a powerful force that can drive positive change and fuel the motivation to overcome challenges. Resilience, on the other hand, is the ability to bounce back from adversity and navigate life's difficulties.

Understanding Hope

Hope can be defined as the optimistic belief that positive outcomes can be achieved, even in the face of adversity. It is a sense of agency, where individuals believe that their actions can make a difference and create a better future. Hope is not only about wishful thinking but involves setting realistic goals, developing strategies, and taking steps towards achieving them.

The Power of Hope Hope has a profound impact on mental health and well-being. Research has shown that hopeful individuals are more likely to experience lower levels of depression, anxiety, and stress. They also tend to have better coping strategies and a greater sense of life satisfaction.

Building Hope As mental health professionals, we can play a crucial role in cultivating hope in individuals. Here are some strategies for building hope:

- **Promoting a sense of purpose:** Helping individuals identify their values, strengths, and goals can provide a sense of purpose and direction in life. Encourage them to reflect on their passions and find meaning in their daily lives.

- **Establishing realistic expectations:** Assisting individuals in setting achievable goals and understanding that progress may be gradual can prevent feelings of frustration and disappointment. Emphasize the importance of small steps and celebrate even the smallest victories.

- **Fostering a positive support system:** Encourage individuals to surround themselves with supportive and positive people who believe in their abilities and provide encouragement and validation.

- **Helping individuals reframe negative thoughts:** Assist individuals in challenging negative thoughts and replacing them with more positive and realistic ones. This cognitive restructuring process can help individuals develop a more hopeful mindset.

- **Encouraging self-care:** Emphasize the importance of self-care activities that promote relaxation, happiness, and personal well-being. This can include engaging in hobbies, spending time in nature, practicing mindfulness, or engaging in physical exercise.

Resilience: Bouncing Back from Adversity

Resilience is the capacity to adapt and recover from significant stress, trauma, or adversity. It is not about avoiding or eliminating challenges but rather developing the skills and resources to cope effectively with them. Resilient individuals have a greater ability to maintain their mental health and well-being in the face of adversity.

Factors Influencing Resilience Several factors contribute to the development of resilience in individuals:

- **Positive relationships:** Having stable and supportive relationships with family, friends, and community members can provide a strong sense of belonging and help individuals navigate difficult times.

- **Emotional regulation:** The ability to manage and regulate emotions effectively is essential in building resilience. This involves recognizing and acknowledging emotions, practicing self-compassion, and developing healthy coping mechanisms.

- **Problem-solving skills:** Resilient individuals possess strong problem-solving abilities, allowing them to approach challenges with a solutions-oriented mindset. They are flexible and adaptable in finding effective strategies to overcome obstacles.

- **Self-efficacy:** Believing in one's ability to overcome challenges and accomplish goals is a central component of resilience. Developing self-efficacy involves setting realistic goals, recognizing personal strengths, and celebrating achievements.

- **Optimism:** Maintaining a positive outlook and finding meaning in adversity can enhance resilience. Optimistic individuals are more likely to view setbacks as temporary and controllable, allowing them to bounce back more effectively.

Promoting Resilience As mental health practitioners, we can foster resilience in individuals and communities through various interventions and approaches:

- **Psychoeducation:** Providing individuals with knowledge and understanding of resilience can empower them to develop coping skills and enhance their ability to navigate challenges.

- **Teaching coping strategies:** Equipping individuals with effective coping mechanisms, such as problem-solving skills, emotional regulation techniques, and relaxation strategies, can promote resilience and facilitate their ability to bounce back from adversity.

- **Supportive interventions:** Offering support groups, individual counseling, and psychotherapy can provide individuals with a safe space to share their experiences, seek guidance, and build a support network.

- **Strength-based approaches:** Focusing on individuals' strengths and resources instead of solely on their deficits can empower them and enhance their resilience. Encourage individuals to identify and utilize their strengths in overcoming challenges.

- **Community engagement:** Creating and fostering supportive communities that promote resilience is vital. Encouraging community involvement, organizing events, and facilitating peer support groups can enhance social connections and provide a sense of belonging.

Promoting Hope and Resilience Together

Hope and resilience are interconnected and complementary. By nurturing hope, we can inspire individuals to believe in their abilities and strive for positive change. Simultaneously, building resilience equips individuals with the skills and resources to navigate challenges and setbacks effectively.

CHAPTER 5: CONCLUSION: TOWARDS A SUSTAINABLE MENTAL HEALTH FUTURE

Integrating Hope and Resilience in Mental Health Care Incorporating hope and resilience into mental health care involves:

- **Strength-based assessments:** Conducting assessments that focus on individuals' strengths, resources, and aspirations, rather than solely on symptoms and deficits, can foster a sense of hope and agency.

- **Goal setting and monitoring:** Collaboratively establishing realistic goals and regularly reviewing progress with individuals can maintain hope and enhance resilience. Celebrate achievements and adapt goals as needed to ensure continuous growth.

- **Promoting self-care:** Emphasize the importance of self-care practices in maintaining well-being and building resilience. Encourage individuals to engage in activities that promote physical, emotional, and mental well-being.

- **Building supportive networks:** Facilitating opportunities for individuals to connect with others who have similar experiences can foster hope and provide a strong support system. Peer support groups and mentoring programs can be invaluable in this regard.

- **Providing psychoeducation:** Educating individuals about the concepts of hope and resilience can empower them to actively participate in their mental health journey. Offer resources, workshops, and educational materials that promote hope and resilience.

Conclusion

Inspiring hope and resilience is a vital aspect of fostering sustainable mental health. By building hope, individuals can cultivate a positive outlook and maintain motivation in the face of adversity. Simultaneously, developing resilience equips individuals with the skills and resources to navigate challenges and bounce back from setbacks. Integrating hope and resilience into mental health care is a collaborative effort that empowers individuals and promotes their overall well-being. Let us continue our journey towards a sustainable mental health future by embracing hope, resilience, and the transformative power they hold.

Index

-doubt, 284
-up, 126, 212, 225, 527

abandonment, 149
abdomen, 416
ability, 1, 5, 38, 49, 51, 53, 54, 59, 77, 106, 112, 137, 189, 194, 204, 213, 235, 243, 259, 280, 282, 298, 305, 317, 322, 334, 337, 363–369, 371, 372, 374–377, 380, 382, 385, 389, 391, 394, 403, 410, 412, 413, 415, 416, 418–420, 423, 429, 434, 447, 448, 459, 464, 467, 469, 471, 532, 547, 548
ableism, 44
absence, 1, 3, 33, 54, 176, 370
absenteeism, 334, 342, 344, 345
abstinence, 83, 129, 130
abuse, 40, 44, 49, 66, 70, 82, 83, 96, 104, 106, 111, 123, 124, 126, 128, 136, 165, 168, 202, 210, 212, 217, 220, 283, 355, 423, 426, 445
academic, 103, 136, 149, 204, 376, 382, 390, 411, 421–426, 431
acamprosate, 127
acceptability, 459
acceptance, 8, 34, 39, 84, 149, 298, 305, 320, 395, 396, 415, 416, 418, 419, 437, 460, 501
access, 2, 8, 11–13, 20, 33–35, 37–42, 46, 47, 53–55, 60, 62, 63, 70, 75, 78, 96, 99, 128, 130, 131, 169, 218, 224, 225, 228, 229, 235, 236, 262, 323, 325, 326, 333, 348, 352, 354–357, 360, 364, 367, 369, 393, 395, 396, 401, 403, 424, 446, 448–450, 452, 457, 458, 460, 461, 468, 471, 472, 477, 478, 480–484, 498, 500, 501, 503, 505, 509, 510, 512, 513, 518, 520, 524, 527, 528, 532, 534, 535, 539, 540, 542, 545, 546
accessibility, 44, 45, 48, 60, 63, 74, 326, 330–332, 345, 355, 358, 400–403, 447, 481, 502, 505, 507, 509, 534

accident, 115
accomplishment, 221, 222, 259, 261, 263, 281, 283, 299, 334, 373
account, 3, 10, 35, 98, 124, 138, 173, 176, 188, 227, 234, 309, 338, 352, 461, 534
accountability, 62, 158, 166
accuracy, 370, 534
achievement, 425, 431, 444
acknowledging, 153, 312, 314, 417–419, 437, 440, 480
act, 1, 25, 43, 62, 71, 264, 283, 299, 371
action, 244, 313, 322, 326, 372, 414, 444, 473–475, 527, 539, 542, 543
activism, 474
activity, 56, 58, 62, 169, 182, 245, 258–270, 413, 431
actualization, 317
acupuncture, 27, 232, 241, 243, 545
Adam, 128
adaptability, 449, 478
adaptation, 370, 459, 469, 472, 474, 475
addiction, 57–59, 83, 96, 119–123, 125, 130, 131, 315
addition, 12, 51, 57, 91, 127, 133, 143, 144, 193, 198, 215, 260, 263, 275, 285, 295, 301, 325, 347, 361, 367, 370, 415, 421, 499, 500
address, 2, 9, 11, 16, 19, 20, 23, 27, 33, 36, 38, 40, 41, 44, 45, 49, 54, 60–64, 66, 74, 75, 77, 84, 96, 98, 104, 106, 114, 115, 121, 125–128, 136, 142, 144, 154, 158–160, 163, 166, 169, 171, 172, 176, 181, 189, 196, 206, 223, 224, 228, 231, 233, 235–237, 241, 245, 246, 263, 265, 266, 275, 281, 282, 284, 285, 316, 318, 325, 330, 331, 333, 336, 337, 339, 341, 348, 356, 360, 389, 397, 406, 412, 413, 421, 422, 426, 432, 446, 447, 458, 460, 461, 464, 466, 468, 474, 477, 481, 482, 484, 485, 489, 492, 495, 499, 500, 503–506, 519, 525, 528, 533–535, 539, 540, 542, 544, 545
adherence, 53, 54, 58, 62, 128, 129, 260, 262, 266, 314, 484, 517
adjunct, 77
adjustment, 44, 243
admiration, 154
adolescence, 1, 155, 189, 408
adoption, 23, 52, 54, 62
adrenaline, 413
adult, 128, 387, 431
adulthood, 1, 25, 155, 189, 433–436, 442
advance, 59, 331, 398
advancement, 52, 56, 61, 79, 229, 495
advantage, 482
advent, 23, 31, 52, 220
adversity, 18, 112, 204, 274, 317, 319, 320, 322, 363, 364, 366–369, 371, 373–376, 380, 382–385, 389, 391, 394, 397, 410–412, 415,

Index

416, 418, 420, 421, 423, 429, 434, 440, 448, 449, 453, 457–459, 461, 464, 467, 469, 471, 478, 547, 548, 550
advice, 53, 171, 330, 331, 333, 371, 391
advocacy, 8, 24, 36, 71, 79, 143, 206, 355, 361, 430, 460, 461, 474, 475, 480, 501, 522–526, 528, 534, 535, 538–540
advocate, 8, 82–84, 224, 369, 452, 460, 478, 480, 491, 501, 519, 520, 522, 534
affect, 43, 51, 55, 81, 83, 112, 194, 213, 245, 309, 401, 441, 445, 477, 527
affection, 295
affirming, 40
affordability, 38, 354, 355, 481
aftermath, 369, 396
age, 41, 54, 96, 367, 369, 387, 443, 445, 447, 448, 518, 519
ageism, 450
ageist, 450
agency, 27, 60, 479, 533, 542–544, 547
agenda, 482
aggression, 25, 40, 57
aging, 437, 443–448, 450
agriculture, 474
aid, 97, 371, 396, 414, 467, 473
aim, 72, 78, 83, 95, 129, 131, 134, 139, 141, 143, 161, 169, 183, 196, 221, 224, 227, 233, 241, 245, 354, 368, 429, 431, 453, 464, 514, 534, 545, 546

air, 70, 457
Albert Bandura, 374
alcohol, 82, 96, 106, 119, 123, 124, 127, 128, 191
Alex, 158
alliance, 160, 227
allocation, 12, 106, 357, 361, 400, 413, 486, 489, 500, 501, 503–505, 521
allow, 97, 279, 388, 416, 490, 493, 518
alternative, 27, 91, 232, 234, 236, 240–244, 322, 364, 372, 415, 421, 430, 478, 545
ambiguity, 337
ambivalence, 127
amnesia, 202, 203
amount, 165
analysis, 24, 25, 36, 99, 370, 482
Anderson, 421
anger, 57, 111, 190, 437
angle, 414
animal, 295–301, 304, 305, 478, 480
anonymity, 63, 326, 330
answer, 281
antidepressant, 22, 78, 128, 261
antipsychotic, 22, 160
anxiety, 4, 18, 25, 35, 37–40, 45, 47, 48, 59, 61, 62, 81, 84, 86–88, 98, 114, 115, 122, 141, 160, 168, 169, 171, 180, 181, 183–185, 192, 194, 202–205, 212, 213, 232, 233, 235, 240, 241, 245, 253, 256, 258–261, 263, 264, 266, 267, 274, 275, 279, 281, 283–285, 295, 297–301, 304, 307, 313, 317, 320, 322, 330,

345, 371, 383, 390, 409,
430, 441, 445, 446, 467,
472, 473, 547
apnea, 196, 446
appearance, 165
appetite, 91, 111, 165, 168
application, 128, 231, 236, 266, 284,
289, 291, 340, 493, 495
appointment, 451
appreciation, 288, 318, 321, 369,
459
apprehension, 84
approach, 2–4, 9–11, 15, 16, 18–23,
26–28, 33–36, 40, 42, 44,
45, 48, 49, 51, 58, 63, 66,
69, 70, 75–78, 83, 91,
95–97, 99, 101, 103–106,
110, 112, 114, 116, 123,
124, 126, 128–131,
134–137, 139, 141, 142,
144, 147–150, 157–160,
163, 165, 168–170, 172,
174–178, 181, 185, 188,
189, 193, 201–203, 217,
218, 220, 221, 224,
226–228, 231–236, 243,
244, 246, 247, 249, 252,
256, 258, 262, 263, 266,
267, 270, 271, 275, 276,
278–281, 288, 291, 294,
295, 297, 301, 305, 308,
312, 315, 316, 331, 333,
335, 337, 344, 345, 347,
348, 352, 357, 366, 367,
370, 372, 373, 376, 385,
391, 393, 400, 403, 404,
415, 418, 421, 423–425,
427, 431, 436, 441, 445,
447, 448, 453, 456, 461,
464, 467, 470, 471,
481–485, 489–492, 495,
499, 509, 511, 512,
516–518, 521, 526, 527,
530, 533, 534, 536,
544–546
appropriateness, 300, 301, 461
approval, 325
area, 59, 75, 281, 333, 453, 467, 475
Aristotle, 15, 16
aromatherapy, 243, 415
arousal, 113, 245
array, 242
art, 276, 282–285, 288, 396, 415,
461, 478, 480, 482
arthritis, 445, 447
artwork, 282, 284
ASPD, 159
aspect, 1, 3, 70, 75, 172, 183, 228,
270, 282, 312, 316, 319,
322, 326, 337, 366, 374,
394, 410, 414, 440, 449,
451, 455, 520, 533, 535,
542, 550
assertiveness, 296
assessment, 12, 45, 83, 90, 95, 97,
101, 107–109, 111, 125,
128, 136, 142, 144, 148,
155–159, 163, 169,
201–203, 211, 215, 223,
226, 262, 266, 344, 409
assignment, 412
assistance, 127, 226, 295, 296, 315,
356, 367, 371, 389, 394,
396, 447, 461, 473, 474
assisted, 99, 128, 296–305, 478, 480
association, 24, 25
asylum, 28, 217, 218, 220

Index

asylums, 21, 28, 66–68, 217, 218, 220, 222, 223, 479
atmosphere, 280
attachment, 300, 312, 320
attack, 181
attainment, 38
attempt, 166
attendance, 424
attention, 24, 56–58, 66, 135, 136, 142, 216, 240, 243, 260, 272, 273, 279, 283, 312–314, 368, 382, 414–417, 440, 477, 516
attentiveness, 516
attitude, 313, 314, 417
audience, 126, 330, 517
author, 369
authority, 500
autism, 256
autonomy, 19, 27, 33, 34, 60, 61, 116, 218, 312, 334, 442, 449, 479, 517, 533, 542
availability, 8, 33, 38, 40, 131, 205, 226, 330, 356–358, 367, 400, 402, 424, 481, 502, 505, 506, 520
aversion, 312
avoidance, 82, 111, 115
awareness, 8, 19, 24, 32, 34, 40, 55, 71, 74, 88, 96, 99, 104, 141, 143, 149, 154, 160, 169, 175, 195, 224, 225, 233, 234, 243, 245, 273–275, 282, 298, 299, 312, 314, 317, 322, 330, 356, 372, 377, 379, 395, 403, 415, 416, 418, 420, 421, 444, 473, 480, 481, 493, 501, 516, 518–521, 523, 526, 528, 533, 534, 538, 540, 542–545
axis, 185, 253

b, 356, 357
baby, 213
background, 107, 138, 221, 227, 228, 396, 509, 517, 529, 539, 541
balance, 15, 16, 21, 22, 34, 56, 58, 59, 153, 186, 218, 275, 279, 322, 337, 345–348, 440–442, 471, 542–544
bargaining, 437
barrier, 8, 98, 225, 339, 357, 513, 520
base, 389, 485–489
basis, 114, 242, 244
bathing, 16
beach, 279
beauty, 40, 165
bed, 189
bedtime, 191, 195, 280
beginning, 84
behalf, 452
behavior, 1, 11, 21, 24, 25, 81, 91, 92, 96, 105, 127, 131, 133, 137, 138, 144, 154, 159, 168, 233, 424
behavioral, 28, 35, 45, 64, 71, 78, 106, 128, 133, 136, 137, 142, 144, 155, 158, 162, 166, 176, 180, 185, 188, 189, 246, 366, 369, 370, 382, 423, 425, 428, 447, 490
being, 1–4, 6–8, 11, 14–16, 19, 21, 24, 26, 28, 35, 36, 39, 43–46, 49, 58–60, 63, 67,

69, 70, 77–79, 84, 88, 91, 92, 107, 111–116, 119, 120, 122–124, 127–131, 133, 134, 136, 141–143, 149, 154, 159, 161, 164, 167, 168, 172, 174, 176, 181–183, 185, 186, 189, 191, 194–196, 198, 199, 202, 209, 215–217, 222–224, 226, 228, 231–237, 240, 241, 243–247, 249, 251–253, 255, 256, 258–261, 263, 264, 266, 267, 269, 270, 272, 274–277, 279, 282, 284, 285, 288, 291, 295, 297–301, 305, 308, 309, 311–313, 315, 316, 322, 325–327, 331, 334, 336–338, 340–342, 344, 345, 347, 348, 352, 355, 357, 361, 363–367, 369, 371–374, 377, 379, 383–385, 387, 388, 391, 392, 394, 396, 397, 400, 407, 409, 410, 412, 414–418, 420, 423, 425, 426, 428–433, 440, 442–453, 455–458, 461, 462, 464, 466, 467, 469, 472, 473, 475, 482–486, 490, 492, 499, 501, 504, 513–516, 519–522, 526, 528, 533–535, 539, 541, 544, 546–548, 550

belief, 22, 66, 179, 220, 223, 364, 365, 367, 374, 391, 418, 422, 547

belonging, 4, 8, 18, 44, 45, 55, 114, 166, 221, 260, 287, 296, 309, 315, 318, 320–322, 330, 338, 367, 369, 371, 372, 385, 388, 389, 394–396, 414, 419, 452, 457, 461, 473, 520

belongingness, 320, 449

benefit, 45, 59, 124, 125, 127, 133, 136, 246, 274, 281, 296, 326, 393

betterment, 54

bias, 62, 486

bile, 15

biloba, 242

binge, 82, 149, 164–168

biodiversity, 472

biofeedback, 534

biology, 35

biopsychiatry, 26

birth, 39, 133, 213

bite, 314, 417

blame, 543

blindness, 176

blood, 97, 182, 233, 260, 264, 275, 296, 299, 413

blur, 345

body, 15, 16, 26, 82, 99, 103, 161, 164–168, 176, 178, 182, 183, 185, 186, 205, 233, 234, 237, 241, 243–247, 255, 259, 261, 262, 267, 274–276, 279–281, 296, 312, 314, 415, 416, 478, 480, 516

bond, 295, 297, 304, 390

bonding, 295–297

book, 388

boost, 245, 261, 264, 280, 295

brain, 26, 112, 119, 122, 133, 139, 165, 185, 195, 204, 205, 234, 247–250, 253, 255, 258–260, 263, 264, 408, 446, 449
branch, 21
break, 58, 203, 253, 266, 372, 418, 519
breath, 246, 314, 416, 417
breathing, 114, 169, 243, 275, 276, 279, 281, 314, 365, 390, 413, 415–417
bridge, 53, 60, 356, 357, 482, 483, 505, 518, 540, 546
brief, 57, 190
Briquet, 173
broom, 278
Buddha, 312
budget, 33, 501, 503
buffer, 320, 385, 389, 394
building, 52, 57, 60, 127, 154, 226, 228, 287, 297–299, 305, 319, 321, 322, 325, 337, 355, 364, 365, 367, 371–373, 377, 379, 380, 382, 384, 385, 388, 391, 394–396, 410–412, 416, 418, 420, 422, 429–431, 434, 436, 442, 451, 457–459, 468, 469, 472–474, 477–479, 484, 485, 488, 489, 501, 519, 521, 526, 541, 542, 544, 547, 549, 550
bulimia, 82, 165–167
bullying, 165
buprenorphine, 127
burden, 11, 22, 36, 53, 169, 228, 347, 348, 351, 446, 468, 509
burnout, 333–337, 342, 345, 440

caffeine, 191
call, 88, 539
calm, 70, 275, 279, 281, 282, 299, 304, 416
calmness, 413
calorie, 166
camaraderie, 395
campaign, 330, 399, 475
campus, 412
capacity, 44, 225, 322, 363, 366, 369, 382, 391, 430, 453, 457, 464, 467, 468, 473, 521, 548
car, 115
care, 2–5, 7–9, 11–14, 16, 18–23, 27, 28, 30–36, 38, 40–45, 47, 49, 51–54, 56, 59–63, 66–71, 74–79, 81–83, 92, 95, 96, 98, 102, 105, 106, 110, 112, 115–119, 121–123, 126, 129, 132, 133, 137, 150, 158, 163, 169, 178, 186, 202, 208, 209, 213, 215–229, 231–233, 235–241, 243, 245–247, 249, 261–267, 276, 282, 284, 285, 287–289, 291, 297, 305, 308, 311, 312, 316, 319, 326, 332, 333, 336, 337, 347, 348, 352–361, 364, 372, 373, 385, 389, 391, 397, 400–407, 415, 440, 442, 446, 447, 449–456, 458, 460, 467, 473, 477–486, 489–491,

493–495, 500–507,
509–513, 518, 526–529,
532–535, 539–542,
544–547, 550
career, 78, 191, 437, 443
caregiver, 451
caregiving, 40, 347, 451
Carol Dweck, 418
case, 38, 45, 91, 95, 99, 106, 114,
115, 124, 125, 127, 128,
136, 142, 158, 166, 184,
185, 188, 191, 202, 224,
226, 261, 262, 266, 267,
269, 284, 287, 340, 343,
387, 409, 425, 442, 447,
459, 461, 504, 511, 512,
544
catalyst, 299
cataplexy, 189–191
category, 172
causation, 37
cause, 15, 37, 133, 139, 146, 176,
177, 180, 189, 192, 195,
204, 207, 210, 309, 337,
437
caution, 109, 243, 258
center, 71, 75, 442, 511, 512
century, 22, 26, 28, 31, 66, 69, 71,
217, 220, 223, 364, 368,
479
ceremony, 6
certification, 298, 300
chair, 278
challenge, 8, 33, 40, 41, 54, 79, 96,
111, 170, 171, 181, 185,
225, 345, 365, 369, 370,
376, 397, 450, 477, 478,
481, 494, 501, 504,
513–515, 518, 533, 534,
540
change, 127, 131, 157, 180, 221,
325, 372, 423, 430, 437,
471–475, 478, 480, 481,
501, 513, 514, 516, 519,
522, 523, 526, 532–536,
538, 539, 547, 549
channel, 283
chapter, 231, 363, 477
character, 96, 213
charge, 170, 332, 478
chatbot, 63
check, 124, 170, 172
checking, 204, 347, 390
chemistry, 165
chest, 181
child, 142, 144, 170, 368, 425
childbirth, 213, 215
childcare, 347
childhood, 1, 12, 21, 25, 26, 83, 111,
135–137, 168, 202, 204,
408, 409
choice, 51, 82, 110, 160, 316, 424,
480
choose, 19, 372
circle, 321
circulation, 243
circumstance, 186
clarity, 243, 275, 280, 281, 312, 313
class, 421, 455
classification, 67, 96
classroom, 421, 423–425
cleaning, 347
cleanliness, 203
client, 287
climate, 425, 471–475
clinic, 484
clock, 63
closure, 22, 33

Index

club, 388
co, 83, 98, 104–106, 123–126, 129, 131, 141, 169, 171, 205, 473, 520
cognition, 57, 82, 113
cohesion, 325, 457, 458, 464, 468, 473
collaboration, 6, 19, 20, 32, 34, 36, 51, 61, 63, 74, 75, 82, 106, 110, 132, 143, 144, 154, 225, 226, 235, 263, 267, 316, 345, 352, 356, 361, 395, 396, 399, 400, 409, 425, 426, 431, 461, 466, 468, 472, 474, 480, 482, 483, 485, 489–491, 494, 501, 517, 519, 527–529, 531–535
collaborative, 19, 20, 23, 31, 45, 77, 110, 144, 161, 172, 202, 227, 267, 352, 431, 447, 478, 483, 484, 490, 491, 519, 521, 527–529, 541, 544, 547, 550
collage, 284
collapse, 190
collection, 62, 482
college, 103, 166, 281, 330, 411, 417, 438
colonization, 6
color, 540
combat, 8, 49, 218, 513
combination, 14, 78, 89–92, 94, 95, 97, 100, 114, 115, 127, 133, 136, 137, 147, 152, 155, 160, 161, 168, 173, 180, 181, 188, 200, 203, 204, 206, 207, 211, 214, 262, 268, 270, 275, 276,
301, 370, 384, 393, 415, 436, 447
comfort, 17, 18, 296, 297, 299, 300, 305, 315, 322, 326, 371, 414, 420, 453, 494
commitment, 22, 34, 127, 153, 344, 478, 482
communicating, 498, 517
communication, 44, 52, 132, 133, 137, 144, 154, 160, 170, 182, 253, 255, 274, 282, 288, 298, 299, 305, 314, 336, 338, 372, 379, 389–391, 394, 415, 425, 429, 452, 453, 467, 468, 490, 491, 493, 495, 496, 498, 516–519, 527, 529
community, 2, 6, 7, 14, 17, 19, 20, 22, 23, 28, 31–34, 55, 71–75, 78, 99, 103, 106, 112, 125, 126, 128, 132, 143, 160, 164, 166, 215, 218, 221–227, 255, 262, 286, 296, 315, 316, 318, 320–322, 325, 326, 333, 348, 361, 363, 369, 371, 372, 388, 394–396, 399, 400, 409, 414, 421, 423–425, 430, 431, 446, 447, 449, 452, 457–461, 464, 466–469, 471–475, 479, 482, 501, 505, 511, 512, 518–521, 523, 527–529, 532–535, 540, 543–545
commute, 347
comorbidity, 121
companionship, 295, 296, 298, 305, 320, 388

company, 340, 343, 344, 438, 442
comparison, 55, 370, 387
compassion, 71, 150, 154, 223, 274, 312–314, 416–419, 516, 542
competence, 5, 6, 16, 20, 42, 75, 374, 403–407, 459, 461, 518, 519
competency, 7, 14, 509, 513, 540
competition, 431
complement, 18, 169, 261, 283, 300, 332, 384
complex, 2, 11, 18, 23, 27, 34–37, 39, 41, 43, 45, 55–57, 67, 78, 86, 91, 96, 99, 101, 104, 111, 119, 122–124, 126, 127, 130, 132, 135, 141, 147, 150, 154, 156, 157, 159–161, 164, 169, 172, 176, 178, 181, 195, 202, 203, 206, 209, 210, 213, 224–227, 234, 235, 247, 255, 283, 311, 312, 364, 369, 372, 429, 430, 445, 446, 456, 457, 472, 489, 491, 517, 519, 526, 529, 530, 545
complexity, 4, 10, 128, 129, 131, 175, 229, 364, 370
component, 77, 129, 166, 170, 192, 223, 267, 322, 352, 374, 376, 377, 379, 391, 403, 411, 416, 420, 440, 516
composition, 253, 256
computer, 62
concentration, 280, 423
concept, 1, 4, 15, 24, 25, 66, 67, 195, 199, 223, 231, 245, 267, 312, 313, 337, 347, 363, 364, 366–369, 374, 377, 388, 391, 413, 418, 423, 457, 466, 474
conceptualization, 176
concern, 9, 60, 348, 492
conclusion, 8, 25, 32, 41, 45, 49, 71, 99, 111, 154, 161, 169, 172, 176, 186, 206, 209, 229, 236, 276, 291, 297, 311, 351, 357, 369, 418, 429, 445, 456, 466, 478, 489, 495, 535, 546
condition, 8, 15, 43, 45, 48, 86, 101, 119, 120, 130, 137, 138, 150, 153, 154, 159, 166, 172–176, 178, 179, 181, 185, 195, 203, 206, 209–211, 213, 214, 218, 221, 241, 246, 300, 452
conduct, 136, 142, 158, 173, 204, 207, 211, 300, 421, 483, 528
conferencing, 52, 518
confidence, 88, 259, 262, 280–283, 285, 287, 295, 296, 330, 367, 376, 377, 421, 425, 429
confidentiality, 54, 60–62, 330, 345
confinement, 217, 218, 221
conflict, 7, 176
confusion, 149, 177
congestion, 471
conjunction, 181, 276
connectedness, 3, 322, 457, 458, 520
connection, 6, 14–17, 44, 55, 83, 119–122, 178, 182, 183, 185, 186, 202, 233, 234, 241, 244–249, 252, 253, 255, 258, 267, 297, 298,

300, 304, 309, 312, 315–320, 367, 377, 390, 394, 450, 452, 478, 516, 533
connectivity, 62, 345
consciousness, 199, 483
consensus, 422
consent, 22, 27, 60, 61, 63, 300, 517, 518
consideration, 34, 63, 466
consistency, 76, 136, 415, 423
construct, 39
construction, 471
consultation, 202
consumption, 83, 130
contact, 132, 515, 516, 527
containment, 217
contamination, 203
contemplation, 313
content, 58, 63, 459, 461, 494, 517
contentment, 320
context, 1, 4, 7, 13, 15–17, 20, 28, 36, 60, 111, 138, 212, 217, 219, 227, 232, 236, 244, 272, 285, 314, 316, 363, 366–368, 370, 376, 453, 455, 461, 464, 466, 467, 477, 516, 519, 520, 527, 543
contingency, 131
continuity, 225
continuum, 1, 106
contrast, 16, 35, 38, 210, 418
contributing, 2, 33, 37, 77, 90, 124, 126, 163, 165, 166, 185, 189, 204, 213, 297, 479
contribution, 24, 348
control, 15, 16, 45, 91, 103, 112, 115, 131, 135, 136, 165, 167, 168, 181, 189, 191, 233, 246, 261, 262, 264, 304, 334, 337, 368, 388, 414, 423, 424, 429, 442
controversy, 148
conversation, 62, 298
conversion, 176–178
cooking, 347, 417
coordination, 34, 106, 225, 352, 402
coping, 17, 19, 25, 36, 45, 61, 77, 88, 91, 98, 103, 106, 124, 128, 136, 159, 161, 166, 167, 169–172, 181, 185, 202, 215, 224, 228, 234, 275, 283, 284, 288, 291, 301, 304, 307, 311, 315, 317, 319, 320, 326, 330–332, 335, 364, 367, 370–372, 389–392, 394–396, 408–412, 414, 419–421, 425, 429, 436–440, 451, 458, 459, 461, 467, 472, 475, 478, 542, 544, 547
cord, 45
core, 132, 142, 159, 369, 373, 377, 416, 478, 492, 495, 533
corner, 280
cornerstone, 222, 519, 527
correlation, 122
cortex, 135, 204
cortisol, 245, 295, 413
cost, 40, 482, 486
counseling, 27, 40, 75, 78, 128, 130, 136, 165, 166, 170–172, 176, 224, 268, 315, 344, 396, 408, 492, 532, 544
counselor, 128
country, 72, 499
couple, 213

course, 372, 376, 414
coverage, 8, 354–356, 401, 481
craft, 221
creation, 8, 221, 471, 489, 491
creativity, 57, 294, 372, 431
credit, 154
crime, 38, 457
criminalization, 33
crisis, 99, 224, 226, 424, 472
criterion, 370
criticism, 25, 26
critique, 27
cultivation, 313, 382
culture, 2, 4–7, 27, 154, 228, 309, 336–338, 340, 341, 344, 367, 422, 423, 426, 442, 452, 467, 483, 491, 501, 543, 544, 546
cure, 190, 191, 193
curiosity, 417, 418, 420
curricula, 424, 481, 494, 501
curriculum, 143, 420, 494, 543
cutting, 468, 483
cyberbullying, 55, 60
cycle, 189, 195, 481
cycling, 260, 262, 266

d, 356, 357
dance, 222, 294, 431
dancing, 262, 446
data, 53, 60, 62, 64, 79, 370, 422, 460, 482, 489, 490, 540
date, 12, 21, 494
day, 23, 187, 191, 263, 314, 389, 412, 416, 417
daycare, 442
daytime, 188–191, 194
deadline, 382
death, 113, 115, 162, 318, 437

debate, 148, 309
decision, 45, 119, 204, 224, 227, 365, 424, 425, 430, 431, 473, 486, 489, 505, 517, 519, 527, 528, 535, 536
decline, 342, 421, 446, 448
decrease, 263, 315, 421, 425
dedication, 418, 419
deepening, 134, 317
defense, 25
deficiency, 15, 195
definition, 1, 2, 4, 49, 161, 172, 367, 369
Deinstitutionalization, 31–33
deinstitutionalization, 22, 28–34, 71, 218, 223, 479
delay, 214
delivery, 7, 12, 44, 52–54, 222, 225, 227–229, 352, 355, 358, 360, 432, 459, 509
demand, 225, 337
demeanor, 298
dementia, 445
denial, 25, 437
department, 422
departure, 67
dependability, 423
dependence, 106, 114
dependency, 25, 128, 543
depersonalization, 334
depression, 3, 4, 15, 35, 37–40, 45, 47, 48, 55, 59, 78, 91, 98, 106, 122, 124, 128, 141, 160, 168, 169, 171, 181, 183, 192, 194, 202, 205, 209, 213–216, 232–236, 245, 253, 256, 258–261, 263, 264, 266, 269, 270, 274, 275, 283, 284, 287,

288, 295, 297, 299, 313, 317, 320, 322, 345, 371, 383, 390, 437, 441, 445–447, 472, 547
deprivation, 37, 194
depth, 97, 161, 315, 370, 460
description, 190
design, 60, 62, 63, 66, 331, 344, 421, 432, 460, 468
designing, 134, 140, 268, 459, 489
desire, 165, 203, 422
destigmatization, 19, 225, 481
destruction, 472
detachment, 368
detection, 61, 82, 169, 397
determinant, 47, 48, 160
determination, 34, 227, 369, 373, 429
deterrent, 7
devaluation, 513
development, 12, 13, 21, 22, 24–27, 35, 37, 40, 44, 49, 50, 52, 54, 67, 69, 71, 72, 82–84, 86, 90, 92, 99, 100, 112, 119, 120, 123, 133, 135, 142, 144, 146, 154, 155, 162, 165, 168–170, 177, 178, 180, 182, 183, 185, 187, 192, 195, 200, 204, 206, 210, 213, 218, 220, 222, 225, 233, 236, 248–250, 253, 299, 325, 332, 352, 355, 363, 364, 368, 372, 373, 382, 394, 407–409, 420, 421, 423, 425, 429, 431, 432, 440, 445, 446, 468, 471, 474, 475, 483, 489, 494, 495, 499, 501, 515, 528, 548

diabetes, 445
diagnosing, 114, 115, 158, 214
diagnosis, 11–13, 21, 22, 53, 61, 64, 66, 76, 79, 82–84, 91, 93, 96, 97, 104, 107, 108, 126–129, 134, 136–138, 142, 146, 150, 154, 155, 157, 158, 161, 163, 164, 167, 169, 172–174, 176, 178, 181, 182, 189–191, 195, 197, 199, 209, 211, 213, 223, 243
dialogue, 19, 20, 315, 474, 520, 528, 533, 543
diary, 190
diet, 98, 114, 249, 250, 252, 253, 255–258, 373, 413, 448
dietary, 15, 171, 250–256, 258
dieting, 161
dietitian, 103, 166, 258
difference, 318, 429, 547
difficulty, 75, 91, 111, 113, 124, 128, 132, 142, 176, 186, 188, 189, 287, 317, 330, 376
digestion, 247
dignity, 34, 69, 218, 223, 479
dimension, 36
direction, 373, 430, 499
disability, 43–46, 48, 49, 84, 123, 137–141, 406, 509, 539
disadvantage, 426
disappointment, 438
disaster, 396, 466–468
discipline, 222, 491, 527
discomfort, 194
discovery, 22, 233, 282, 283, 287, 294, 317
discrimination, 2, 6–8, 18, 34, 36, 37, 44, 47–49, 98, 123,

141, 158, 227, 321, 325,
355, 395, 396, 460, 477,
479, 481, 509, 513, 533,
539, 540, 542, 546
disease, 181, 233, 296, 348, 445
disharmony, 14
disorder, 3, 81, 82, 86, 88, 90, 91, 93,
97, 99, 102–104, 119, 123,
124, 126, 128, 132–135,
137, 141, 142, 144, 156,
157, 160, 161, 163–166,
168–172, 176–179, 185,
186, 189, 191, 195, 197,
199, 201, 205, 208–213,
216, 240, 256, 261, 262,
269, 275, 300, 348
disparity, 506
displacement, 25, 472
displeasure, 13
disregard, 158, 159
disruption, 15, 446
dissatisfaction, 165, 168
dissemination, 355, 483, 488, 489,
495–498
dissociation, 423
distance, 53, 75, 321, 534
distraction, 57, 221, 261, 299
distress, 8, 25, 37, 44, 47, 48, 55, 77,
84, 96, 99, 103, 122, 146,
149, 159, 167, 174–176,
181, 183, 185, 192, 194,
203, 204, 233, 309, 371,
444, 453, 458, 472, 516
distribution, 38, 99, 355, 360, 458,
495, 501, 503, 505, 509,
529, 540
district, 425
disturbance, 165
diversion, 299

diversity, 3, 14, 98, 228, 424, 477,
478, 483, 519, 539–541
divide, 54, 60, 61
divorce, 322
doctor, 181
dog, 296, 300, 305, 307
door, 33
dopamine, 35, 195, 253, 255, 259
dosage, 77
doubt, 284
down, 253, 266, 280, 282, 314, 372,
412, 414, 416, 418, 420,
519, 533, 534
drainage, 473
drawing, 19, 233, 317
dream, 24, 25, 438
driving, 115, 480, 534
drop, 213
drowsiness, 194
drug, 99, 119, 129–131
duration, 95, 193, 209, 210, 263,
416
duty, 34
dynamic, 36, 233, 288, 316, 370,
373, 385, 517, 519
dysbiosis, 253, 256
dysfunction, 195, 426
dysregulation, 150, 423

ear, 320, 321, 451
earthquake, 467
ease, 269, 281, 300, 388, 400, 416
eating, 82, 99–104, 149, 161,
164–172, 274, 283, 313,
314, 413, 414, 417, 448
echinacea, 242
eco, 472, 473
ecotherapy, 473
edge, 115, 468, 483

Index

education, 7, 8, 19, 20, 37, 38, 40, 41, 43, 44, 54, 75, 78, 92, 96, 98, 99, 112, 130, 131, 134, 139, 143, 149, 164, 171, 175, 176, 178, 215, 218, 224, 235, 262, 316, 334, 344, 357, 361, 376, 391, 395, 400, 420, 421, 424, 425, 437, 447, 458, 472, 473, 481, 484, 489–492, 494, 499, 501, 509, 517, 519, 520, 528, 529, 533, 534, 540, 543

effect, 57, 296, 462

effectiveness, 12, 27, 60, 74, 99, 125, 129, 136, 149, 170, 225, 229, 241, 244, 261, 267, 275, 282, 284, 287, 305, 307, 331, 340, 341, 367, 373, 374, 393, 405, 409, 432, 459–461, 475, 485, 515, 521, 526

efficacy, 127, 131, 212, 228, 244, 264, 364, 367, 374–377, 389, 424, 429, 431, 448, 458, 473

efficiency, 53, 54, 60, 352, 471

effort, 8, 260, 321, 326, 337, 340, 365, 377, 389, 412, 418, 419, 422, 469, 483, 505, 513, 550

ego, 25

Egypt, 21

electrolyte, 166

element, 515

emergence, 21–23, 26, 217, 220

emergency, 224, 467, 468

Emily, 88, 166, 167, 281

Emma, 149

Emmy Werner, 364, 368

emotion, 149, 245

empathy, 63, 149, 150, 154, 174, 175, 227, 287, 296, 298, 314, 321, 331, 371, 372, 379, 389, 391, 394, 395, 397, 417, 420, 425, 451, 481, 515, 516, 518, 519, 522, 526, 542, 544

emphasis, 3, 16, 25, 67, 71, 75, 217, 221, 227, 294, 479

employee, 336, 337, 340, 341, 344, 442

employment, 8, 32, 34, 38, 41, 43, 44, 141, 149, 175, 226, 235, 458, 461, 520, 528, 534

empowerment, 8, 44, 51, 82, 110, 116, 264, 287, 291, 304, 305, 333, 356, 404, 429–433, 480, 543

emptiness, 149, 287, 317, 440

encounter, 266, 389, 422

encouragement, 98, 166, 171, 266, 287, 315, 321, 330, 347, 372, 388, 419, 420, 430, 431, 452, 453, 522

end, 33, 62, 437, 453, 455

endeavor, 318, 423

endocrine, 253

endorphin, 269

endurance, 262

energy, 91, 128, 243, 262, 263, 269, 276, 287, 296, 345, 373, 421, 422, 440, 471, 473

enforcement, 75, 110, 355

engage, 1, 18, 19, 51, 58–60, 91, 124, 125, 128, 130, 131, 154, 158, 160, 161, 204,

241, 246, 259, 264, 279, 280, 282, 300, 321, 322, 337, 390, 392, 430, 431, 446, 447, 449, 450, 452, 459, 494, 505, 517, 519, 521, 528, 540
engagement, 54, 55, 58, 60, 61, 78, 132, 148, 259, 262, 299, 308, 318, 321, 326, 344, 386, 388, 409, 425, 428, 430, 445–447, 458, 459, 468, 474, 489, 517–519, 521, 539
enhance, 4, 7, 18, 20, 32, 44, 45, 57–59, 61, 74, 106, 127–129, 133, 136, 139, 144, 147, 160, 161, 168, 169, 186, 198, 199, 203, 221, 222, 227–229, 231, 234, 235, 241, 243–247, 258–264, 266, 267, 274, 276, 279, 280, 284, 285, 287, 288, 298, 299, 308, 316, 317, 320, 322, 366, 367, 369, 371, 373, 375, 378, 379, 381, 382, 385–388, 391–393, 404, 405, 407, 409–412, 415, 420, 424, 429–435, 440, 442, 444, 447–450, 453, 457, 459, 467–469, 471–473, 475, 479, 482, 483, 493, 494, 506, 507, 516–519, 526, 534, 542
enhancement, 128, 296, 364
enjoyment, 58, 59, 222
entertainment, 56
entirety, 370
environment, 15, 16, 19, 38, 44, 45, 51, 63, 66, 67, 69–71, 75, 82, 105, 109, 112, 116, 119, 128, 136, 143, 154, 160, 181, 195, 203, 216, 221, 279, 287, 298–300, 315, 322, 326, 329, 331, 333, 336–342, 379, 387–394, 396, 404, 405, 409, 415, 417, 419, 423–425, 446, 447, 449–453, 457, 458, 469, 471, 491, 494, 498, 501, 513, 515, 516, 519, 520, 522, 539, 542–544, 546
epidemic, 99
episode, 95, 166, 167
equal, 8, 38–40, 43, 60, 143, 354, 355, 491, 509, 532, 539
equality, 8, 41, 535
equanimity, 312
equation, 370
equilibrium, 440
equine, 298, 301, 304
equipment, 130
equipping, 420, 452, 495, 544
equity, 6, 40–43, 49, 61, 354, 355, 357, 367, 460, 482, 507, 509–513, 520, 540
era, 21, 28, 66, 67, 217, 220, 221, 326
erosion, 474
error, 77
escalation, 397
escapism, 57
establishment, 28, 33, 67, 68, 71, 72, 82, 217, 218, 479
esteem, 8, 37, 44, 51, 70, 111, 136, 160, 164–166, 168, 221, 222, 258–261, 264, 266,

283, 284, 287, 295, 299, 320, 331, 429, 431
estrogen, 213
Ethan, 144
ethnicity, 12, 41, 43, 46, 47, 49, 355, 406, 509, 519, 539
etiology, 147, 150, 209, 213
evacuation, 467
evaluation, 62, 76, 93, 97, 115, 163, 165, 184, 189–191, 202, 207, 211, 215, 262, 340, 345, 432, 459–461, 521
evening, 192
event, 49, 50, 82, 106, 107, 111, 113, 115, 116, 186, 203, 475
evidence, 2, 7, 12, 14, 18–20, 23, 63, 67, 76, 77, 99, 106, 111, 112, 129–131, 143, 144, 160, 165, 168–170, 176, 179, 204, 213, 224, 229, 232, 236, 240, 241, 244, 255, 258, 270, 276, 285, 298, 305, 312, 352, 355, 376, 409, 429, 480, 483, 485–490, 495, 498–500, 505, 506, 515, 517, 528, 532, 539, 540, 545, 546
evolution, 13, 14, 16, 220, 478, 483
exacerbation, 50, 120, 183, 233, 367
exam, 281, 417
examination, 163, 173, 262
example, 3, 4, 6, 12, 15, 17–19, 25, 35, 46–48, 62, 75, 78, 88, 95, 99, 101, 122, 124, 125, 127, 142, 154, 182, 203, 233–236, 241, 245, 246, 248, 275, 278, 281, 296, 300, 307, 315, 330, 346, 347, 354, 369, 376, 379, 396, 409, 425, 428, 438, 471, 490, 492, 493, 527, 528, 532, 534, 539, 543
excess, 15
exchange, 52, 83, 131, 516
exclusion, 2, 7, 34, 44, 218, 481, 513, 533
exercise, 4, 15, 53, 58, 78, 98, 109, 112, 114, 164–166, 258–271, 296, 347, 373, 413, 446, 448, 478, 480, 482
exhaustion, 213, 334
existence, 312, 316–319, 355, 529
exorcism, 16
expansion, 481
expectation, 383
experience, 3, 8, 18, 36, 37, 44, 47–49, 58, 61, 62, 82, 90, 92, 111, 136, 141, 149, 160, 173, 175, 179, 189, 196, 203, 209, 210, 213, 216, 221, 263, 270, 274–276, 280, 281, 283, 295, 298, 300, 301, 304, 309, 312, 313, 316, 317, 320, 331, 332, 334, 335, 345, 348, 355, 371, 383, 405, 412, 415, 416, 422, 423, 435, 437, 438, 446, 453, 458, 459, 472, 474, 488, 509, 526–529, 534, 542, 547
expertise, 227, 284, 304, 333, 393, 474, 489–491, 520, 527–529, 535
explanation, 18, 173, 176
exploration, 21, 25, 84, 213, 283, 285, 316, 318, 373, 516

exposure, 38, 55, 61, 88, 111, 123, 133, 139, 168, 181, 203, 266, 423, 426, 457
expression, 6, 41, 55, 233, 282–285, 288, 291, 294, 298, 431
eye, 132, 516

fabric, 321
face, 8, 9, 37–40, 43, 47, 48, 54, 58, 74, 125, 128, 141, 149, 158, 174, 205, 223, 225, 226, 228, 235, 265, 321, 336, 337, 342, 355–357, 364, 366–369, 371, 373, 374, 382, 385, 388, 397, 400, 410, 412, 415, 416, 418–420, 422, 423, 426, 429, 433, 440, 442, 448, 449, 453, 457, 464, 466, 467, 472, 473, 475, 481, 482, 504, 526, 539, 540, 547, 548, 550
fact, 261
factor, 176, 235, 320, 363, 370–373, 383, 391, 394, 457, 458, 479
failing, 96, 218
failure, 218, 418
fair, 509
faith, 17–20, 315, 316, 501, 520
fall, 34, 188, 191
family, 8, 35, 36, 39, 44, 55, 95, 103, 106, 108, 114, 123, 124, 144, 158, 160, 161, 170, 181, 191, 207, 210, 211, 222, 224, 235, 320, 321, 347, 367, 371, 388–391, 394, 395, 397, 407, 414, 424–426, 440, 449, 451, 467
farming, 222
fatigue, 166, 190, 194, 263
fatty, 232, 258
fear, 7, 8, 22, 63, 81, 84, 98, 103, 104, 111, 149, 161, 164, 179, 326, 372, 390, 395
feature, 179
feedback, 62, 154, 287, 331, 365, 418, 420, 422, 460, 521
feeling, 1, 167, 187, 189, 213, 281, 385, 413, 421, 425
fellow, 388
fetch, 296
field, 13, 14, 21, 23–28, 59, 61, 63, 71, 76, 79, 95, 134, 143, 148, 169, 203, 205, 209, 218, 220, 245, 249, 250, 253, 258, 279, 285, 309, 313, 331, 364, 366, 368, 479–481, 489, 490, 494–496, 516, 529, 532, 535
fight, 413
figure, 69
Fiji, 474
financing, 361, 468, 501, 502, 505
finding, 56, 77, 167, 322, 384, 436, 542, 543
fire, 467
fishing, 474
fitness, 62, 259, 262, 269, 278, 296, 446, 448
flaw, 213, 418
flexibility, 135, 243, 313, 366, 372, 416, 418, 449
flight, 413
flood, 467

Index

flow, 243, 260, 264, 278, 313
focus, 10, 22, 24, 27, 35, 38, 40, 58, 71, 75, 83, 84, 109, 129, 136, 154, 157, 164, 170, 178, 185, 217, 222, 223, 228, 272, 279–281, 283, 305, 313, 314, 356, 357, 373, 410, 412, 413, 416–419, 421, 429–431, 450, 460, 480, 521, 533, 540, 546, 547
fog, 202
follow, 97, 126, 136, 212, 225, 437, 527
following, 10, 65, 101, 105, 114, 137, 167, 179, 193, 214, 237, 251, 256, 282, 288, 304, 308, 322, 342–344, 347, 352, 353, 382, 399, 401, 402, 428, 503, 504, 506–508, 535
food, 103, 164–168, 170–172, 253, 314, 467, 484
footprint, 471
force, 7, 313, 547
forefront, 132, 474, 483
forest, 279
forgiveness, 419
form, 56, 57, 280, 282, 285, 294, 298, 305, 321, 334, 392
formation, 468
forum, 330
Foster, 321, 395, 420, 468
foster, 13, 20, 40, 222, 282, 288, 291, 299, 315, 316, 318, 321, 322, 332, 341, 365, 372, 385–387, 391, 394, 396, 407, 414, 421–423, 429, 431, 448–450, 452, 457, 469, 473, 479, 489, 517–520, 529, 533, 534, 539, 540, 543, 549
foundation, 12, 14, 16, 52, 67, 69, 71, 218, 222, 395, 400, 420, 429, 485
fragmentation, 484
framework, 17, 18, 36, 112, 129, 231, 233–236, 284, 309, 312, 352, 355, 406, 499, 544, 545
freedom, 316
frequency, 191, 193, 210, 262, 474
Freud, 21, 24, 25
friend, 115, 451
frustration, 44, 57, 136, 177, 194, 446
fulfillment, 3, 317, 321, 373, 440
fullness, 166
function, 132, 137, 182, 194, 195, 233, 243, 245, 250, 253, 255, 258, 260–264, 446, 448, 449
functionality, 202
functioning, 12, 38, 43, 49, 70, 74, 82, 84, 88, 90, 95, 112, 113, 116, 123, 133, 136–138, 142, 147, 153, 157, 159, 160, 167, 173, 174, 176, 177, 180, 189–191, 195, 199, 209, 211, 222, 234, 259, 262, 263, 409, 413, 441, 445
funding, 22, 33, 34, 70, 72, 74, 141, 225, 226, 357–361, 432, 481, 491, 500–503, 505, 529, 534, 540, 542, 546
furniture, 467
future, 8, 11, 13, 23, 28, 30, 31, 39,

41, 43, 52, 59, 61–63, 66, 67, 69, 79, 84, 92, 104, 132, 150, 154, 182, 186, 206, 209, 213, 267, 271, 280, 285, 322, 326, 331, 333, 341, 352, 355, 357, 361, 366, 367, 373, 383, 385, 388, 391, 397, 400, 410, 418–420, 422, 426, 429, 430, 432, 433, 438, 442, 448, 459, 469, 471, 475, 477–481, 483, 485, 490, 498, 501, 505, 509, 515, 521, 526, 532, 533, 535, 538, 539, 541–544, 547, 550

gain, 24, 25, 46, 66, 77, 165, 185, 233, 264, 283, 312, 315, 318, 364, 370, 371, 395, 451, 478, 482, 490, 526
Galen, 15
gambling, 149
game, 57–59, 390
gamification, 59
gaming, 57–59
gap, 356, 357, 482, 483, 495, 506, 509, 540, 546
garden, 388
gardening, 70, 222, 260
gas, 474
gathering, 224
gender, 12, 39–41, 46–49, 355, 367, 406, 424, 455, 509, 519, 539
gene, 190
generation, 22, 429, 471
genetic, 3, 35, 86, 89, 92, 96, 100, 123, 133, 135, 139, 147, 152, 155, 156, 162, 165, 168, 189, 190, 192, 200, 204, 207, 210, 211, 231, 234
geography, 13
Gerald Epstein, 281
ginkgo, 242
girl, 136
given, 4, 66, 284
go, 313, 417, 437, 451
goal, 31, 45, 90, 130, 133, 141, 147, 153, 168, 171, 177, 180, 222, 224, 226, 266, 267, 282, 400, 431, 470, 489
governance, 458
government, 358, 395, 468, 498–501, 504, 520
graduate, 330, 438
graduation, 424
grandiosity, 154
gratitude, 280, 366, 385, 412, 417
Greece, 21
green, 457, 471
greenhouse, 474
grief, 78, 437, 438, 440, 443, 453, 472, 473
grip, 203
grooming, 304
ground, 314
groundwork, 67, 221
group, 48, 83, 88, 92, 96, 103, 106, 124, 149, 159, 161, 199, 221, 224, 260, 262, 266, 267, 274, 276, 287, 307, 320, 321, 372, 391, 393–395, 397, 412, 424, 426, 457, 461, 479
growth, 9, 58, 154, 160, 260, 264, 282–285, 288, 291, 292,

Index 571

296, 301, 305, 316, 317, 332, 363, 365, 366, 368, 379, 384, 388, 393, 414, 418–420, 422, 423, 431, 440, 458, 478, 542–544
guarantee, 157
guidance, 18, 58, 78, 103, 166, 168, 169, 215, 232, 233, 281, 282, 288, 300, 304, 308, 309, 315, 316, 318, 321, 331–333, 357, 371, 389, 392–394, 396, 414, 430, 431, 435, 522, 527
guide, 107, 117, 142, 148, 222, 223, 237, 251, 285, 289, 291, 297, 301, 307, 369, 391, 422, 431, 478, 489, 499, 521
guilt, 91, 111, 113, 166, 309, 315
gut, 185, 247–249, 253, 255, 256, 258

half, 31
hall, 281
hand, 15, 24, 29, 37, 40, 43, 47, 55, 57, 186, 243, 280, 309, 317, 331, 332, 367, 376, 383, 417, 440, 443, 457, 458, 495, 539, 547
handicrafts, 70
handwashing, 204
happiness, 261, 280, 297, 299, 320, 385, 449
harassment, 55
hardship, 366, 394, 458
harm, 22, 34, 67, 83, 99, 123, 129–132, 157–159, 203, 300
harmony, 15, 313

head, 217, 366, 416
healing, 6, 44, 51, 52, 83, 109, 111, 115, 116, 183, 203, 221, 232, 233, 241, 243, 247, 282, 283, 285, 288, 291, 292, 304, 305, 332, 396, 404, 407, 423, 425, 437, 440, 461, 473
health, 1–28, 30–69, 71–79, 81–84, 87, 88, 90–93, 96–99, 104–112, 115, 116, 119–129, 131, 132, 141, 148, 150, 154, 156, 158–161, 163, 164, 166–170, 172, 178, 181, 182, 185, 186, 195, 196, 199, 201, 203–207, 212, 213, 215–229, 231–272, 274–276, 279–283, 285–291, 295–302, 305, 306, 308–323, 325–327, 331–334, 336–345, 347–361, 363–369, 371, 373, 374, 377, 383–385, 388, 390, 391, 394–407, 409, 410, 412, 416, 418, 420, 421, 424, 426, 428, 429, 433, 435, 436, 440–453, 455–462, 464, 466, 468, 469, 472–475, 477–487, 489–496, 498–524, 526–550
healthcare, 8, 12, 37–39, 41, 42, 44, 48, 52–54, 61, 74, 91, 102, 106, 110, 112, 130, 141, 143, 163, 164, 166, 169, 171–175, 177, 178, 182, 186, 189, 193, 195, 197, 199, 202, 211, 212, 215,

216, 224, 227, 228, 232, 235, 236, 241, 244, 247, 258, 260, 262, 263, 266, 288, 334, 336, 337, 345, 348, 395, 400, 446, 448, 449, 452, 453, 455, 468, 481–484, 486, 488, 499, 502, 505, 509, 520, 526–529, 531, 534, 540, 543, 545, 546

hearing, 4, 369
heart, 62, 181, 182, 275, 296, 299
Helen Keller, 369
help, 2, 7, 8, 12, 15, 18–20, 38, 40, 41, 44, 45, 47, 51, 52, 58, 61, 63, 77, 88, 91, 95, 97, 98, 102, 103, 105, 108, 112, 114, 115, 125, 128, 133, 136, 143, 150, 153, 154, 160, 166–169, 171, 172, 175, 181, 185, 186, 189–191, 195, 202, 203, 205, 213, 215, 224, 228, 233, 235, 243, 253–255, 260–262, 264, 266, 273, 276, 279–281, 283, 284, 295, 296, 298, 299, 304, 315, 316, 319, 321, 326, 330–332, 335, 336, 339, 356, 365, 366, 370, 371, 373, 376, 377, 379, 380, 385, 388, 389, 397, 399, 400, 402, 409–411, 413, 414, 417–419, 423, 425, 429, 430, 435–437, 443, 444, 446, 447, 449–451, 453, 455, 460, 469, 481, 482, 484, 501, 505–507, 509, 513, 515–518, 520, 528, 529, 534, 535, 540, 542–544

helplessness, 111, 446
helpline, 167
highlight, 8, 13, 14, 55, 121, 182, 255, 312, 331, 422, 525
history, 13, 35, 69, 71, 96, 97, 123, 155, 158, 163, 168, 173, 176, 190, 202, 207, 210, 211, 213, 217, 220, 223, 262, 295, 309, 364, 368, 369, 407, 477–480
hoarding, 205
home, 144, 274, 280, 447
homelessness, 22, 33, 355
hope, 17, 209, 213, 301, 309, 311, 331, 332, 367, 391, 451–453, 458, 518, 521, 547, 549, 550
hopelessness, 37, 213
hormone, 295
horror, 111
horse, 301, 304
horticulture, 415
hospital, 336
hospitalization, 22, 71, 123, 170
house, 21, 217
household, 347, 389
housing, 32, 34, 37, 127, 226, 447, 471, 484, 499, 520, 528
hub, 223
human, 1, 11, 21, 24–26, 31, 62, 63, 66, 221, 295–297, 305, 309, 316, 318, 320, 369, 458, 472, 479, 480, 500, 528
humor, 414
hunger, 166, 314
hurricane, 396

Index 573

husband, 447
hygiene, 98, 189, 191, 195, 196, 198, 199
hyperactivity, 136, 137, 142
hyperarousal, 115, 423
hypervigilance, 82, 111, 113, 304, 423
hypothesis, 37, 122, 135

idea, 4, 391
ideal, 66
ideation, 39
identification, 84, 95, 141, 144, 215, 228, 527
identity, 6, 39, 41, 48, 149, 199, 202, 295, 309, 317, 396, 444, 457, 474, 509, 539
illness, 1, 3, 4, 13, 14, 18, 21–23, 26–28, 31–33, 35, 36, 41, 66–69, 95, 123, 125, 126, 186, 209, 217, 218, 220–223, 226–229, 234, 241, 245, 339, 366, 369, 401, 407, 437, 453, 479, 481, 499, 501, 509
image, 103, 161, 164–168, 259, 279, 419, 425, 450
imagery, 279, 281, 282
imaging, 53
imbalance, 14, 253, 345, 441
impact, 2–7, 9, 12, 13, 15–17, 19, 20, 24, 28, 29, 32, 36, 37, 39–41, 44–49, 51, 52, 55–57, 60, 71, 75, 79, 81, 82, 88, 91, 92, 95, 96, 99, 107, 111, 112, 116, 119, 126, 128, 135, 136, 141, 154, 158, 159, 166, 172, 184, 186–191, 193–196, 199, 204, 217, 218, 222, 225, 226, 235, 245, 246, 250, 252, 253, 255, 256, 259–261, 263, 264, 267, 279, 280, 282, 295–297, 299, 305, 311, 317, 319, 320, 330, 332, 334, 337, 340, 342, 345, 348, 355–357, 363, 367, 372, 383, 385, 388, 389, 396, 399, 402, 404–407, 409, 412, 416, 419, 423–426, 432, 433, 435, 437, 440–443, 445, 448, 450–453, 455–458, 460, 461, 466, 467, 474, 475, 478–480, 484, 486, 491, 492, 494, 495, 498, 501, 514, 515, 519–521, 525, 526, 528, 539, 540, 542, 546, 547
impairment, 58, 82, 84, 96, 137, 146, 159, 167, 173, 176, 204
impermanence, 368
implement, 12, 75, 136, 154, 189, 218, 254, 336, 340, 343, 347, 372, 398, 407, 421, 468, 501
implementation, 12, 29, 33, 34, 54, 64, 66, 70, 117, 129, 297, 325, 331, 348, 349, 352–355, 357, 432, 442, 460, 461, 480, 489, 499, 520, 543
importance, 1, 3, 4, 12, 14–16, 19, 21, 26–28, 36, 49, 67, 69–71, 88, 103, 104, 115, 116, 130, 154, 167, 171, 218, 221–223, 225–229,

232, 236, 241, 252, 258, 267, 285, 311, 312, 316, 319, 337, 340, 345, 348, 352, 363, 364, 368, 380, 385, 388, 395, 397, 403, 406, 407, 409, 426, 430, 440, 442, 464, 469, 477–480, 483, 485, 489–492, 499, 501, 512, 522, 533, 535, 542, 543, 545

improvement, 67, 70, 76, 157, 205, 284, 399, 419, 422, 469, 483, 521, 528

impulse, 91, 135, 165, 168

impulsivity, 136, 137, 142, 149, 150, 160

in, 1–4, 6–9, 11–28, 31, 33–36, 38–47, 49–67, 69–79, 81–84, 88, 91, 92, 95–99, 103, 104, 106, 109–117, 119, 121–126, 128–137, 139, 141–144, 146, 148, 149, 153, 154, 158–161, 163–173, 175, 176, 178, 181–183, 185, 186, 188–192, 194–196, 199, 202–206, 208–215, 217, 218, 220–229, 231–238, 240–243, 245–253, 255, 256, 258–264, 266–270, 272–276, 278–289, 291, 294–301, 304–306, 308, 309, 311–322, 325, 326, 329–334, 336–342, 344, 346–348, 352–357, 360, 361, 363–377, 379, 380, 382–385, 388, 390–397, 399–401, 403–405, 407, 409, 410, 412–427, 429–440, 442–453, 455–462, 464, 466–469, 471–475, 477–496, 498–501, 503, 505–507, 509–524, 526–529, 532–535, 537, 539–550

inability, 190

inadequacy, 55, 136, 165, 309, 387

inattention, 136, 137

incarceration, 22, 355

incidence, 12, 164, 484

incident, 344

inclusion, 8, 141, 145, 221, 241, 355, 477, 483, 501, 539–541

inclusivity, 20, 39, 75, 84, 227, 326, 331, 395, 432, 466

income, 9, 38, 46, 356, 401, 458, 472, 481, 482, 511

incompetence, 376, 418

inconsistency, 486

increase, 40, 74, 86, 104, 123, 124, 129, 133, 141, 160, 165, 204, 205, 213, 245, 259, 262, 267, 284, 295, 299, 313, 344, 356, 372, 395, 413, 416, 421, 426, 441, 445, 448, 501, 534, 540, 545

independence, 45, 84

India, 275

individual, 1–4, 6, 8, 9, 16, 18, 19, 22, 25, 27, 34, 36, 39, 43–46, 48–51, 64, 76–78, 88, 90, 93, 94, 96–98, 101, 103, 104, 106–108, 110–116, 119, 123, 124, 126, 127, 132–134, 136, 138, 142, 146, 148, 149,

Index   575

    153–155, 158, 160, 161,
    170, 172, 173, 175, 181,
    188, 189, 191, 194–196,
    199, 201, 203, 205, 207,
    215, 218, 221, 223, 224,
    227, 228, 231, 234, 243,
    244, 251, 255, 262, 268,
    270, 276, 286, 289,
    298–301, 309, 316, 317,
    319, 320, 322, 331, 334,
    335, 345, 348, 363, 364,
    366–371, 374–376, 387,
    388, 401, 408, 410, 415,
    424–426, 436–438, 441,
    448, 451, 452, 455,
    457–459, 464, 467–469,
    472, 477, 490, 491, 518,
    521, 523, 527, 533, 539,
    542–545
individuality, 449
industry, 336
inequality, 458, 546
inevitability, 368
influence, 1, 2, 4, 7, 14–16, 18,
    24–27, 35, 38, 47, 60, 71,
    99, 139, 141, 165, 168,
    182, 222, 228, 231, 234,
    235, 244, 253, 267, 335,
    356, 367, 370, 405, 406,
    457, 482, 484, 491, 501,
    519, 536
information, 8, 11, 24, 52, 54, 60,
    62, 63, 97, 102, 104, 108,
    130, 142, 149, 167, 181,
    204, 215, 224, 262, 266,
    288, 308, 389, 395, 400,
    450, 452, 468, 482, 501,
    515–517, 520
infrastructure, 106, 225, 356, 357,

    361, 467, 468, 471, 473,
    482, 491, 546
inhalation, 233
inhibition, 135
initiative, 428
injection, 129, 130
injury, 45, 113
innovation, 13, 59, 468, 534, 535,
    546, 547
input, 227, 460
insecurity, 37, 46
insertion, 243
insight, 24, 25, 34, 77, 157, 233,
    283, 312, 315, 317, 318
insomnia, 186–189, 192, 196, 446
inspiration, 372, 395
inspiring, 425, 478, 547
instability, 38, 149, 425
instance, 6, 35, 40, 47, 48, 64, 235,
    364, 459, 471, 490, 491,
    540
institutionalization, 22, 28, 218, 223
instruction, 294
insurance, 8, 354–356, 358, 360,
    401, 468, 481
intake, 164, 166
integrating, 7, 19, 79, 112, 131, 186,
    223, 228, 244, 246, 263,
    265, 266, 276, 311, 318,
    333, 351, 404, 417, 422,
    474, 475, 481, 484, 485,
    490, 492, 494, 495, 501,
    513, 527, 543
integration, 19, 22, 27, 32–34, 36,
    53, 59, 61, 63, 66, 78, 134,
    218, 221, 224–228, 235,
    246, 264, 267, 278, 285,
    301, 347, 352, 355, 361,
    481–483, 490, 494, 495,

499, 505, 508, 526, 534, 545
integrity, 329, 518
intelligence, 63, 137, 154, 364–366, 372, 373, 377–379, 418, 420, 422, 430, 482, 534
intensity, 111, 193, 209, 263, 266
intention, 276, 279, 336
interaction, 2, 63, 70, 96, 114, 132, 133, 135, 142, 147, 182, 210, 221, 222, 233–235, 259, 262, 266, 304, 307, 308, 431, 446
interconnectedness, 3, 10, 48, 78, 182, 228, 231, 234, 237, 241, 313, 348, 431, 478, 482, 483, 499, 534, 544, 546
interest, 60–62, 91, 113, 124, 241, 252, 266, 269, 309, 320, 322
internet, 52, 62, 326
interplay, 2, 27, 35, 36, 41, 46, 78, 86, 127, 178, 185, 195, 233, 236, 312, 530
interpretation, 53, 459, 461
interrelationship, 267
intersect, 49, 406, 455, 456
intersection, 18, 20, 43, 315
intersectionality, 46, 48, 49, 355, 406, 455–457, 539
intervention, 12, 64, 75, 76, 83, 84, 95, 96, 102, 103, 106, 108, 111, 112, 126, 130, 133, 141–145, 164, 167, 169, 213, 224, 226, 228, 236, 268, 288, 300, 352, 354, 356, 357, 370, 397, 407–410, 426–429, 478, 482, 484, 485, 493, 520, 527, 528, 532, 545–547
interview, 155, 202, 204, 331
interviewing, 127, 128
intimacy, 320
intuition, 63
invalidation, 174
invest, 321, 505, 529
investigation, 194
involvement, 59, 124, 131, 134, 170, 221, 222, 224, 425, 451, 519
iron, 193, 195
irritability, 111, 113, 188, 189, 441
island, 474
isolation, 8, 33, 38, 44, 48, 57, 66, 106, 114, 175, 220, 221, 225, 235, 260, 298, 315, 321, 331, 371, 387, 389, 391, 414, 441, 443, 446–449, 513
issue, 2, 9–11, 33, 75, 99, 154, 169, 400, 443, 542

Jake, 304
jargon, 517
job, 38, 46, 91, 334, 336, 337, 342, 344, 437–439
jogging, 262, 263
John, 330
Johnson, 447
join, 106, 266, 321, 449, 475, 480
joint, 243
journal, 280, 412, 494
journaling, 169, 318, 365, 366, 414
journey, 2, 84, 103, 117, 125, 127, 149, 167, 172, 216, 225, 227, 301, 304, 315, 331–333, 376, 378, 379,

391, 436, 438–440,
451–453, 455, 477, 483,
505, 515, 522, 542, 547,
550
joy, 280, 297–299, 373, 449
judgment, 8, 98, 240, 273, 275, 294,
314, 321, 326, 372, 390,
395, 414–417
jurisdiction, 499
justice, 33, 36, 79, 112, 355, 458,
474, 477, 482–484, 507,
539–541

kindness, 69, 221, 321, 416, 419
knowledge, 11–15, 19, 26, 112, 209,
213, 242, 315, 316, 331,
371, 372, 389, 396–400,
403, 404, 420, 452, 458,
461, 468, 473, 474,
489–495, 498, 521,
526–528, 535, 544, 545

labeling, 516
labor, 222, 347
laboratory, 97
lack, 3, 7, 8, 22, 33, 34, 38, 39, 48,
62, 63, 67, 101, 142, 149,
154, 157, 165, 167, 169,
175, 189, 213, 217, 218,
235, 236, 263, 317, 334,
337, 356, 369, 402, 441,
444, 458, 460, 481, 509,
539
land, 6
landscape, 23, 79, 534
language, 142–144, 401, 459–461,
491, 498, 516, 517, 519,
540
laughter, 190, 415

law, 75, 110
laziness, 189
leader, 154
leadership, 154, 379, 430, 432
learning, 31, 61, 62, 64, 98, 137,
149, 260, 288, 296, 316,
363, 366, 372, 393,
418–422, 424, 436, 446,
449, 483, 492–495
leave, 336, 450
legacy, 67, 68, 223, 450
legislation, 71, 356, 468, 500, 501,
540, 546, 547
leisure, 56, 222, 347, 440
lens, 4, 14, 18, 26
lesson, 479, 480, 483, 484
level, 163, 262, 266, 269, 322, 331,
337, 357, 363, 370, 399,
402, 467, 468, 472, 477,
521, 533, 545
leverage, 245, 326, 332, 357, 500,
520
liberation, 312
life, 1, 3, 8, 12, 15, 16, 18, 44, 45, 51,
61, 77, 78, 81, 82, 88, 91,
92, 96, 97, 103, 111, 113,
115, 116, 119, 122, 125,
128, 133, 136, 137, 139,
146, 149, 157, 159, 164,
165, 167, 170, 173, 175,
176, 181, 184, 187–191,
193–196, 199, 202, 204,
206, 210, 211, 213, 225,
226, 236, 252, 254, 260,
273–276, 278, 281, 282,
284, 285, 296, 297, 309,
313, 314, 316–320, 322,
326, 337, 345–348, 355,
363, 365–369, 373, 374,

377, 381–385, 387, 388, 394, 407, 410, 412, 417–420, 431, 433, 435–445, 447, 448, 450, 453, 455, 471, 478, 545, 547
lifespan, 291
lifestyle, 15, 16, 27, 28, 78, 83, 90, 97, 188, 189, 191, 195, 249, 260, 296, 413
lifetime, 137
light, 1, 12, 14, 247
likelihood, 76, 123, 129, 394
limit, 27, 54, 194, 225
line, 26, 136, 160, 278
link, 247, 284
linkage, 128
list, 412
listener, 299, 321
listening, 287, 314, 320, 388, 417, 516, 519
literacy, 54, 60, 62, 323, 356, 397–400, 444, 445, 478, 483, 484, 543, 545, 547
literature, 7, 388
living, 34, 38, 45, 70, 133, 202, 213, 217, 221, 279, 326, 356, 447
location, 54, 279, 281, 322, 355, 400, 482, 509
loneliness, 55, 260, 295, 298, 315, 320, 371, 387, 441, 446, 447
look, 74, 81, 377, 481
loss, 91, 92, 124, 161, 170, 176, 189, 190, 202, 269, 322, 436–440, 443, 446, 448, 472
love, 295, 320, 389, 420

loyalty, 295, 298

machine, 61, 62, 64
maintenance, 27, 35, 99, 165, 168–170, 177
major, 33, 128, 269, 445, 481
making, 7, 45, 88, 92, 104, 119, 132, 136, 149, 168, 181, 204, 224, 227, 258, 278, 281–283, 285, 287, 296, 309, 318, 321, 365, 380, 408, 416, 424, 425, 430, 431, 450, 473, 485, 486, 489, 505, 517, 519, 527, 528
malnutrition, 163, 170
man, 158, 184
management, 45, 76, 78, 79, 83, 91, 95, 114, 115, 127, 131, 135, 142, 144, 148, 154, 160, 161, 165, 166, 169, 170, 172, 178, 182, 185, 188, 209, 211, 212, 224, 226, 229, 243, 246, 247, 250, 251, 253, 255, 270, 296, 332, 336, 347, 377, 379, 396, 412–415, 421, 424, 435, 442, 447, 452, 453, 471, 544
managing, 1, 27, 53, 58, 92, 96, 106, 124, 137, 153, 157, 160, 170, 172, 183, 185, 188, 191, 211, 240, 245, 258, 264, 266, 275, 282, 283, 301, 304, 315, 397, 410, 412–415, 436, 440, 446, 447, 453, 455
mangrove, 474
mania, 91, 209

Index 579

manifestation, 3, 49, 133, 185
manipulation, 243
manner, 53, 111, 121, 182, 228, 284, 397, 410, 414, 416, 421, 498, 547
manual, 222, 243
Marcus Aurelius, 15
marginalization, 37, 44, 47, 513
Marie, 38
Mark, 184, 185
mark, 25, 218
market, 344
marketing, 346
marriage, 78
massage, 16, 233, 241, 243
mastery, 259, 261
material, 37
math, 376
matter, 355
Max, 300
Maya, 45
meal, 166, 171, 172, 417
meaning, 17, 18, 20, 112, 120, 309, 311, 316–319, 373, 385, 414, 444, 448, 450, 453, 455
means, 15, 218, 240, 282, 285, 312, 380, 418, 429, 458, 535
measure, 370, 521
measurement, 369, 370
mechanism, 37, 414
media, 54–56, 60, 62, 168, 284, 321, 330, 332, 387, 388, 399, 489, 515
medicalization, 23, 26–28, 136
medicate, 106
medication, 18, 27, 28, 53, 62, 77, 78, 83, 90, 91, 94–96, 99, 106, 114, 115, 122, 127, 128, 130, 131, 136, 137, 147, 160, 161, 172, 176, 180, 181, 188, 189, 191, 203, 206, 207, 224, 226, 235, 259, 261, 263, 268, 275, 276, 447, 451
medicine, 21, 232, 233, 236–242, 244, 276, 482, 492, 545
meditation, 17, 91, 232, 233, 240, 241, 243, 245–247, 272–276, 312–315, 318, 347, 365, 412–417
medium, 283, 340
meeting, 75, 88
melancholia, 15
member, 451
memory, 1, 112, 135, 199, 202, 260, 382
mentoring, 331–333, 391, 395
mentorship, 521
Mesopotamia, 21
messaging, 62
metaphor, 297
methadone, 127
methylphenidate, 136, 190
Mia, 387, 388
Michael Rutter, 364, 368
microbial, 253
microbiota, 253, 255, 256
midlife, 442–445
migration, 461, 472
milestone, 223
mind, 1, 11, 15, 16, 21, 24–26, 62, 178, 182, 183, 185, 186, 233, 234, 237, 241, 243–247, 261, 267, 270, 272, 275, 279–281, 312, 331, 416, 478, 480, 518

mindful, 56, 58, 59, 267, 274, 310, 314, 321, 365, 414, 416, 417, 518
Mindful Multitasking, 417
mindfulness, 27, 61, 91, 114, 149, 169, 170, 185, 202, 232, 240, 241, 243, 245, 270, 272–275, 279, 283, 312–315, 319, 365, 368, 382, 385, 390, 412, 415–418, 436, 473, 482, 545
Mindfulness Apps and Resources, 417
mindset, 244, 281, 365, 367, 377, 383–385, 411, 412, 416, 418–420, 422, 452, 473, 543
minority, 47, 48, 539
mirror, 299
misinformation, 7, 60
mismatch, 334
mistreatment, 66–68, 479
misunderstood, 172, 203, 395, 533
misuse, 122, 165
mitigation, 474
mix, 438
Mobile, 53
mobile, 52, 57, 144, 229, 356, 432, 534
mobility, 37, 46, 53, 326, 447, 518
modality, 21, 27, 160, 298, 305
model, 2–4, 15, 23, 26–28, 35, 36, 226, 231, 233–236, 245, 356, 478, 480, 545, 547
modeling, 370, 452
moment, 240, 273–275, 283, 312, 313, 318, 414–416, 516
momentum, 31, 71, 223

money, 91
monitor, 53, 62, 158, 262, 263
monitoring, 52, 53, 95, 99, 124, 166, 170, 212, 267, 340, 499
month, 113
mood, 47, 57, 62, 81, 82, 88–92, 106, 113, 124, 160, 165, 171, 209–211, 213, 253, 255, 258–264, 266, 267, 269, 270, 275, 276, 280, 287, 295, 298, 413, 446, 448
morale, 154
morning, 188, 412, 417
mother, 38
motherhood, 214, 216
motivation, 45, 58, 59, 119, 127, 131, 262, 263, 266, 267, 280, 299, 301, 372, 373, 419, 452, 547, 550
motor, 133, 176
mouth, 416
movement, 22, 28–31, 69–71, 176, 217, 218, 220–223, 246, 260, 267, 294, 314, 479
multidimensionality, 2
multitasking, 417
multitude, 276, 342
muscle, 184, 185, 189–191, 214, 233, 245, 247, 413
music, 222, 233, 285–288, 294, 431, 478
mutuality, 526

naloxone, 99, 131
narcolepsy, 189–191, 196
narrative, 319, 533, 535
nation, 9

nature, 1, 6, 11, 14, 27, 36, 49, 55, 58, 76, 104, 107, 111, 157, 173, 194, 197, 204, 233, 266, 297, 298, 312, 313, 316, 318, 364, 367, 370, 440, 455, 457, 473, 480, 526, 529
neck, 243
need, 3, 7, 9, 11, 16, 18, 34, 36, 53, 56, 60, 62, 67, 74, 75, 98, 99, 105, 121, 127, 154, 158, 175, 176, 178, 218, 223, 224, 236, 316, 320, 326, 331, 333, 338, 348, 354, 356, 357, 370, 396, 400, 401, 403, 406, 420, 423, 429, 431, 437, 454, 469, 479–481, 483, 484, 491–494, 504, 521, 524, 526, 528, 542, 546, 547
needle, 83, 131
neglect, 44, 49, 66, 111, 217, 220, 222, 423
neighborhood, 38, 468, 511
nerve, 247, 248, 255
nest, 443
network, 1, 106, 114, 247, 255, 320, 326, 330, 371, 385, 388, 394, 412, 419, 452, 519, 542, 544
neurobiology, 96
neurofeedback, 534
neuroplasticity, 266
neuroscience, 22, 489
neurostimulation, 178
neurotransmitter, 35, 210, 234, 261, 264
newborn, 213, 215
news, 86

nicotine, 119
night, 188, 189, 192
non, 19, 57, 63, 105, 128, 130, 186, 232, 241, 273, 282–284, 294, 295, 298, 299, 305, 312–314, 332, 451, 452, 468, 479, 516, 531
nonprofit, 399
nonreactivity, 415
nose, 416
notice, 255, 282
notion, 8, 222
novel, 212, 534
number, 356, 506
numbness, 111
nursing, 527
nurture, 246, 318, 321, 385
nurturing, 4, 40, 66, 216, 221, 228, 249, 315, 316, 318, 320–322, 394, 420, 449, 478, 549
nutrient, 258
nutrition, 53, 171, 250, 252, 255, 413, 478, 480, 482
nutritionist, 266

objective, 64
observation, 417
obstacle, 34
occupational, 71, 82, 133, 139, 142–144, 221, 222, 333–337, 484, 490, 527
occurrence, 83, 104, 123, 126
offer, 17, 18, 20, 63, 73, 125, 130, 169, 209, 213, 215, 223–226, 234, 244, 274, 276, 279, 281, 288, 296, 298, 309, 315, 316, 318, 320, 321, 326, 327, 331,

344, 357, 388, 391, 395, 396, 420, 424, 431, 432, 438, 451, 460, 482, 519, 528, 532, 534
offering, 27, 32, 53, 54, 59, 104, 263, 299, 301, 330, 332, 431, 451
on, 1–10, 12–19, 21, 22, 24–28, 31, 32, 35, 36, 38–41, 43–45, 47, 49–53, 55–58, 60, 64, 66, 67, 70, 71, 75, 78, 79, 82–84, 88, 92, 93, 95, 96, 99, 103, 107–109, 111, 112, 114–116, 119, 125–127, 129–131, 135–137, 144, 154, 158, 160, 161, 164–172, 175, 176, 178, 185–188, 190, 191, 193–195, 199, 201, 202, 204, 213, 215, 217, 218, 220–223, 226–228, 231, 233, 235, 236, 243, 244, 247, 250, 252, 253, 255, 256, 258–264, 266, 267, 269, 275, 276, 279–285, 287, 291, 294–301, 304, 305, 309–311, 314, 316–320, 330–335, 344, 345, 347, 348, 355–357, 363–371, 373, 383, 385, 389, 391, 394–396, 399, 404, 406, 407, 410, 412, 414, 416, 417, 419–426, 428–432, 440, 442, 443, 448–450, 452, 453, 457–462, 467–469, 472–475, 477, 479, 480, 482–484, 486, 491, 494, 495, 499, 500, 513, 515–517, 519, 525–528, 534, 539, 540, 543–547
one, 1, 25, 29, 36, 51, 55, 57, 75, 91, 94, 112, 113, 126, 160, 176, 221, 240, 241, 243, 256, 295, 312, 313, 316–318, 321, 322, 330, 331, 364, 367, 369, 372–374, 383, 391, 395, 403, 410, 415, 417–420, 436, 437, 469, 472, 475, 479, 522, 542–544
onset, 12, 135, 189, 211, 224, 236, 367
openness, 326, 417, 491, 543
operation, 72
opioid, 99, 122, 127, 130, 131
opportunity, 32, 98, 160, 259, 307, 418, 426, 482
oppression, 48, 116, 455, 456
optimism, 301, 365–367, 373, 383–385, 418, 452, 473
order, 3, 11, 13, 69, 113, 316, 352, 358, 418, 433, 459, 485, 489, 492–495, 501, 505, 519, 529
orderliness, 203
organization, 136, 142, 344, 399, 475
orientation, 355, 430, 509, 539
other, 4, 15, 24, 27, 34, 37, 40, 43, 45, 47, 55, 57, 58, 62, 70, 74, 75, 77, 98, 101, 104, 106, 108, 111, 114, 120, 126, 130, 131, 133, 136, 163, 165, 168, 173, 186, 190, 193, 201, 202, 205, 207, 221, 224, 225, 228,

232, 235, 241–243, 261, 266, 268, 270, 275, 276, 279, 282, 283, 296, 301, 309, 315, 317, 321, 331, 332, 359, 363, 367, 376, 383, 384, 395, 412, 417, 426, 431, 440, 443, 453, 457, 458, 471, 472, 479, 482, 486, 490, 491, 495, 508, 519, 527, 533, 539, 546, 547
outcome, 266, 280, 282, 419, 422
outlet, 431
outline, 499
outlook, 1, 280, 285, 363, 365–367, 383, 410, 411, 414, 439, 448, 450, 550
outpatient, 106
outreach, 19, 75, 224, 226, 356, 400
overcrowding, 70, 222
overdose, 130, 131
overlap, 104, 128, 201, 455
overreliance, 28
oversight, 67
ownership, 520, 543, 544
oxygen, 260
oxytocin, 295, 320

Pacific Island, 474
Pacific Islander, 474
pain, 44, 173, 176, 181, 184, 214, 243, 246, 247, 259, 274, 447, 453
painting, 233
panacea, 18
panic, 81, 275
paper, 53
paradigm, 31, 78, 119
paralysis, 176, 190, 191

parent, 136, 143
parenthood, 437
parenting, 12
Paris, 217
parity, 354–356
part, 45, 54, 222, 270, 275, 280, 282, 332, 348, 372, 437, 452, 501
participation, 43, 59, 124, 320, 326, 425, 447, 460, 468, 520
partnership, 75, 227, 425, 517
passion, 388
past, 31, 50, 67, 69, 106, 124, 202, 263, 478, 479, 483, 485
path, 440
pathologist, 144
pathway, 253
patience, 125, 314
patient, 33, 53, 54, 64, 70, 76, 181, 218, 240, 241, 246, 282, 336, 453, 489, 517, 545
pattern, 149, 153, 159
peace, 274, 282, 283, 312, 313, 453, 455
pediatrician, 144
peer, 8, 44, 45, 125, 127, 149, 165, 169, 171, 331–333, 391, 393, 394, 397, 426, 479, 489, 521–528, 532, 544
people, 2, 17, 22, 41, 44, 45, 55, 56, 84, 113, 119, 129, 186, 189, 278, 282, 297, 315, 321, 326, 348, 368, 369, 371, 388, 391, 429–433, 458, 474, 475, 479, 498
perception, 7, 18, 55, 67, 71, 82, 92, 96, 165, 167, 185, 217, 218, 221, 228, 259, 374, 482, 533

perfectionism, 165, 203, 417
performance, 103, 136, 194, 260, 280, 281, 334, 421, 424
period, 67, 69, 165, 167, 217, 220, 222
perpetuation, 2, 185
perseverance, 364, 422
persistence, 125, 376, 419
person, 1–4, 36, 43, 45, 49, 53, 71, 81, 90, 92, 113, 114, 120, 137, 138, 173, 199, 203, 204, 209, 213, 221–224, 226, 227, 229, 232, 235, 237, 241, 245, 246, 282, 321, 330, 388, 417, 423, 426, 432, 436, 438, 440, 451, 453, 483, 490, 516, 526, 527, 529, 533, 535, 542
personality, 24, 151, 159–161, 203, 221, 234, 335
personnel, 218
perspective, 1, 4, 9, 13, 16, 26, 147, 186, 309, 315, 319, 332, 368, 369, 373, 414, 480
pet, 295, 296
phase, 172, 209, 210
phenomenon, 33, 227
philanthropic, 360
Philippe Pinel, 66, 69, 217
philosophy, 15, 16, 217, 276, 313, 316, 318, 368
phone, 88, 388
physician, 21, 217, 447
place, 28, 54, 62, 279
plan, 28, 78, 87, 91, 99, 103, 106, 114, 115, 128, 142, 144, 160, 172, 175, 189, 191, 197, 199, 202, 215, 233, 240, 241, 244, 246, 263, 264, 266, 267, 269, 284, 300, 308, 331, 447, 467, 471, 490
planet, 475
planning, 34, 101, 108, 142, 150, 163, 224, 460, 471, 472, 494, 503, 505, 517, 520, 527, 533
plant, 242
platform, 36, 55, 294, 329, 330, 393, 501, 521
Plato, 15, 16
play, 6, 8, 17, 20, 35, 41, 46, 47, 64, 71, 96, 98, 131, 133, 136, 142, 143, 165, 171, 172, 182, 183, 191, 199, 204, 210, 215, 223–226, 233, 251, 253, 263, 298, 315, 318–320, 329, 331, 344, 348, 361, 364, 365, 373, 380, 385, 388, 394, 395, 397, 420, 425, 429, 430, 440, 446, 448, 449, 451–453, 457, 462, 464, 466, 467, 469, 473, 477, 482, 492, 495, 498, 501, 505, 519, 522, 527, 533, 542, 543, 546, 547
playfulness, 299
playing, 296, 493
pleasure, 269
point, 150, 255, 348, 527
policy, 8, 12, 13, 36, 44, 131, 141, 337, 352–356, 400, 432, 458, 474, 475, 480, 481, 486, 489, 499, 501, 520, 526, 528, 534–538, 541, 546, 547

Index 585

popularity, 53, 62, 272, 282, 415
population, 9, 39, 357, 425, 448, 459, 460, 464, 486, 499, 500
portion, 171
position, 315
positive, 1, 4, 12, 17–19, 29, 32, 39, 45, 57–59, 67, 76, 77, 113, 123, 125, 131, 164, 170, 172, 206, 218, 228, 245, 255, 256, 258–261, 263, 264, 267, 275, 279–281, 284, 285, 287, 295–299, 305, 309, 310, 320, 322, 333, 336–338, 341, 344, 363–367, 369–373, 377, 379, 383–385, 389, 394, 408, 410–412, 414, 416, 417, 419–421, 423–426, 429, 430, 439, 442, 448–450, 452, 469, 473, 478, 480, 501, 515, 516, 519, 520, 522, 523, 526, 537, 538, 542, 547, 549, 550
positivity, 385
possess, 63, 300, 316, 367, 371
possession, 15, 18, 66, 221
possibility, 332
post, 396, 399
postpartum, 213–216
potential, 17–19, 27, 34, 36, 54, 56–61, 63, 64, 66, 67, 114, 125, 126, 130, 133, 136, 139, 141, 142, 144, 158, 172, 178, 186, 192, 200, 201, 212, 222, 223, 226, 227, 232, 240, 244, 266, 269, 270, 275, 288, 297, 300, 310, 311, 315, 316, 330, 333, 360, 365, 367, 370, 407, 414, 418, 419, 423, 426, 429, 431, 437, 467, 468, 478, 481, 486, 515, 518, 532, 534, 535, 545
poverty, 38, 49, 325, 355, 368, 457, 458, 499, 509, 546
power, 12, 61, 103, 233, 282, 285, 288, 291, 313, 331, 333, 368, 369, 385, 388, 391, 394, 399, 418, 467, 473, 474, 479, 480, 482, 491, 501, 513, 515, 517, 518, 521, 539, 550
powerlessness, 37
practice, 12, 13, 20, 23, 27, 71, 76, 77, 79, 119, 131, 217, 237, 241, 243, 272–282, 285, 289, 291, 297–299, 312–314, 318, 319, 331, 346, 365, 377, 378, 390, 403–405, 412, 415–420, 430, 446, 449, 452, 467, 474, 475, 480, 483, 485, 486, 489, 491, 493, 494, 528, 544
practicing, 16, 70, 112, 169, 189, 191, 216, 275, 279–281, 312, 347, 373, 379, 385, 412, 416, 436, 473, 519, 542
praise, 25, 154
prayer, 17
pre, 260
precipitation, 472
precursor, 15
predisposition, 3, 123, 156, 165,

168, 204, 211, 383
pregnancy, 133, 215
prejudice, 7, 44, 481
preoccupation, 82, 165, 181
preparedness, 396, 466–468
prescribing, 53, 262
prescription, 99, 119, 123
presence, 37, 82, 97, 104, 128, 137, 146, 155, 173, 176, 185, 201, 211, 295–300, 305, 307, 308, 314, 370, 445, 451
present, 11, 18, 23, 60, 69, 113, 118, 156, 163, 170, 181, 182, 240, 273–275, 280, 283, 300, 312, 313, 318, 414–416, 451, 471, 516, 528
preservation, 218, 474
pressure, 40, 47, 165, 182, 233, 275, 296, 299, 334, 337, 411–413, 426
prevalence, 9, 11, 12, 104, 112, 356, 480
preventing, 12, 130, 211, 363, 367, 407, 409
prevention, 11–13, 21, 99, 104, 106, 124, 128–130, 161, 164, 172, 226, 236, 250, 255, 283, 348, 352, 409, 478, 482, 485, 534, 545, 546
principal, 421
principle, 60, 241, 279, 297, 305, 391, 464
prioritization, 413
priority, 297, 300, 521, 539, 546
privacy, 53, 54, 60–63, 79, 331, 333, 482, 518
probiotics, 258

problem, 1, 57, 137, 260, 280, 365, 367, 372, 373, 380–382, 394, 411, 412, 414, 421, 422, 429, 430, 449, 458, 473
process, 26, 31, 33, 34, 44, 45, 77, 98, 104, 106, 109, 114, 116, 124, 136, 142, 166, 167, 170, 171, 181, 190, 195, 202, 222, 224, 232, 247, 266, 282–285, 298, 299, 301, 303, 308, 316, 317, 340, 370, 373, 375, 377, 385, 390, 412, 418, 419, 422, 429, 436–438, 440, 445, 448, 451, 452, 460, 461, 469, 495, 503, 517, 521, 527
processing, 203, 516
production, 255, 259, 261, 266
productivity, 154, 194, 342, 344, 345, 355, 413, 442
professional, 18, 45, 58, 88, 90, 93, 102, 103, 115, 150, 156–158, 160, 166, 171–173, 188, 197, 199, 204, 207, 211, 258, 260, 281, 298, 305, 316, 321, 322, 330–332, 334, 337, 346, 409, 435, 436, 440, 447, 451, 458, 483, 492–495, 518, 542
professionalization, 218
proficiency, 54
profile, 367
progesterone, 213
prognosis, 453
program, 19, 20, 75, 99, 124–126, 166, 262, 268, 274, 275,

409, 421, 428, 432, 442, 459–461, 532
progress, 13, 14, 59, 74, 144, 153, 157, 159, 205, 263, 266, 418, 420, 422, 452, 481, 499, 535
progression, 182, 224, 437, 484, 545
project, 382, 417, 421, 422, 475, 532
projection, 25
prominence, 78, 364, 368, 479
promise, 61, 66, 79, 159, 206, 212, 249, 466, 480, 534
promotion, 60, 235, 288, 340, 348, 498, 519–521, 526, 533, 545
proposal, 75
protection, 53, 60, 217, 458
provide, 3, 4, 8, 13–19, 23, 28, 31, 36, 39, 40, 44, 45, 51, 54, 55, 57, 58, 60–64, 66, 69, 71, 72, 75, 78, 81–84, 95, 97, 98, 102, 114, 115, 125–128, 130, 136, 142–144, 158, 160, 161, 166–169, 171, 178, 181, 202, 204, 215–217, 221, 223, 224, 226, 229, 232, 233, 236, 244, 255, 260–263, 270, 276, 279–282, 287, 288, 291, 294–300, 305, 308, 309, 311, 312, 315, 316, 318, 320–322, 326, 331–333, 338, 347, 357, 358, 367, 370, 372, 373, 385, 387, 388, 390, 391, 394–397, 403, 404, 414, 417, 419, 420, 422, 424, 426, 430–432, 435, 436, 440, 446–453, 458, 460, 461, 467–469, 471, 473, 474, 479–481, 483, 484, 490, 491, 493, 494, 499, 501, 505, 518–522, 526, 529, 533–535, 546
provider, 166, 227, 258, 262, 263, 266, 517
provision, 12, 32, 71, 112, 217, 218, 352, 458, 499, 505
proximity, 54, 224
psychiatrist, 66, 69, 124, 128, 156, 207, 211, 490, 527
psychiatry, 21–24, 26, 27, 67, 250, 252, 253, 258, 489, 527
psychoanalysis, 23–25
psychoeducation, 28, 45, 229, 267, 408, 409, 517, 519
psychologist, 45, 144, 156, 211, 374, 418, 490, 527
psychology, 24, 25, 44, 45, 313, 364, 368, 415, 422, 489, 490, 492, 527
psychopathology, 370
psychopharmacology, 23, 35, 77, 79
psychosis, 92, 95
psychosocial, 23, 27, 28, 71, 94–96, 135, 137, 155, 207, 226, 228, 448, 453
psychotherapy, 21, 23, 25, 27, 77–79, 90, 91, 94–97, 114, 115, 147, 159–161, 165, 172, 176, 180, 181, 203, 275, 276, 282, 490
public, 16, 22, 71, 169, 175, 225, 348–351, 356, 468, 469, 471, 480, 481, 484, 489, 495, 501, 508, 509, 518, 535

punishment, 18, 21, 70, 217, 221
purging, 15
purity, 130
purpose, 1, 17, 18, 70–72, 218, 221, 295, 299, 309, 316–319, 321, 373, 385, 396, 429, 430, 444, 448, 450, 453, 458
purposelessness, 443
pursuit, 444, 539, 542
push, 22, 149, 420
puzzle, 57

quality, 2–4, 13, 33, 38, 42, 44, 45, 47, 48, 51, 70, 74, 77, 79, 88, 103, 106, 113, 122, 125, 129, 133, 136, 139, 141, 149, 157, 159, 173, 175, 176, 189–191, 193, 195, 196, 198, 199, 206, 211, 213, 225, 226, 252, 260, 261, 263, 276, 280, 284, 321, 336, 347, 355, 358, 371, 390, 445, 447–449, 453, 455, 458, 471, 477, 482, 485–489, 498, 499, 501, 502, 505, 506, 509, 512, 528, 535, 540, 541, 546
quest, 383
question, 281
quirk, 203

race, 12, 41, 43, 46, 49, 355, 406, 455, 509, 539
racing, 241, 280
racism, 6, 47
range, 1, 17, 50, 53, 73, 74, 79, 88, 106, 111, 112, 127, 131, 132, 143, 151, 162, 223, 225, 226, 232, 238, 241, 244, 283, 286, 290, 293, 357, 393, 395, 423, 457, 458, 496, 499, 525, 539, 545, 546
rapport, 109, 460
rate, 62, 182, 275, 299
rationality, 15
re, 51, 447
reach, 167, 326, 330, 332, 357, 422, 432, 488, 498, 500
reactivity, 113
readiness, 241
reading, 446, 449, 494
reality, 63, 66, 92, 144, 203, 229, 312, 318, 357, 384, 453, 482, 534, 535
realization, 284
realm, 282, 319
reason, 221
reasoning, 137, 222
reassurance, 149, 204
recognition, 16, 27, 31, 58, 71, 164, 169, 222, 227, 275, 282, 295, 337, 348, 364, 415, 464, 479, 480, 501, 513, 542
recommendation, 256
record, 158, 280
recovery, 8, 12, 32, 44, 51, 55, 70, 83, 95, 96, 98, 102–104, 106, 109, 112, 114, 117, 122, 124–129, 132, 148, 150, 161, 164, 166, 167, 169, 171, 172, 181, 209, 215, 221–229, 315, 332, 333, 357, 396, 413, 437, 451, 452, 467, 468, 478, 481,

515, 526
recreation, 218, 431
recruiting, 357
redirection, 33
reduction, 3, 57, 78, 83, 99, 115, 129–132, 158, 189, 206, 243, 245, 246, 269, 275, 283, 284, 295, 298, 299, 301, 304, 415, 442, 468, 474, 513–515
reductionism, 27
reference, 280
refining, 515
reflection, 282, 285, 316, 318, 319, 365, 373, 377–379, 412, 436, 450, 493, 542, 544
reform, 66, 68, 534–538
reformation, 220
reframing, 366, 414, 419, 533
refugee, 461
refusal, 25
regimen, 222, 260
region, 475
regulation, 67, 111, 116, 134, 147, 149, 165, 168, 170, 210, 245, 253, 296, 298, 299, 313, 366, 367, 372, 394, 410, 412, 415, 416, 418, 420, 421, 423–425, 430, 445, 449, 499, 501, 544
rehabilitation, 44, 45, 71, 166, 217, 218, 226, 283, 286
reimbursement, 481
reinforcement, 131
reintegration, 128, 222
rejection, 321, 372
relapse, 90, 95, 98, 104, 106, 123, 124, 126, 128, 129, 163, 172, 211, 283

relation, 6
relationship, 17, 37–39, 41, 43, 46, 55–57, 60, 119, 120, 122, 148, 166, 168, 171, 172, 182, 184, 222, 244, 247, 250, 253, 287, 295, 297, 309, 311, 331, 377, 379, 391, 412, 425, 437, 445, 472, 517, 518, 527
relativism, 4, 7
relaxation, 57, 58, 91, 112, 114, 185, 189, 191, 222, 232–234, 243, 246, 247, 261, 275, 279, 280, 283, 295, 297, 298, 373, 413, 416, 446
release, 185, 259, 261, 264, 267, 269, 282, 288, 294, 295, 299, 320, 413
relevance, 312, 432, 459
relevancy, 520
reliability, 370
reliance, 27, 53
relief, 22, 57, 77, 195, 203
reliever, 283
religion, 18–20, 309–312
reminder, 67, 479
reminiscence, 450
remorse, 158
removal, 217
replacement, 276
report, 18, 108, 204, 336, 364, 370, 421
reporting, 97
representation, 515
repression, 25
research, 2, 7, 11–13, 20, 23, 25–27, 40, 57, 59, 67, 69, 76, 77, 79, 86, 89, 92, 96, 123, 126, 129, 132–134, 136,

143, 145, 146, 149, 155, 156, 169, 178, 182, 186, 195, 204–206, 209, 210, 212, 213, 244, 247–249, 261, 297, 357, 361, 368, 369, 421, 432, 460, 468, 475, 480, 482, 483, 485, 487–491, 494–498, 500, 528, 534, 546, 547
resilience, 1, 4, 6, 12, 15, 16, 44, 45, 49, 51, 52, 79, 82, 103, 109, 111, 112, 114, 115, 119, 203, 206, 223, 227, 228, 231, 234, 236, 247, 258, 274–276, 279, 284, 288, 297, 313, 316, 317, 319, 320, 322, 331–333, 335, 361, 363–382, 384–397, 404, 407–413, 415–420, 422–425, 429–434, 436, 440, 442–445, 447–455, 457–462, 464, 466–469, 471–475, 477–480, 484, 519, 521, 522, 534, 539, 543, 547–550
resistance, 153, 313, 325
resource, 12, 218, 226, 357, 361, 400, 482, 486, 489, 500, 501, 503–505, 532
respect, 18–20, 39, 61, 69, 221, 227, 297, 331, 333, 371, 414, 423, 438, 457, 459, 479, 491, 516, 517, 519, 526
respite, 57, 447
response, 28, 31, 49, 71, 106, 113, 186, 205, 212, 223, 255, 275, 334, 344, 369, 375, 376, 413, 416, 425, 467, 468, 473, 474, 479
responsibility, 34, 158, 215, 298, 299, 316, 415, 430, 477, 498, 500, 542–544
rest, 195, 413
restoration, 170, 221, 474
restriction, 164, 166
restructuring, 414
result, 2, 8, 23, 28, 33, 36, 49, 66, 69, 82, 106, 111, 116, 136, 152, 159, 168, 188, 189, 207, 344, 413, 423, 425, 447
retention, 442
retirement, 446
reversal, 131
review, 155, 158, 163, 450, 500
revolution, 217
reward, 119, 122, 168
riding, 304
right, 19, 34, 60, 77, 87, 149, 191, 214
rigor, 67
rise, 28, 54, 472
risk, 2, 11, 12, 27, 35, 37, 44, 51, 53, 58, 63, 72, 86, 95, 99, 100, 104, 114, 123, 128, 130, 131, 133, 144, 156, 158, 164, 165, 168, 169, 192, 200, 204, 206, 210, 213, 224, 235, 256, 296, 320, 407, 426–429, 445, 468, 479, 482, 484, 545
roadmap, 499
role, 1, 2, 4, 8, 11, 12, 16, 17, 19–21, 24–26, 35, 39, 41, 44–47, 49, 51–53, 64, 66, 71, 78, 98, 99, 125, 131, 133, 136, 141, 142, 144, 165, 170,

171, 182, 183, 186, 191,
199, 204, 210, 215,
222–226, 233, 245, 247,
250, 251, 253, 255, 259,
260, 263, 267, 275, 298,
309, 315–320, 325, 329,
331, 337, 344, 348, 352,
354, 355, 361, 363–367,
369, 371, 373, 375–377,
380, 382, 383, 385, 388,
390, 391, 394, 395, 397,
407, 413, 420, 422, 425,
426, 429–431, 434, 440,
446–449, 451–453, 457,
459, 462, 464, 466, 467,
469, 472, 473, 478, 480,
482, 489, 492, 493, 495,
498, 501, 505, 513, 516,
519, 521, 522, 526, 527,
533, 535, 542, 543, 546,
547
Roman Empire, 21
root, 40, 188, 338, 474
routine, 58, 70, 95, 191, 195, 196,
260, 262, 265, 266, 269,
280, 282, 314, 347, 417,
446, 484
rule, 173, 181, 193, 201
rumination, 415
run, 168, 204

sadness, 15, 91, 128, 213, 269, 287,
447
safeguard, 60
safer, 130, 131
safety, 22, 51, 110, 158, 212, 244,
297, 298, 300, 329–331,
356, 372, 404, 423, 447,
457, 467, 480

Samoa, 474
San Francisco, 75
Sarah, 91, 103, 106, 115, 124, 125,
136, 181, 188, 189, 191,
202, 263, 266, 269, 270,
284, 285, 287, 288, 300,
301, 346, 347, 379, 390,
411, 412, 417, 438, 439
Sarah, 191
satiety, 314
satisfaction, 18, 259, 317, 320, 331,
334, 336, 342, 344, 345,
385, 440, 442, 453, 517,
547
scale, 9, 71, 217
scan, 274
scenario, 115, 136, 154, 346, 381
scene, 203
schedule, 191
scheduling, 451
schemas, 159
schizophrenia, 82, 206–209, 234,
261, 262, 322, 516
school, 136, 166, 399, 421,
423–425, 428, 437, 481,
501
science, 221, 421, 473
scope, 1, 2, 25, 477
screen, 215, 388
screening, 12, 97, 409, 484
sculpting, 233
sea, 284, 472, 474
search, 316, 318
season, 417
section, 9, 14, 17, 21, 24, 28, 33, 39,
43, 49, 52, 61, 71, 76, 84,
88, 96, 99, 104, 115, 126,
129, 161, 169, 172, 186,
189, 195, 199, 223, 227,

237, 245, 250, 252, 255,
261, 263, 267, 272, 276,
279, 282, 289, 295, 301,
305, 312, 316, 319, 322,
333, 337, 345, 352, 358,
371, 377, 380, 385, 388,
391, 394, 397, 403, 407,
412, 420, 423, 426, 436,
440, 442, 445, 448, 451,
457, 466, 469, 472, 479,
481, 483, 485, 489, 495,
498, 501, 509, 516, 519,
522, 526, 535, 542
sector, 336
security, 53, 54, 60, 62, 79, 296, 320,
333, 389, 437, 482
seeking, 2, 7, 8, 18, 38, 40, 47, 51,
58, 60, 61, 63, 79, 98, 105,
112, 119, 129, 149, 150,
153, 167, 199, 204, 216,
224, 228, 237, 281, 284,
288, 315, 316, 319, 321,
322, 327, 330, 331, 333,
339, 356, 365, 372, 399,
402, 418, 419, 435, 436,
453, 481, 484, 501, 509,
513, 515–517, 520, 527,
534, 542–544
segregation, 217
selection, 37, 148
self, 8, 15, 16, 34, 37, 44, 45, 51, 55,
56, 62, 70, 97, 106, 108,
111, 112, 114, 115,
122–124, 127, 128, 131,
133, 134, 136, 137, 147,
149, 154, 160, 164–166,
168–170, 202–204, 215,
216, 221, 222, 227–229,
233, 234, 243, 245, 246,
258–262, 264, 266, 274,
275, 280, 282–285,
287–289, 291, 294, 295,
298, 299, 312–314,
316–320, 322, 331, 332,
336, 337, 347, 364, 365,
367, 370, 372–379, 385,
389, 391, 397, 412, 413,
415–425, 429, 431, 435,
436, 440, 442, 448–453,
458, 467, 473, 493, 494,
534, 542, 544
sensation, 176, 314, 417
sense, 1, 4, 8, 17, 18, 39, 44, 45, 55,
70, 103, 111, 112, 114,
115, 131, 149, 160, 165,
166, 169, 171, 202, 203,
218, 221, 222, 259–264,
267, 274, 275, 279–283,
287, 288, 295–301, 304,
305, 309, 311–313,
315–322, 330, 332, 334,
338, 367, 369, 371–373,
385, 388, 389, 394–396,
414, 418–420, 423, 424,
429, 430, 440, 443, 444,
448–452, 457, 458, 461,
473, 516, 518, 520, 533,
542–544, 547
sensitivity, 7, 18, 109, 355, 414, 426,
457, 518, 519, 540
series, 49, 116, 195, 442
Serotonin, 259
serotonin, 35, 165, 204, 205, 234,
236, 253, 255, 259, 261,
320
service, 7, 12, 106, 112, 355, 403,
430, 500
session, 284

set, 100, 123, 126, 142, 199, 266, 363, 366, 380, 418, 436, 452, 490, 513, 542
setback, 376
setting, 45, 61, 70, 228, 266, 267, 305, 332, 347, 373, 385, 413, 422, 430, 431, 442, 547
severity, 49, 94, 111, 132, 160, 166, 172, 176, 181, 190, 193, 197, 204, 210, 215, 217, 262, 484
sex, 39
sexuality, 406, 455
shadow, 347, 348
Shakti Gawain, 281
shame, 8, 44, 111, 113, 128, 166, 218, 309, 315
shape, 2, 4, 6, 24, 26, 59, 82, 99, 165, 168, 234, 367, 369, 385, 404, 408, 423, 455, 464, 539, 542
share, 54, 55, 149, 169, 205, 287, 300, 307, 315, 326, 331, 333, 347, 388, 392, 395, 396, 450, 461, 479, 493, 518, 520–522, 526, 528
sharing, 53, 129, 171, 468, 474, 481, 543
shelter, 468
shift, 3, 22, 23, 28, 31, 33, 58, 66, 67, 69, 71, 78, 119, 218, 223, 227, 279, 281, 344, 413, 416, 437, 479, 480, 543
shock, 438
shortage, 22, 356, 400, 481
show, 79, 153, 212, 321, 451
Siddhartha Gautama, 368
side, 27, 67, 77, 125, 232

sight, 369
Sigmund Freud, 24, 26, 176
Sigmund Freud, 21
sign, 181, 213, 220, 418
significance, 119, 311, 316, 322, 369, 388, 477
silence, 8
simplicity, 313
sister, 202
site, 442
situation, 280, 368
size, 165, 168, 221, 256, 298, 367
skepticism, 174
skill, 314, 371, 413, 415, 416, 420, 431, 475, 490, 516
sleep, 4, 62, 91, 98, 111–114, 186–199, 211, 243, 261–264, 274, 280, 282, 373, 413, 441, 446, 448, 449
sleepiness, 188–191
smartphone, 281, 417, 481
smell, 279
smoke, 467
Snapchat, 54
sobriety, 131
socialization, 57, 221
socializing, 190
society, 1, 4, 7, 8, 14, 15, 28, 31, 33, 39, 44, 46, 52, 56, 76, 84, 99, 126, 128, 141, 143, 159, 164, 172, 175, 176, 218, 221, 222, 247, 295, 315, 333–335, 337, 345, 347, 348, 355, 391, 397, 400, 410, 412, 423, 450, 478, 481, 492, 501, 514–516, 518, 519, 524,

525, 533, 539, 540,
542–544
socio, 2, 461, 529
solace, 17, 20, 298, 315, 317, 330
solution, 217, 421, 422
solve, 1, 137, 372, 410
solving, 57, 137, 260, 280, 365, 367, 372, 373, 380–382, 394, 411, 412, 414, 421, 422, 429, 430, 449, 458, 473
somatization, 185
Somatization Disorder, 175
somatoform, 182
song, 287
songwriting, 287
soul, 15
sound, 255, 353
source, 17, 25, 299, 304, 309, 320, 372, 388, 431
space, 20, 55, 130, 169, 171, 280, 281, 284, 285, 287, 294, 301, 307, 315, 326, 327, 390, 392, 416, 451, 452, 461, 526
speaker, 369, 516
specialist, 53, 189–191, 197, 199
specialty, 22, 23, 26, 224, 225
specific, 2, 12, 25, 26, 35, 44, 45, 48, 51, 58, 64, 78, 81, 84, 90, 93, 94, 97, 114, 125, 126, 128, 137, 142, 144, 148, 156, 157, 159, 160, 163, 167, 172, 181, 186, 187, 189, 190, 195, 197, 201, 204, 221, 241, 243, 253, 257, 262, 275, 281, 286, 298, 299, 314, 330, 331, 333, 334, 347, 356, 367, 370, 374, 405, 413, 422,
426, 432, 448, 459–461, 486, 491, 498, 500, 517, 519, 520, 533
spectrum, 256
speech, 139, 142–144
spending, 320, 321, 347, 417
spine, 243
spirit, 237, 241, 312, 369
spirituality, 19, 20, 478, 480
spontaneity, 313
spread, 129
St. John's, 232, 242
stability, 15, 91, 130, 210, 226, 309, 320, 370, 458
staff, 70, 106, 217, 225, 423–425
stage, 1, 25, 236, 370, 443
stakeholder, 61, 352
stance, 417
standardization, 76
standing, 159, 278
start, 241
starting, 130, 150, 255, 258, 260, 416, 438
state, 3, 58, 243, 259, 267, 273, 283, 299, 312, 316, 348, 413
status, 8, 12, 27, 35, 37–39, 41, 46, 48, 49, 53, 54, 78, 213, 235, 355, 357, 458, 479, 482, 484, 509, 519, 539
step, 33, 218, 247, 280, 337, 353, 355, 413, 417, 451, 488, 492, 514, 516, 532
stigma, 2, 7, 8, 18, 34, 38–40, 44, 48, 63, 96, 98, 104–106, 123, 126, 128, 129, 132, 141, 149, 150, 158, 169, 175, 176, 205, 213, 218, 221, 222, 224–227, 236, 315, 325, 326, 331, 339–341,

356, 395–397, 399–402,
444, 477, 478, 480, 481,
483, 484, 494, 501, 509,
513–520, 528, 534, 535,
538, 540, 542–547
stigmatization, 479
stillness, 313
stimulant, 136
stimulation, 243, 298, 450
storage, 62
story, 103, 149, 369
storytelling, 6, 461, 474, 519
strain, 22, 91, 334
strategy, 130, 131, 418, 475, 517
stream, 243
strength, 15, 17, 36, 112, 191, 243,
262, 263, 298, 316, 317,
364, 368, 373, 391, 395,
396, 445, 455
strengthening, 23, 32, 373, 473, 484
stress, 1, 3, 18, 36, 38, 47, 57, 61, 62,
78, 91, 103, 112, 114, 120,
166, 169, 182, 184–186,
190, 210, 213, 233, 235,
243, 245, 246, 255, 259,
261, 263, 264, 266, 267,
274–276, 279, 282–285,
295, 297–299, 301, 309,
313, 314, 320, 333–338,
341, 343, 345, 347, 363,
365, 366, 369, 371–373,
377, 383–385, 388, 389,
394, 396, 397, 410–417,
419, 421, 423, 430,
435–437, 440–442, 448,
452, 457, 458, 467, 472,
479, 540, 544, 547, 548
stroke, 445
structure, 112, 221, 234

struggle, 128, 132, 195, 225, 241,
345, 440
student, 103, 166, 281, 376, 382,
411, 412, 417, 421, 424,
425
study, 99, 114, 115, 245, 267, 269,
287, 336, 364, 368, 376,
409, 442, 461, 478, 511,
512
suasion, 222
subconscious, 282
subject, 66, 136, 217, 309
substance, 40, 82, 83, 96–99,
104–106, 119, 123–131,
205, 210, 212, 283, 355,
426, 445
substitute, 63, 258, 316
success, 40, 160, 161, 225, 265, 280,
341, 342, 344, 345, 377,
385, 419, 422, 423, 425
suffering, 15, 18, 26, 66, 312, 368
suicide, 40, 123, 355
summary, 2, 4, 13, 61, 112, 452, 458,
498, 529
sunlight, 70
supervision, 130, 270
supervisor, 347
supplement, 204
supplementation, 195, 258
support, 1–4, 7, 8, 12, 17–20,
22–24, 32–34, 36, 38–41,
43–46, 48, 51, 52, 54, 55,
58–60, 62, 63, 67, 71, 72,
75, 78, 79, 81, 83, 84, 87,
88, 91, 95, 97–99,
102–104, 106, 107, 111,
112, 114, 115, 117, 119,
124–128, 130–132,
134–137, 139–141, 143,

144, 147, 149, 150, 153,
159–161, 166, 167,
169–172, 175, 176, 179,
181, 189, 191, 202, 203,
206, 207, 213–216,
222–226, 229, 232–236,
244, 247, 249, 252, 253,
258, 259, 262, 266, 270,
278, 281, 283, 288, 291,
295–301, 303–305,
307–309, 311, 313, 315,
316, 318–323, 325–333,
336, 337, 339, 343, 345,
347, 357, 358, 361, 364,
366, 367, 369–373, 385,
387–397, 400, 402–404,
407, 411, 412, 414, 417,
419, 420, 424–426,
429–432, 435–437,
439–441, 446–453, 455,
457–461, 464, 466–469,
471, 473, 478–480,
482–484, 490–494,
499–501, 505, 516–529,
532–534, 539, 540,
542–544, 546, 547
surprise, 190
surrounding, 7, 13, 22, 27, 33, 38,
44, 98, 105, 137, 148, 150,
178, 225, 315, 385, 401,
415, 481, 494, 513, 533
survey, 331, 344
susceptibility, 245, 317
sustainability, 4, 54, 141, 225, 262,
265, 319, 322, 337, 344,
348, 358, 363, 366, 403,
432, 445, 466, 471, 475,
478, 501, 505, 515, 521,
526

swimming, 446, 448
symmetry, 203
symptom, 3, 94, 148, 172, 175, 179,
181, 185, 190, 195, 206,
229
symptomatology, 182
syndrome, 173, 196, 443
synthesis, 266
system, 22, 28, 33–35, 53, 54, 83,
97, 122, 127, 132, 135,
144, 168, 181, 182, 185,
190, 218–220, 245, 253,
255, 275, 312, 320, 367,
372, 423, 480, 483–485,
505, 513, 519, 526, 529,
540, 541, 543

table, 527
tai, 233
Tai Chi, 246, 276–279
tailor, 36, 78, 172, 181, 270, 374,
451, 519
tailoring, 45, 221, 512
taking, 3, 112, 124, 132, 188, 191,
266, 281, 347, 388, 501,
534, 547
tale, 67, 218
talk, 7, 21, 283, 413, 419, 420, 449
tap, 59, 282
target, 12, 25, 26, 35, 38, 126, 143,
245, 257, 330, 398, 459,
496, 517
task, 280, 369, 417
taste, 279
teaching, 45, 143, 421, 422, 430
team, 45, 106, 121, 126, 128, 139,
142, 144, 154, 166, 226,
260, 262, 332, 379, 446,

Index 597

447, 453, 490, 491, 527, 546
teamwork, 57, 154, 336, 379, 431
tech, 340, 344
technique, 275, 281
technology, 45, 54, 56, 59–63, 79, 143, 229, 321, 326, 331, 333, 343, 345, 361, 387, 432, 450, 481, 483, 518, 519, 534, 535
teenager, 390
telecommunication, 52
telehealth, 75, 356
telemedicine, 52–54, 60, 481
tension, 185, 233, 243, 245, 247, 413, 414, 416
term, 22, 27, 31, 71, 83, 95, 106, 111, 112, 114, 126, 128, 129, 136, 148, 153, 167, 172, 176, 186, 188, 202, 211, 226, 260, 262, 344, 407, 409, 426, 430, 432, 461, 469, 484
test, 281
testament, 369
testing, 130, 190
text, 313
textbook, 478
The Pacific Islands, 474
the Pacific Islands, 474
the United States, 71
theater, 431
theory, 15, 21, 24, 26
therapist, 77, 88, 103, 115, 128, 144, 149, 159–161, 166, 181, 202, 203, 263, 266, 269, 282, 284, 287, 298, 300, 304, 307, 392, 393, 490
therapy, 18, 21, 36, 45, 61, 69–71, 77, 78, 83, 84, 88, 91, 103, 106, 115, 124, 127, 128, 133, 136, 137, 143, 144, 149, 153, 159–161, 166, 169, 181, 185, 189, 191, 202, 203, 206, 218, 222, 224, 233, 235, 240, 241, 243, 246, 259, 261, 263, 267–271, 275, 276, 282–288, 294, 296–305, 307, 308, 319, 322, 330, 390–397, 415, 424, 447, 450, 451, 461, 478–480, 482, 490, 527, 534
thinking, 35, 82, 92, 96, 113, 185, 235, 236, 365–367, 372, 382–385, 416, 458, 547
thought, 15, 34, 185, 195, 243, 261
threshold, 370
thyroid, 163
time, 1, 9, 14, 22, 28, 58, 62–64, 66, 69, 70, 76, 88, 96, 103, 114, 115, 126, 128, 142, 155, 160, 166, 181, 189, 202, 204, 217, 255, 266, 267, 285, 287, 304, 314, 320, 321, 330, 334, 337, 345, 347, 363, 370, 382, 387, 388, 390, 412, 413, 416, 417, 433, 437, 440, 442, 451, 453, 455, 469, 472, 491, 494, 518, 544
tissue, 243
tobacco, 96
today, 54, 333, 342, 387, 415, 440
toll, 166, 194, 473
tone, 189, 190
tool, 57–60, 63, 276, 282, 284, 285, 288, 384, 392, 416, 420,

450, 517, 523
top, 300, 416
topic, 83, 148
touch, 92
track, 53, 62, 169, 190, 370, 499
tracking, 53, 59, 229
tract, 248, 255
tradition, 314
train, 275
training, 7, 79, 106, 127–129, 131, 136, 143, 144, 178, 225, 262, 263, 272, 280, 297, 298, 300, 304, 315, 316, 332, 357, 366, 382, 396, 409, 424, 425, 446, 450, 459, 461, 473, 481–483, 490–495, 521, 529, 540, 541
trait, 363, 366, 385
tranquility, 279, 313, 368
transcendence, 319
transformation, 294, 480
transgender, 39
transition, 34, 144, 433, 437–439, 442
translation, 490, 495–498
transmission, 130, 131
transparency, 62, 63
transportation, 40, 75, 224, 266, 356, 389, 447, 471, 518, 534
trauma, 6, 40, 44, 47, 49–52, 82, 83, 98, 99, 107–112, 115–119, 168, 183, 202, 204, 283, 356, 363, 366, 368, 369, 396, 403–407, 410, 423–426, 461, 472, 473, 477, 479, 480, 548
traumatization, 51

travel, 75, 186, 326, 356
treat, 82, 127, 159, 160, 205, 217, 242, 316, 407, 416, 495
treatment, 7–9, 11–14, 16, 18, 19, 21–24, 26–28, 31, 33, 38, 41, 53, 58–61, 64, 66–71, 76–79, 82–84, 86–88, 90–92, 94–99, 101–112, 114, 115, 119, 121–131, 136, 137, 139, 142, 147–150, 153, 154, 157–161, 163–172, 174, 175, 177, 178, 180–182, 186, 188–191, 193–199, 201–203, 205, 208, 209, 211–213, 215–218, 220–224, 226–228, 233, 235, 240, 241, 243, 245–247, 250, 255, 261, 263, 264, 266–270, 275, 283–285, 288, 298–301, 304, 308, 356, 389, 391, 392, 401, 409, 451, 452, 481–484, 486, 491, 506, 509, 513, 517, 527, 533, 534, 540, 545, 546
triaging, 54
trial, 77
trigger, 109, 181, 187, 210, 261
trust, 51, 54, 60, 109, 227, 297–299, 304, 305, 333, 356, 371, 404, 423, 426, 458, 460, 491, 516, 517, 540
trusting, 222, 423
trustworthiness, 51, 110, 480
turmoil, 166
turn, 122, 371, 477
turnover, 334, 345
type, 201, 320

Index 599

uncertainty, 318, 438, 475
underdiagnosis, 47, 169
underfunding, 8
understanding, 1–4, 6–9, 11, 13–18,
    20, 21, 23–28, 35, 36, 39,
    40, 44, 46, 49, 68, 70, 71,
    76, 78, 82–84, 88, 95–99,
    108, 111, 112, 114, 132,
    134, 137, 141, 142, 144,
    149, 150, 161, 164, 166,
    169, 171, 174–176, 178,
    181, 185, 186, 194, 195,
    205, 209, 216, 220, 221,
    231, 233–236, 267, 276,
    283, 284, 289, 309, 312,
    315, 316, 319, 321, 326,
    330, 331, 333, 337, 340,
    357, 364, 365, 367–372,
    385, 389, 391, 393–395,
    397, 400, 404, 410, 416,
    418, 419, 423–425, 437,
    440, 451, 452, 456, 459,
    460, 468, 473, 474,
    478–482, 489–493, 501,
    515–518, 520, 522, 526,
    527, 529, 532, 539–542,
    544–546
undertreatment, 47
underutilization, 401
uneasiness, 81
unemployment, 33, 37
uniqueness, 4, 221
unit, 394
universe, 316
up, 12, 33, 126, 188, 190, 212, 218,
    225, 376, 396, 494, 527,
    535
urbanization, 9, 217
urge, 195

urine, 97
use, 22, 27, 52, 54, 56–63, 70, 76,
    77, 79, 82, 83, 96–99,
    104–106, 108, 114, 119,
    122–131, 155, 158, 163,
    164, 171, 181, 201, 203,
    205, 232, 233, 241, 243,
    268, 282, 286, 370, 371,
    387, 388, 410, 420, 422,
    424, 432, 478, 481, 482,
    486, 501, 517, 539
user, 330, 450

validation, 45, 160, 169, 171, 320,
    321, 330, 332, 371, 385,
    390, 391, 394, 395, 418,
    449
validity, 370
value, 16, 23, 221, 422, 533, 543
variability, 175, 244, 486, 489
variety, 101, 213, 281, 289, 292, 334,
    423, 494
vehicle, 282
veteran, 307, 308
vice, 15, 104, 245, 247, 267
video, 52, 56, 57, 518
view, 2, 14, 98, 227, 365, 376, 418,
    422
vigilance, 67
violence, 22, 40, 47, 49, 106, 111,
    113, 116, 423, 425, 426,
    457
virtue, 15, 16, 368
visit, 222
visualization, 279–282, 366
vitality, 243, 279
voice, 62, 424, 474
volunteer, 468
volunteering, 318, 395, 449

vomiting, 164, 165
vulnerability, 36–38, 426, 464

wait, 33, 63
waiting, 278, 402
wake, 189, 190, 195, 396
wakefulness, 190
walking, 260, 262, 263, 266, 269, 274, 296, 313, 314, 414, 417, 446, 448
wall, 278
war, 82, 106, 111, 113
warning, 91, 172, 468
waste, 471
watching, 202
water, 467
way, 1, 4, 14, 21, 24, 25, 52, 54, 56, 63, 67, 71, 76, 83, 120, 166, 176, 218, 222, 280, 283, 287, 294, 312, 385, 404, 414–416, 420, 451, 483, 517, 545
weakness, 66, 96, 101, 176, 190, 213, 220
weather, 472, 474
wedding, 202
week, 165, 167, 187, 263, 266, 269, 347
weight, 82, 99, 103, 133, 161, 163–165, 170, 296
welfare, 297, 300, 301
well, 1–4, 6, 8, 11, 14–16, 19, 21, 24, 35, 36, 39, 43–46, 49, 52, 58–60, 63, 67, 69–71, 77–79, 84, 88, 91, 92, 107, 111–116, 119, 120, 122–124, 127–131, 133, 134, 136, 141–143, 149, 154, 159, 161, 164, 167, 168, 172, 174, 176, 181–183, 185, 186, 189, 191, 193–196, 198, 199, 202, 209, 215, 216, 221–224, 226, 231–237, 240, 241, 243–247, 249, 251–253, 255, 256, 258–261, 263, 264, 266, 267, 269, 270, 272, 274–277, 279, 282, 284, 285, 288, 289, 291, 295–301, 305, 308, 309, 311–313, 315, 316, 322, 325–327, 331, 334, 336–338, 340–342, 344, 345, 347, 348, 352, 355, 361, 363–367, 369, 371–374, 377, 379, 383–385, 387, 388, 391, 392, 394, 396, 397, 400, 407, 409, 410, 412, 414–418, 420, 423, 425, 426, 428–433, 440, 442–453, 455–458, 461, 462, 464, 466, 467, 469, 472, 473, 475, 481–486, 489, 490, 492, 499, 501, 513–515, 519–522, 526–528, 533–535, 539, 541, 544–548, 550
wellbeing, 17, 18, 20, 27, 55–59, 102, 103, 213, 227–229, 279–282, 312–314, 316–320, 322, 331, 333, 366, 388, 389, 391, 403, 433–436, 462, 467, 477–480, 492, 505, 516, 519, 542–544
wellness, 16, 53, 72, 75, 172, 231,

Index

284, 316, 433, 442, 501
whole, 2, 52, 99, 175, 232, 241, 245, 267, 334, 348, 355, 369, 391, 448, 485, 525, 542, 544
will, 9, 14, 21, 24, 33, 39, 43, 49, 52, 61, 71, 76, 82, 84, 86, 88, 96, 99, 106, 126, 129, 133, 154, 156, 161, 169, 172, 186, 189, 195, 199, 204, 207, 211, 223, 227, 231, 250, 253, 255, 257, 261, 263, 267, 272, 276, 279, 282, 289, 299, 301, 312, 322, 331, 333, 337, 345, 348, 352, 355, 358, 363, 371, 376, 377, 380, 383, 385, 388, 394, 397, 403, 407, 412, 423, 426, 436, 445, 447, 448, 451, 457, 466, 469, 472, 479, 481, 483, 485, 495, 498, 501, 509, 519, 522, 535
willingness, 128, 160, 175, 241, 318, 399, 542
willpower, 101
wisdom, 318, 393, 474
withdrawal, 122
witness, 264, 472
woman, 45, 91, 106, 115, 124, 149, 181, 191, 202, 213, 263, 266, 269, 284, 287, 300, 447
work, 11, 13, 21, 23, 36, 39, 41, 43, 45, 46, 52, 61, 69, 75, 77, 84, 87, 88, 92, 99, 106, 136, 149, 150, 154, 160, 164, 170, 182, 184, 188, 190, 191, 194, 204, 209, 213, 215, 218, 221, 225, 226, 244, 255, 262, 263, 266, 267, 271, 299, 307, 316, 332–334, 336–338, 340–342, 344–348, 355, 357, 361, 364, 368, 379, 400, 410, 412, 418, 419, 436, 440–442, 453, 469, 471, 475, 478, 485, 486, 489–492, 499–501, 509, 513, 515, 520, 521, 527, 528, 535, 539–541, 544, 547
worker, 447, 490, 527
workforce, 74, 225, 226, 334, 336, 344, 345, 357, 361, 437, 541, 546
working, 45, 104, 135, 158–160, 188, 190, 283, 297, 305, 336, 337, 344, 347, 395, 417, 483, 520, 526, 528, 535, 546
workload, 334, 413
workplace, 8, 154, 334, 337–341, 344, 379, 501
workspace, 347
world, 11, 14, 57, 70, 113, 136, 309, 312, 316, 379, 380, 410, 415, 429, 440, 472, 475, 478, 483, 493, 495
worry, 81, 84, 181
worsening, 195, 409
wort, 232, 242
worth, 188, 244, 260, 276, 295, 299, 320, 385, 389, 419
worthlessness, 91
Wu Wei, 313

year, 45, 91, 106, 115, 124, 136, 149,

158, 166, 181, 184, 188, 191, 202, 263, 266, 269, 284, 287, 300, 447
yoga, 27, 232, 233, 241, 246, 247, 269, 270, 274–276, 312, 448
youth, 426–433

Zimbabwe, 532
zone, 322, 420

Milton Keynes UK
Ingram Content Group UK Ltd.
UKHW021124111124
451035UK00016B/1209